Neglected and Emerging Tropical Diseases in South and Southeast Asia and Northern Australia

Neglected and Emerging Tropical Diseases in South and Southeast Asia and Northern Australia

Special Issue Editors

Patricia Graves
Thewarach Laha
Peter A. Leggat
Khin Saw Aye

MDPI • Basel • Beijing • Wuhan • Barcelona • Belgrade

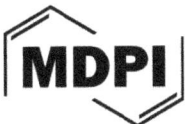

MDPI

Special Issue Editors

Patricia Graves
James Cook University
Australia

Thewarach Laha
Khon Kaen University
Thailand

Peter A. Leggat
James Cook University
Australia

Khin Saw Aye
Ministry of Health and Sports
Republic of the Union of Myanmar

Editorial Office
MDPI
St. Alban-Anlage 66
Basel, Switzerland

This is a reprint of articles from the Special Issue published online in the open access journal *Tropical Medicine and Infectious Disease* (ISSN 2414-6366) from 2017 to 2018 (available at: http://www.mdpi.com/journal/tropicalmed/special_issues/neglected_emerging_tropical_diseases)

For citation purposes, cite each article independently as indicated on the article page online and as indicated below:

LastName, A.A.; LastName, B.B.; LastName, C.C. Article Title. *Journal Name* **Year**, *Article Number*, Page Range.

ISBN 978-3-03897-089-7 (Pbk)
ISBN 978-3-03897-090-3 (PDF)

Cover image courtesy of Jan Douglass.

Contents

About the Special Issue Editors

Patricia Graves, MSPH, PhD, is a specialist in the epidemiology of malaria, filariasis, and other vector-borne diseases, with extensive experience in applied research and consulting in the Pacific, Africa, and Asia. From 2007 to 2011, she worked as an epidemiologist for The Carter Center, Atlanta, GA, USA, conducting program implementation as well as monitoring and evaluation of integrated control programs for malaria, filariasis, and other neglected tropical diseases in Ethiopia and Nigeria. She has been an advisor to the Pacific Regional Filariasis Elimination program since 2000, especially on survey design and evaluation of control programs. She joined the James Cook University in 2012 as the Director of the WHO Collaborating Centre for Lymphatic Filariasis, Soil-Transmitted Helminths, and other Neglected Tropical Diseases, where she manages a serology laboratory for lymphatic filariasis. This center has now been renamed the WHO Collaborating Centre for Vector-Borne and Neglected Tropical Diseases.

Thewarach Laha is an Associate Professor in Parasitology and the Head of the Department of Parasitology, Faculty of Medicine, Khon Kaen University, Khon Kaen, Thailand. Dr. Laha's research focuses on the molecular pathogenesis of liver fluke infection and liver fluke-induced bile duct cancer.

Peter A. Leggat, AM, is Professor and co-Director of the World Health Organization Collaborating Centre for Vector-borne and Neglected Tropical Diseases, College of Public Health, Medical and Veterinary Sciences, James Cook University, Australia. He is a consultant for various organizations, including the Australian Defence Force, the Therapeutic Goods Administration (Australia), and the World Health Organization. He is currently President of The Australasian College of Tropical Medicine and Secretary-Treasurer of the International Society of Travel Medicine. Professor Leggat holds honorary and adjunct Professorial positions in six universities in five countries. A former Fulbright Scholar and Fulbright Ambassador, he has published more than 500 journal papers, 30 books, and 90 chapters and has presented more than 400 papers at national and international meetings. He was admitted as a Member of the General Division of the Order of Australia in 2013 and promoted to Commander of the Order of St John in 2016.

Khin Saw Aye is Deputy Director General of the Department of Medical Research, Ministry of Health and Sports, Republic of the Union of Myanmar. She is involved in research focused on immunology, pathology, and the molecular mechanisms of malaria, tuberculosis, dengue, and hepatitis.

Tropical Medicine and Infectious Disease

MDPI

Editorial

Neglected and Emerging Tropical Diseases in South and Southeast Asia and Northern Australia

Peter A. Leggat [1,2,*], **Patricia Graves** [1], **Thewarach Laha** [3] and **Khin Saw Aye** [4]

1   World Health Organization Collaborating Centre for Vectorborne and Neglected Tropical Diseases, College of Public Health, Medical and Veterinary Sciences, James Cook University, Townsville, QLD 4811, Australia; patricia.graves@jcu.edu.au
2   Faculty of Science, University of Nottingham Malaysia Campus, Jalan Broga, Semenyih 43500, Selangor Darul Ehsan, Malaysia
3   Department of Parasitology, Faculty of Medicine, Khon Kaen University, Khon Kaen 40002, Thailand; thewa_la@kku.ac.th
4   Department of Medical Research, Ministry of Health and Sports, Yangon 11191, Myanmar; ksadmr@gmail.com
*   Correspondence: Peter.Leggat@jcu.edu.au; Tel.: +61-7-4781-6108

Received: 19 June 2018; Accepted: 20 June 2018; Published: 22 June 2018

This Special Issue focuses on recent research on the important emerging and neglected tropical diseases (NTDs) in South and South East Asia and Northern Australia. This region stretches from Pakistan in the west to the Philippines in the east, and includes Afghanistan and countries to the east, the Indian subcontinent, mainland South-East Asia, and the tropical regions of Australia. Many of these areas are highly endemic for important NTDs and other tropical diseases, including lymphatic filariasis (LF), soil-transmitted helminthiases (STH) such as hookworm infection, trichuriasis, ascariasis, and strongyloidiasis, rickettsial diseases and arboviral diseases. Several of these diseases are targeted for elimination or enhanced control by the World Health Organization (WHO) in the next 5 to 10 years, although some have chronic lasting sequelae and disability needing lifelong management. Control methods used include preventive chemotherapy, enhanced screening and treatment, intensified disease management, vector control, interruption of human to animal transmission, environmental/sanitation improvements and disability prevention/mitigation. A current list of WHO NTDs is given in Table 1.

Table 1. Neglected Tropical Diseases [1].

Neglected Tropical Diseases
Buruli ulcer
Chagas disease
Dengue and Chikungunya
Dracunculiasis (guinea-worm disease)
Echinococcosis
Foodborne trematodiases
Human African trypanosomiasis (sleeping sickness)
Leishmaniasis
Leprosy (Hansen's disease)
Lymphatic filariasis
Mycetoma, chromoblastomycosis and other deep mycoses
Onchocerciasis (river blindness)
Rabies
Scabies and other ectoparasites
Schistosomiasis
Soil-transmitted helminthiases
Snakebite envenoming
Trachoma
Yaws (Endemic treponematoses)
Taeniasis/Cysticercosis

At the time of publication, there have been 11 papers published upon peer review acceptance in this Special Issue, including eight original papers, two review papers and one perspectives piece. They each contribute to a much better understanding of Neglected and Emerging Tropical Diseases in South and Southeast Asia and Northern Australia. The contributions to these topics can be summarized as follows: four submissions on LFs [2–5], four submissions on STHs [6–9], two submissions on rickettsial diseases [10,11], and one submission on arboviral diseases [12]. A systematic review and meta-analysis leads the opening section on LF [2], which reviews prevalence and disease burden of LF in southeast Asia [2]. Two studies in Myanmar review the utility of dried blood spots on filter paper for sampling for detection Bm14 antibody and Og4C3 antigen in cases of LF [3,4], with the latter indicating need for reconciliation between different sampling methods. A further study in Myanmar examined the usefulness of low-cost devices for measuring tissue compressibility and extracellular fluid, used and accepted in other clinical settings, for objective assessment of lymphedema [5]. A review paper leads the other major section on STH, which focuses on the prevalence of STHs in different groups, including immigrants, travellers, military personnel and veterans in Australia and Asia [6]. This is followed by studies examining an extended period of surveillance data on *Strongyloides stercoralis* [7]; and a study examining the prevalence of STHs in remote Aboriginal communities, both in the Northern Territory, Australia [8]; and a study examining the links between dietary intake, nutritional status, and intestinal parasites, such as *Schistosoma japonicum*, *Ascaris lumbricoides*, *Trichuris trichiura*, and hookworm, in the Philippines [9]. The two rickettsial papers examine hospital admissions for Queensland tick typhus in north Brisbane, Australia [10], and the other study based in Thailand looks at the influence of land use on scrub typhus in rodents [11]. Lastly, a perspective piece reminds us that Australia is home to more than 75 arboviral diseases-, which pose a public health threat to the Australian population [12].

The diversity of papers, the depth of the topics and the relative geographical reach of the authors (including authors from several countries across Asia, as well as authors from Australia and Europe) in this Special Issue confirm the continued collective major interest in this area. This wide-ranging open access collection contributes to a much better understanding on the epidemiology, presentation, diagnosis, treatment, prevention and control of neglected and emerging tropical diseases in South and Southeast Asia and Northern Australia. As the editors of this Special Issue, we trust that you find the content useful, as the authors are pleased to share their knowledge with an international audience. We look forward to future opportunities to update advances in this field and encourage you or publish your work in or propose a Special Issue for *Tropical Medicine and Infectious Disease*.

Funding: This research received no external funding.

Conflicts of Interest: The authors declare no conflict of interest.

References

1. World Health Organization. Neglected Tropical Diseases. Available online: http://www.who.int/topics/tropical_diseases/factsheets/neglected/en/ (accessed on 17 June 2018).
2. Dickson, B.F.R.; Graves, P.M.; McBride, W.J. Lymphatic Filariasis in Mainland Southeast Asia: A Systematic Review and Meta-Analysis of Prevalence and Disease Burden. *Trop. Med. Inf. Dis.* **2017**, *2*, 32. [CrossRef]
3. Masson, J.; Douglass, J.; Roineau, M.; Aye, K.S.; Htwe, K.M.; Warner, J.; Graves, P.M. Concordance between Plasma and Filter Paper Sampling Techniques for the Lymphatic Filariasis Bm14 Antibody ELISA. *Trop. Med. Inf. Dis.* **2017**, *2*, 6. [CrossRef]
4. Masson, J.; Douglass, J.; Roineau, M.; Aye, K.S.; Htwe, K.M.; Warner, J.; Graves, P.M. Relative Performance and Predictive Values of Plasma and Dried Blood Spots with Filter Paper Sampling Techniques and Dilutions of the Lymphatic Filariasis Og4C3 Antigen ELISA for Samples from Myanmar. *Trop. Med. Inf. Dis.* **2017**, *2*, 7. [CrossRef]
5. Douglass, J.; Graves, P.; Lindsay, D.; Becker, L.; Roineau, M.; Masson, J.; Aye, N.N.; Win, S.S.; Wai, T.; Win, Y.Y.; et al. Lymphatic Filariasis Increases Tissue Compressibility and Extracellular Fluid in Lower Limbs of Asymptomatic Young People in Central Myanmar. *Trop. Med. Inf. Dis.* **2017**, *2*, 50. [CrossRef]

6.   Gordon, C.A.; Kurscheid, J.; Jones, M.K.; Gray, D.J.; McManus, D.P. Soil-Transmitted Helminths in Tropical Australia and Asia. *Trop. Med. Inf. Dis.* **2017**, 2, 56. [CrossRef]

7.   Mayer-Coverdale, J.K.; Crowe, A.; Smith, P.; Baird, R.W. Trends in *Strongyloides stercoralis* Faecal Larvae Detections in the Northern Territory, Australia: 2002 to 2012. *Trop. Med. Inf. Dis.* **2017**, 2, 18. [CrossRef]

8.   Holt, D.C.; Shield, J.; Harris, T.M.; Mounsey, K.E.; Aland, M.; McCarthy, J.S.; Currie, B.J.; Kearns, T.M. Soil-Transmitted Helminths in Children in a Remote Aboriginal Community in the Northern Territory: Hookworm is Rare but *Strongyloides stercoralis* and *Trichuris trichiura* Persist. *Trop. Med. Inf. Dis.* **2017**, 2, 51. [CrossRef]

9.   Ross, A.G.; Papier, K.; Luceres-Catubig, R.; Chau, T.N.; Inobaya, M.T.; Ng, S.-K. Poverty, Dietary Intake, Intestinal Parasites, and Nutritional Status among School-Age Children in the Rural Philippines. *Trop. Med. Inf. Dis.* **2017**, 2, 49. [CrossRef]

10.   Stewart, A.; Armstrong, M.; Graves, S.; Hajkowicz, K. Epidemiology and Characteristics of Rickettsia australis (Queensland Tick Typhus) Infection in Hospitalized Patients in North Brisbane, Australia. *Trop. Med. Inf. Dis.* **2017**, 2, 10. [CrossRef]

11.   Chaisiri, K.; Cosson, J.-F.; Morand, S. Infection of Rodents by *Orientia tsutsugamushi*, the Agent of Scrub Typhus, in Relation to Land Use in Thailand. *Trop. Med. Inf. Dis.* **2017**, 2, 53. [CrossRef]

12.   Gyawali, N.; Taylor-Robinson, A.W. Confronting the Emerging Threat to Public Health in Northern Australia of Neglected Indigenous Arboviruses. *Trop. Med. Inf. Dis.* **2017**, 2, 55. [CrossRef]

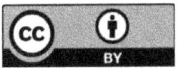

Tropical Medicine and Infectious Disease

MDPI

Review

Lymphatic Filariasis in Mainland Southeast Asia: A Systematic Review and Meta-Analysis of Prevalence and Disease Burden

Benjamin F. R. Dickson [1],*, Patricia M. Graves [2] and William J. McBride [3]

[1] College of Medicine & Dentistry, James Cook University, Cairns, QLD 4870, Australia
[2] College of Public Health, Medical and Veterinary Sciences, James Cook University, Cairns, QLD 4870, Australia; patricia.graves@jcu.edu.au
[3] College of Medicine & Dentistry, James Cook University, Cairns, QLD 4870, Australia; john.mcbride@jcu.edu.au
* Correspondence: benjamin.dickson@my.jcu.edu.au; Tel.: +61-402-597-626

Received: 15 June 2017; Accepted: 17 July 2017; Published: 27 July 2017

Abstract: Accurate prevalence data are essential for the elimination of lymphatic filariasis (LF) as a public health problem. Despite it bearing one of the highest burdens of disease globally, there remains limited reliable information on the current epidemiology of filariasis in mainland Southeast Asia. We conducted a systematic review and meta-analysis of available literature to assess the recent and current prevalence of infection and morbidity in the region. Fifty-seven journal articles and reports containing original prevalence data were identified, including over 512,010 participants. Data were summarised using percentage prevalence estimates and a subset combined using a random effects meta-analysis by country and year. Pooled estimates for microfilaraemia, immunochromatographic card positivity and combined morbidity were 2.64%, 4.48% and 1.34% respectively. Taking into account pooled country estimates, grey literature and the quality of available data, we conclude that Lao People's Democratic Republic (PDR), Myanmar and Northeast India demonstrate ongoing evidence of LF transmission that will require multiple further rounds of mass drug administration. Bangladesh, Malaysia, Thailand and Vietnam appear close to having eliminated LF, whilst Cambodia has already achieved elimination status. We estimate that the burden of morbidity is likely high in Thailand; moderate in Cambodia, Myanmar, and Northeast India; and low in Bangladesh. There was insufficient evidence to accurately estimate the disease burden in Lao PDR, Malaysia or Vietnam. The results of this study indicate that whilst considerable progress toward LF elimination has been made, there remains a significant filariasis burden in the region. The results of this study will assist policy makers to advocate and budget for future control programs.

Keywords: lymphatic filariasis; Southeast Asia; prevalence; infection; morbidity; lymphoedema; hydrocoele

---

1. Introduction

Lymphatic filariasis (LF) is a mosquito-borne tropical disease that affects 67.88 million people in 73 countries worldwide [1–3]. It is caused by infection with the nematodes *Wuchereria bancrofti (Wb)*, *Brugia malayi (Bm)* or *Brugia timori*. Chronic infection causes lymphatic dysfunction, resulting in severe morbidity from progressive, irreversible swelling of the limbs and genitals. LF is a significant cause of permanent disability worldwide, accounting for an estimated 19.43 million cases of hydrocoele, 16.68 million cases of lymphoedema and 2.02 million disability-adjusted life years lost [3,4].

In recognition of the significant worldwide burden of LF, the World Health Organization (WHO) established the Global Program to Eliminate LF (GPELF) calling for the elimination of LF by 2020 [1,5]. The program adopted a two-pronged approach: first, interrupt transmission through annual single-dose mass drug administration (MDA) of entire at-risk populations with albendazole in combination with either diethylcarbamazine (DEC) or ivermectin for a minimum of five years; and, second, alleviate the significant morbidity burden associated with the disease.

Numerous methods are currently used to diagnose LF infection. Traditionally, thick blood smears (TBS) were used to identify microfilaraemia (mf) in the peripheral circulation. TBS have now been largely superseded by more sensitive antigen-based tests but are still used as a measure of potential infectivity and ongoing transmission. Antigen tests include immunochromatographic card tests (ICT) and Og4C3 enzyme-linked immunosorbent assays (ELISA) which use monoclonal antibodies to detect the excretory-secretory antigens produced by adult filarial worm infection [6,7]. Because they detect a different stage of the life-cycle and do not require adult worms to be producing microfilariae, they are two- to fivefold more sensitive than TBS [8]. Antibody-based tests detect circulating IgG4 antibodies against Bm14 antigen (*B. malayi* and *W. bancrofti*) or BmR1 (*B. malayi* only) [9]. Whilst highly sensitive and specific, antibody prevalence cannot prove current infection because antibodies remain elevated for many years after treatment [9]. Urinary antibody tests have been trialled but are less sensitive than blood-based antibody tests [8,10]. PCR assays to detect LF DNA in humans are also available, but are not used routinely because they require advanced laboratory facilities and are less sensitive than other methods [8,10].

LF is endemic in all countries within mainland Southeast Asia [1,2,5]. The geographical region spans both the WHO Southeast Asia and Western Pacific regions and includes Cambodia, Lao People's Democratic Republic (PDR), Myanmar, Thailand, Vietnam and Malaysia. Emerging data suggest a possibly high prevalence of filariasis in Myanmar. Given the country's significant shared border with Northeast India and Bangladesh, both were also included.

The WHO Southeast Asia and Western Pacific regions account for 55.7% of the at-risk population, with 94.6% of reported lymphoedema cases and 85.2% of reported hydrocoele cases globally [2]. The areas considered here (mainland Southeast Asia plus Northeast India and Bangladesh) account for over a fifth of the population of these two regions. Elimination of LF in this area would therefore have a significant impact on the global disease burden. LF in these countries is caused by *W. Bancrofti* and *B. malayi*, and transmitted mainly by *Culex quinquefasciatus*, with some contribution by *Aedes* spp. and *Mansonia* spp. mosquitoes [11].

All countries in this review have commenced elimination programs. Elimination as a public health problem has been validated in Cambodia, whilst Bangladesh, Thailand and Vietnam have transitioned to post-MDA surveillance. The remaining countries are still conducting MDA [1,2,5].

WHO country validation of 'elimination of LF as a public health problem' requires a set of surveys and steps to determine whether the prevalence is below the target level (upper 95% CI of 2% in *Culex* spp. transmission areas such as Southeast Asia) [12]. One important milestone is the passing of three consecutive transmission assessment surveys (TAS) conducted on six- to seven-year-old children in each defined geographical evaluation unit (EU). The TAS survey sets critical cut-off values for the number of positive children that must not be exceeded for the EU to pass [13]. The sample sizes and critical cut-off values for the TAS in *Culex* spp. transmission areas are designed so that an EU has (1) at least a 75% chance of passing if the true prevalence of antigenaemia is 1.0% (half the target level); and (2) no more than a 5% chance of incorrectly passing if the true prevalence of antigenaemia is $\geq$2% [13].

Despite the significant LF burden in this region, there remain limited reliable data on the current prevalence of infection and morbidity. Whilst previous reviews have examined this topic, all are significantly out-dated or incomplete [14–16]. Reliable, current data on the prevalence of LF are required for the implementation and evaluation of elimination programs as well as future advocacy efforts. Accordingly, we conducted a systematic review and meta-analysis of publicly-available data in studies and grey literature to assess the recent (since the early 1990s) and current prevalence of LF infection and morbidity in mainland Southeast Asia, Bangladesh and Northeast India.

2. Materials and Methods

2.1. Protocol

This systematic review is reported using the Preferred Reporting Items for Systematic Reviews and Meta-Analysis (PRISMA) guidelines [17]. A review protocol was registered with PROSPERO international prospective register of systematic reviews, which can be viewed online [18].

2.2. Information Sources

Information was gathered through three sources: (1) a literature search of PubMed and MEDLINE databases; (2) a web-based search of the WHO library for relevant publications; and (3) direct contact with regional and national LF Program directors to obtain National LF Program reports [19]. Countries with National LF Programs submit annual reports to their respective WHO regional office outlining their MDA and surveying activities for the preceding year. A summary of the data is published annually in a regional WHO meeting report. Reference lists of all papers were screened to identify additional publications.

2.3. Search Strategy

A literature search was conducted for available publications on PubMed and MEDLINE via OvidSP up until 11 December 2016 by one investigator. The search strategy used for both databases was: (lymphatic filariasis or Wuchereria bancrofti or Brugia timori or Brugia malayi or lymphoedema or hydrocoele or elephantiasis or microfilariae or microfilaraemia) AND ((Myanmar or Burma or Thailand or Laos or Cambodia or Vietnam or Malaysia or Bangladesh) OR (India and Assam or Meghalaya or Nagaland or Manipur or Tripura or Mizoram or Arunachal Pradesh)). Combinations of the database search terms were used to search the WHO library.

2.4. Study Selection and Inclusion Criteria

The titles, abstracts and if indicated, full text of records from online databases and the WHO library (IRIS) were screened for eligibility. Published studies and reports with original prevalence data on LF infection or morbidity from identified countries were included. Where reports were not available, WHO publications referencing their data were used and recorded.

Only literature available in English and published from 1995 onward was included. There were no restrictions on age, study size, design or power. Any uncertainty regarding the inclusion of a paper was resolved through consensus discussion with other authors.

2.5. Data Collection Process

A standardised data collection form was used to record information from included publications. All data was then entered into a Microsoft Excel spreadsheet for analysis.

2.6. Data Items

Extracted data included study characteristics, sampling method and prevalence data. Data were extracted directly from text and tables within the publications.

Primary outcomes were the prevalence of infection (including measurement method and species) and chronic morbidity (lymphoedema or hydrocoele) in the given population.

Where interventional studies were included, the prevalence data that were most representative of the population were used. That is, when a whole area participated in MDA external to the study, the post-intervention data were used. When an intervention was implemented only on the study sample, baseline data were used.

2.7. Risk of Bias Assessment

A modified bias risk assessment tool was developed to evaluate included studies. It was based on the Crowe and GATE validated critical appraisal tools [20,21]. Risk of bias was assessed by one reviewer on the basis of five independent factors: total sample size (>1000, 300–1000 or <300), sampling of location (representative randomisation, not stated/unclear or non-representative), sampling of participants (representative randomisation, not stated/unclear or non-representative), assessment of infection (internationally accepted methodology, not stated/unclear or non-consensus methods) and assessment of morbidity (independently assessed, not stated/unclear or patient reported). A total risk of bias score was generated by allocating zero, one or two points for each factor. The quality assessment was used to interpret the reliability of each study's results. Because of the limited number and significant quality variation between studies, the bias assessment was not incorporated directly into the meta-analysis.

WHO filariasis publications are based on national LF programs annual reports. WHO Regional Program Review Groups (RPRG) assess annual national LF program surveillance reports during their consideration of the country's request for the donation of MDA drugs. Although general guidelines are provided by WHO, methodology within countries frequently varies substantially and may not be optimal due to poorly resourced programs and frequent personnel changes [22]. Independent assessments of data quality within programs are rarely done.

2.8. Summary Measures and Synthesis of Results

Available data were summarised using percentage prevalence estimates and presented in tables by country and region.

A meta-analysis of primary outcomes from studies was completed using the *metaprop* procedure in STATA version 12.1 to produce overall estimates with exact binomial confidence intervals. A subset meta-analysis of migrant workers in Thailand and India was also done. A random effects model was used to account for the variation in LF prevalence between and within studies. Weighting of studies was done using the method of DerSimonian and Laird [23]. The heterogeneity of data from each meta-analysis was measured using the I^2 statistic [24].

A map of baseline and most recent LF distribution was generated by combining government prevalence maps found in grey literature. Endemicity was classified at implementation unit level by all countries. Recent maps were available for all countries except Malaysia.

3. Results

3.1. Study Selection

The search protocol identified 629 papers (Figure 1). Of these, 554 clearly did not meet the inclusion criteria (i.e., were review articles or did not include original prevalence data on infection or morbidity published since 1995 from the identified areas). From the remaining 75 records, 17 were excluded because they did not contain original prevalence data, and one because the full text was not available after contacting the author. The included 57 papers comprised 38 peer-reviewed journal articles and 19 grey literature reports [5,25–79]. With the exception of Chansiri et al. [30], which contained only polymerase-chain reaction (PCR) infection data, all studies were included in the meta-analysis.

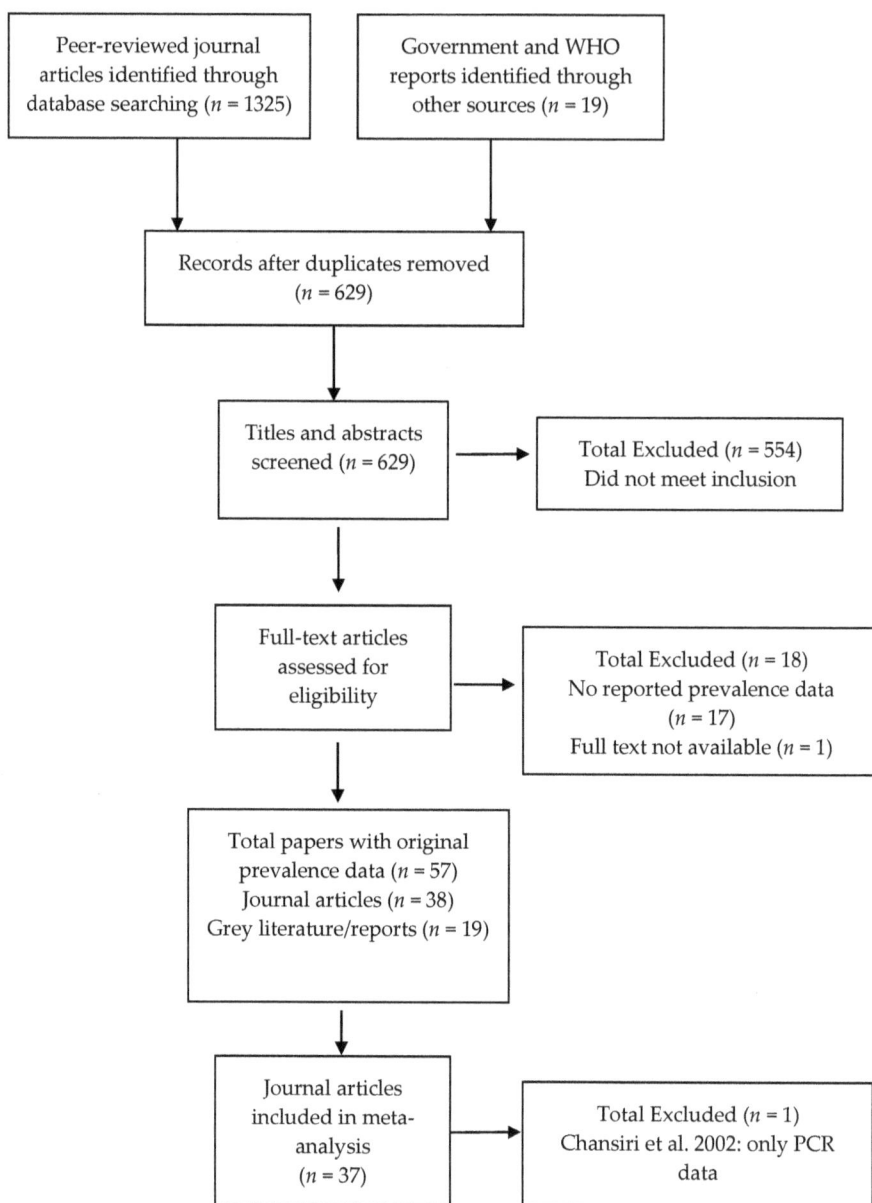

Figure 1. Study selection flow chart.

3.2. Study Characteristics

The characteristics of the 38 included journal articles are summarised by country in Table 1. This includes 17 from Thailand, eight each from Malaysia and Northeast India, three from Bangladesh and two from Cambodia. There were no studies included from Lao PDR, Myanmar or Vietnam.

All articles described primary studies, and included cross-sectional surveys (CSS) (25 studies, 66%), field diagnostic test evaluation studies (FDE) (8, 21%), field drug trials (FDT) (3, 8%) as well as a longitudinal observational and a retrospective cohort study. Publication year ranged from 1995 to 2016.

Together the included studies assessed 382,274 participants with wide variation in sampling unit and sample size (145 to 232,005). Two studies, Saha et al. (2011) and Krairittichai et al. (2012), contributed substantially to overall participant numbers with sample sizes of 232,005 and 102,090, respectively [44,55]. Eleven of the 17 studies from Thailand assessed Myanmar migrant populations, whilst seven of the eight papers from Northeast India examined those living in tea estates.

Studies most frequently assessed infection with the traditional thick blood smear (TBS) method (30 studies, 79%), followed by ICT (10, 26%), IgG4 antibody (10, 26%), Og4C3 ELISA (6, 16%) and PCR (3, 8%) tests. One study used urine rather than blood to detect IgG4 antibodies [56]. Almost half of the studies (16, 42%) used multiple methods. Sixteen studies assessed the prevalence of chronic LF morbidity. Of these, seven (44%) assessed both hydrocoele and lymphoedema.

Table 2 summarises the characteristics of the 19 included grey literature reports. These include 15 WHO publications, three annual national programmatic reports and a report from a non-governmental organisation.With the exception of one WHO report, all papers summarise data from government prevalence surveys conducted as part of their national MDA programs. Whilst only some sample sizes were reported, at least 129,736 individuals were surveyed. Baseline mapping and MDA surveillance surveys predominantly used TBS to diagnose infection, whilst post-MDA TASs used ICT.Some government morbidity information was available for all countries, but the data were very limited.

3.3. Risk of Bias within Studies

The risk of bias assessment of included studies is summarised in Table S1. Overall, study quality was suboptimal. Only seven studies (18%) used fully representative sampling methods and consensus data collection methods.

The sample sizes of published studies were overall acceptable, with 33 studies including greater than 300 participants. However, sample sizes were generally small relative to government surveys.

The sampling of study location introduced a significant risk of bias. Only ten (26%) studies adequately described the random site selection required for regionally representative data. Of the remaining studies, 21 (55%) did not describe the method/reason for study site selection, and seven (18%) intentionally selected study sites.

Participant sampling within study locations also contributed to risk of bias. Only 18 (47%) studies described random participant selection. Eighteen (47%) studies did not clearly state the method of selection, whilst the remaining two studies excluded those with recent diethylcarbamazine treatment.

With the exception of Chansiri et al., all studies used a consensus method for the detection of LF infection [30]. It is unclear whether the TBS samples in Krairittichai et al. were taken at night, which may have affected the sensitivity of their results [44].

Of the fifteen studies that assessed LF morbidity, only four (25%) described examination methods in detail. Of the remaining papers, eight (50%) provided some detail and four (25%) did not state the method used.

Table 1. Included peer-reviewed journal articles.

Study (Publication Date) [Study Period] [Ref.]	Study Design	Sampling Population/Unit (Age of Participants)	Sample Size	Diagnostic Method	
				Infection	Morbidity
Bangladesh					
Hafiz et al. (2015) (2011) [33]	CSS [b]	Households in 30 villages (≥10)	1242	Mf, ICT	Hyd./Lymph. [h]
Saha et al. (2011) [NS [g]] [55]	CSS	Households in 19 unions (≥1)	232,005	-	Lymph.
Samad et al. (2013) [NS] [56]	FDE [a]	School children (5–10)	319	ICT, IgG4 [e]	-
Cambodia					
Leang et al. (2004) (2000–2001) [45]	CSS	83 villages (≥1)	3468	Mf, ICT	Hyd./Lymph.
Priest et al. (2016) (2012) [52]	CSS	2200 households (women 15–39)	2150	IgG4	-
Northeast India					
Dutta et al. (1995) (1992) [32]	CSS	Individuals in 1 tea estate (≥1)	1553	Mf	NS
Khan et al. (1999) [NS] Study 1 [37]	CSS	Individuals in 1 tea estate (≥1)	821	Mf	Hyd./Lymph.
Khan et al. (1999) [NS] Study 2 [40]	CSS	2 communities: tea workers and non-tea workers (≥1)	1446	Mf	NS
Khan et al. (1999) [NS] Study 3 [38]	CSS	1 weaving community (≥1)	446	Mf	-
Khan et al. (2004) [NS] [39]	CSS	Individuals in 1 tea estate (≥1)	656	Mf	Hyd./Lymph.
Khan et al. (2015) (2012–2013) [41]	CSS	Individuals in 1 tea estate (infection ≥2, morbidity ≥18)	634	Mf	Hyd./Lymph.
Medhi et al. (2006) (2002–2003) [47]	CSS	Households in 8 tea estates (≥1)	4016	Mf	Hyd./Lymph.
Prakash et al. (1998) (1994) [51]	CSS	Households in 1 tea estate (≥1)	1105	Mf	Hyd./Lymph.
Malaysia					
Ahmad et al. (2014) [NS] [25]	CSS	Households/schools on 1 island (≥1)	298	Mf	-
Cox-Singh et al. (1999) [NS] [31]	CSS	2 districts (NS)	145	Mf, PCR	-
Hakim et al. (1995) (1992) [34]	FDT [c]	2 villages (≥6 months old)	499	Mf	-
Jamail et al. (2005) (2001–2002) [35]	FDE	7 districts(≥1)	2545	Mf, IgG4	-
Lim et al (2001) [NS] [46]	FDE	5 villages and 2 schools (≥1)	1134	Mf, IgG4	-
Rahmah et al. (2003) [NS] [53]	FDE	16 schools (7–12)	5138	IgG4	-
Rahmah et al. (2010) [NS] [54]	FDE	School children (6–10)	973	IgG4	-
Wan Omar et al. (2001) [NS] [62]	FDE	Migrant workers in palm oil estates (WA [i])	630	Mf	Lymph.

Table 1. *Cont.*

Study (Publication Date) [Study Period] [Ref.]	Study Design	Sampling Population/Unit (Age of Participants)	Sample Size	Diagnostic Method	
				Infection	Morbidity
Thailand					
Bhumiratana et al. (2004) (2002) [28]	FDT	Myanmar workers (WA[i])	860	Mf, ICT, Og4C3	-
Bhumiratana et al. (2005) (1998–2001) [26]	CSS	Myanmars and Thais in multiple villages (≥1)	433	Mf, ICT, Og4C3	-
Bhumiratana et al. (1999) (1998) [27]	FDE	Multiple villages (≥1)	225	Mf, ICT	Hyd.
Bhumiratana et al. (2002) (1999) [29]	CSS	1 village (≥1)	219	Mf, ICT	Hyd.
Chansiri et al. (2002) (1997–2001) [30]	CSS	Migrant workers in 4 provinces (WA[i])	1299	PCR	-
Jiraamonnimit et al. (2009) (2005 to 2006) [36]	LO[d]	3 provinces (≥7)	500	Mf, IgG4	Lymph.
Koyadun et al. (2003) (2001–2002) [43]	FDT	Myanmar migrants and Thais in 3 districts (≥15)	660	ICT	-
Koyadun et al. (2005) (2003) [42]	CSS	Myanmar workers (≥10)	904	Mf	-
Krairittichai et al. (2012) (2010) [44]	RCS[f]	Migrant workers at 1 hospital (WA[i])	102,090	Mf	-
Nuchprayoon et al. (2003) [NS] Study 1 [48]	FDE	Myanmar workers at 2 factories (WA[i])	337	Mf, ICT, Og4C3	Hyd.
Nuchprayoon et al. (2003) [NS] Study 2 [49]	CSS	2 villages (≥1)	433	Mf, Og4C3, IgG4	-
Nuchprayoon et al. (2001) [NS] [50]	CSS	1 sub-district (≥1)	196	Mf, Og4C3, PCR	-
Satimai et al. (2011) [NS] [57]	CSS	Myanmar migrants and Thais in 2 provinces (≥1)	1031	ICT, IgG4	-
Swaddiwudhipong et al. (1996) (1995) [58]	CSS	Myanmar workers and their families (≥1)	8377	Mf	NS
Triteeraprapab et al. (1999) [NS] [61]	CSS	Myanmar workers in 6 industrial plants (WA[i])	654	Mf	-
Triteeraprapab et al. (2001) [NS] Study 1 [59]	CSS	4 districts in 1 province (≥1)	2462	Mf	-
Triteeraprapab et al. (2001) (1999) Study 2 [60]	CSS	Myanmar migrants in 1 community (≥2)	371	Mf, Og4C3, IgG4	-

[a] Field diagnostic test evaluation. [b] Cross-sectional survey. [c] Field Drug trial. [d] Longitudinal observational study. [e] Urine IgG4. [f] Retrospective cohort study. [g] Not stated. [h] Hydrocoele/lymphoedema. [i] Working age.

Table 2. Included grey literature.

Reports [Ref.]	Year	Sample Size	Diagnostic Method Infection	Diagnostic Method Morbidity
Annual Reports				
Myanmar Ministry of Health. National Program to Eliminate LF: Annual Reports [68–70]	2004	23,668	Mf	-
	2011	10,845	Mf	-
	2012	14,649	Mf	Hyd./Lymph. [c]
World Health Organization Reports				
WHO SEARO: Elimination of lymphatic filariasis in the Southeast Asia Region. Reports of the 1st, 7th, 8th, 9th, 10th Meeting of the Regional Program Review Group. [74–78]	2005 2010 2011 2012 2013	NS [b]	Mf (ICT) [a]	Hyd./Lymph.
WHO Regional Office for Southeast Asia: Elimination of lymphatic filariasis in the Southeast Asia Region. Reports of the 5th and 8th Meeting of the Regional Program Managers. [63,64]	2006 2011	NS	Mf (ICT) [a]	Hyd./Lymph.
WHO Regional Office for Southeast Asia: Towards eliminating lymphatic filariasis: Progress in the Southeast Asia Region (2001–2011). [5]	2013	NS	Mf	Hyd./Lymph.
WHO Regional Office for Southeast Asia: Regional Strategic Plan for Elimination of Lymphatic Filariasis (2004–2007). [71]	2004	NS	Mf	Hyd./Lymph.
WHO Western Pacific Region: First Mekong-Plus Program Managers Workshop on Lymphatic Filariasis and Other Helminthiasis. [66]	2009	Cambodia: 23,705 Lao PDR: 9286 Vietnam: 18,302	Mf/ICT	Hyd./Lymph.
WHO Regional Office for the Western Pacific. Reports of the 13th and 14th Meeting of the Western Pacific Regional Program Review Group on Neglected Tropical Diseases. [72,79]	2013 2014	NS	Mf/ICT	Hyd./Lymph.
WHO Malaysia Office. Country Cooperation Strategy 2009–2013. [67]	2010	NS	Mf	-
WHO: Meeting of the Neglected Tropical Disease Strategic and Technical Advisory Group's Monitoring and Evaluation Subgroup on Disease Specific Indicators. [80]	2014	NS	Mf	-
UNDP/World Bank/WHO/UNICEF: Research on rapid geographical assessment of Bancroftian filariasis. [73]	1997	7000	ICT	-
Non-Governmental Organization Reports				
Family Health International 360 and USAID: End Neglected Tropical Diseases in Asia Final Report. [65]	2015	Cambodia: 18,809 Lao PDR:3472 Vietnam: NS	Mf/ICT	Hyd./Lymph.

[a] ICT only used in one survey. [b] Not stated. [c] Hydrocoele/lymphoedema.

4. Prevalence Results and Discussion by Country

4.1. Overview

This systematic review and meta-analysis assessed the prevalence estimates for LF infection and morbidity in mainland Southeast Asia, Bangladesh and Northeast India. These estimates are important for the successful implementation and evaluation of elimination programs. Data on the prevalence and distribution of infection are needed to identify and prioritise regions for inclusion in MDA programs. MDA rounds aim to interrupt LF transmission to prevent new infections, eventuating in LF elimination. Prevalence data are then required following MDA rounds to evaluate their effectiveness and reassess the need for further rounds. However, even after transmission has ceased, those with previous infection may, or will have already developed chronic disease manifestations. National programs therefore require data on the morbidity burden in order to implement alleviation programs.

Prevalence data from included studies and grey literature are summarised by country and region in Tables S2–S3. Figure 2 illustrates the most recent distribution of LF compared to that at baseline (pre-MDA).

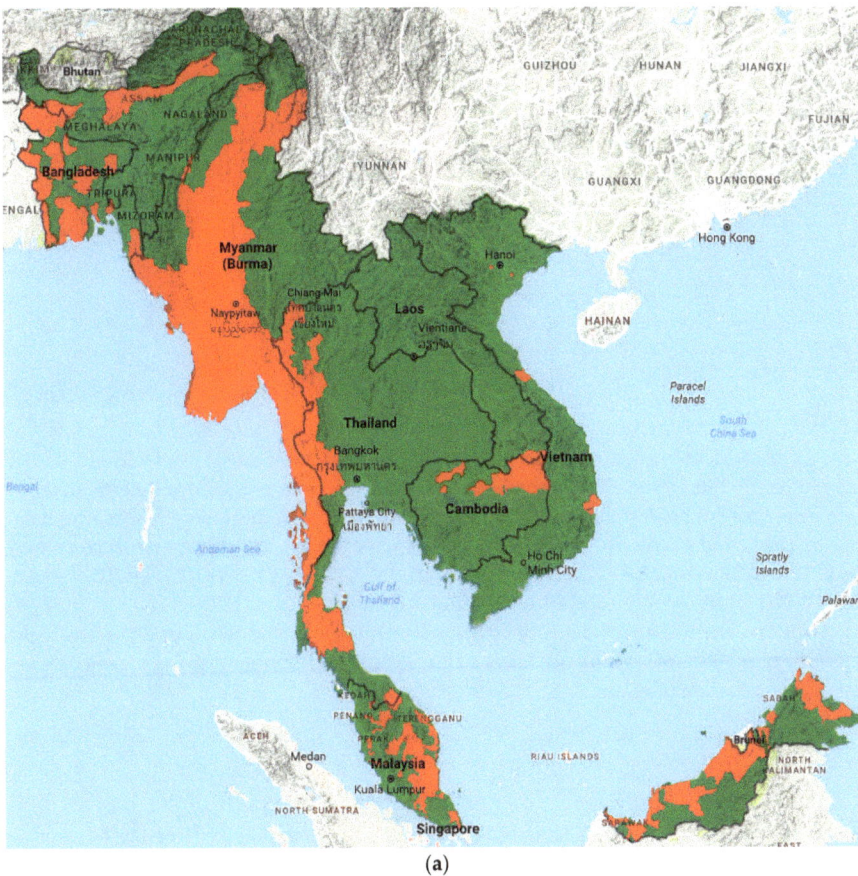

(a)

Figure 2. *Cont.*

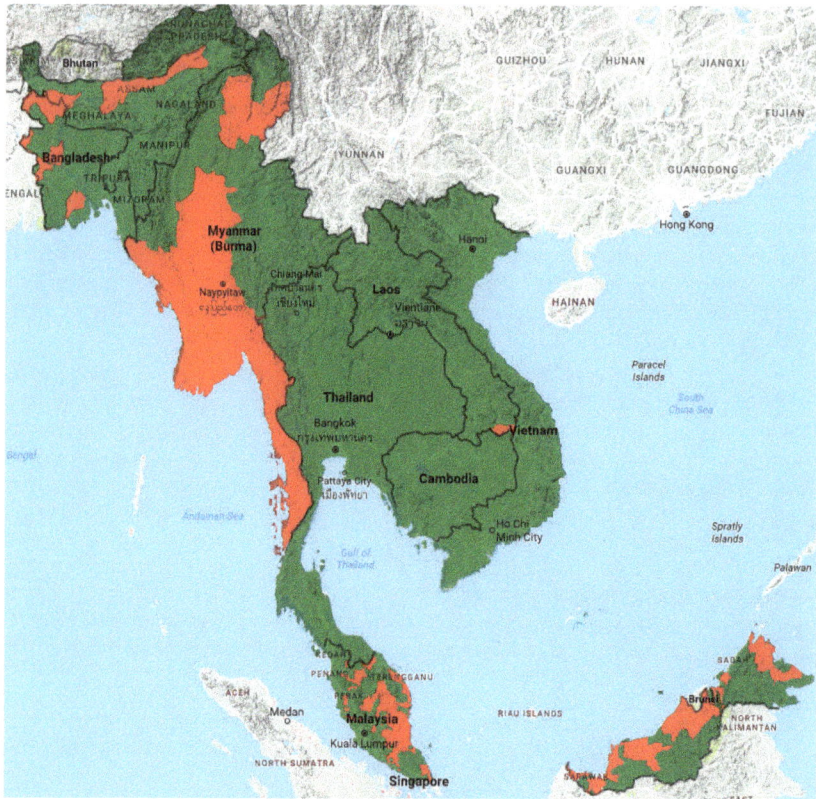

(b)

Figure 2. Distribution of LF endemic areas (red): (**a**) at baseline; and (**b**) based on most recent data.

Exact prevalence estimates cannot be calculated because of the nature of available data. However, we have attempted to estimate the current prevalence of infection and morbidity for each country through assessment of pooled country estimates, grey literature and the quality of available data.

Given the varied sensitivity of detection methods, we defined infection prevalence as low (Mf <0.5%, ICT/Og4C3 <1%, IgG4 <2%), medium (Mf 0.5–1.9%, ICT/Og4C3 1–3.9%, IgG4 2–7.9%), high (Mf 2–3.9%, ICT/Og4C3 4–7.9%, IgG4 8–15.9%) and very high (Mf ≥4%, ICT/IgG4 ≥8%, IgG4 ≥16%). For morbidity, we defined a prevalence of <0.5% as low, Mf 0.5–1.9% as medium, 2–3.9% as high and ≥4% as very high. Baseline prevalence refers to the level of infection prior to the commencement of the national elimination program.

4.2. Bangladesh

4.2.1. Results

Grey literature indicates that bancroftian filariasis was endemic in 34 of the 64 districts of Bangladesh during mapping between 2002 and 2004, with an estimated 75.96 million of the country's 148.77 million at risk [5,65,78]. Fifteen districts were considered low endemic with antigenaemia levels greater than 1% but microfilaraemia less than <0.6% [65,80]. They did not undergo MDA and have now passed two of three TAS, with the last to be completed in 2016 [65]. The remaining 19 districts had initial microfilaraemia prevalences of 0.2–16% [80]. These districts completed MDA rounds in

2014 and have now passed a TAS survey to determine whether MDA can be stopped, with a further TAS planned for 2017 to 2018. National infection prevalence estimates decreased from 1% in 2004 to 0% in 2010 [5].

Three studies from 2011–2013 have assessed infection prevalence in the northern endemic states of Nilphamari and Panchargarh [33,55,56]. They have found prevalences by Mf, ICT and IgG4 of 1.13%, 0.31–1.70% and 2.19%, respectively.

As of 2011, government surveys had identified 23,486 cases of lymphoedema (0.10%) and 65,320 (0.27%) cases of hydrocoele [76]. Two studies have assessed the morbidity prevalence in Bangladesh [33,55]. A large household survey of 232,005 participants reported a lymphoedema prevalence of 0.45%, whilst a smaller survey found a prevalence of lymphoedema and hydrocoele of 2.66% and 4.16% respectively

4.2.2. Discussion

Government data suggests *W. bancrofti* was historically widespread across Bangladesh with a focus in the country's west. Baseline infection prevalence appeared high to very high, consistent with a previous review and a study of Bangladeshi migrants [15,62]. MDA in Bangladesh appears to have been successful with both government data and recent studies demonstrating low to moderate levels of ongoing infection. The country has now transitioned to post-MDA surveillance and will aim to apply for elimination status after TAS in 2018.

Large-scale household surveys and government data suggest an overall low morbidity burden but a high prevalence of lymphoedema and very high prevalence of hydrocoele in Nilphamari District. As Bangladesh approaches LF elimination, resources should be shifted to further quantifying and tackling the morbidity burden.

4.3. Cambodia

4.3.1. Results

Government mapping in 2004 reported 18 endemic districts in four northern and northeastern provinces with 3.61% of the national population at risk (474 800) [5]. Government surveys reported a pre-MDA prevalence of 0.38–2.75% in these provinces (mixed ICT and TBS) [65]. A 2000–2001 study in these endemic provinces showed Mf and ICT prevalence ranging 0–1.13%, and 0–1.94%, respectively [45].

Five rounds of MDA were completed between 2005 and 2009. A post-MDA countrywide serological study in 2012 found a prevalence by IgG4 of 6.60% in this north region and 1.19–1.65% in the rest of the country [52]. All endemic districts passed required TAS by 2015 [65]. In 2016, Cambodia was validated by the WHO as having eliminated LF as a public health problem [2].

In 2001, the government reported 58 cases of LF-related morbidity (40 lymphoedema and 18 hydrocoele) in Cambodia [66]. The highest prevalence was in Stung Treng (10), Takeo (10) and Rattanakiri (9). A study from the same year found the prevalence of lymphoedema and hydrocoele in endemic provinces ranged from 0 to 0.44% and 0 to 2.97% respectively [45].

4.3.2. Discussion

Government baseline mapping indicated *W. bancrofti* and *B. malayi* were endemic at low to moderate levels in four provinces in northern Cambodia. Two representative studies and a prior review confirmed these findings [14]. Cambodia completed post-MDA surveillance in 2015 and WHO validated elimination of LF as a public health problem in 2016.

Whilst LF transmission has now ceased, an overall moderate combined morbidity burden remains in Cambodia. Although the government reported only 58 cases of morbidity in 2001, a representative survey from the same year found a low prevalence of lymphoedema (0.34%) and moderate prevalence of hydrocoele (1.64%) across the four endemic provinces. When the study's results are extrapolated using 1998 census population data [81], case estimates for lymphoedema and hydrocoele are 2800–17,382 and

8474–27,461 in the four provinces, respectively. Now that MDA is complete, efforts in Cambodia need to shift to assessing and alleviating the morbidity burden in the country.

4.4. Northeast India

4.4.1. Results

Filariasis is endemic in 250 districts across 20 states in India, with 617 million individuals at risk [78]. Assam is considered the only endemic state in Northeast India [5].

Baseline government mapping from 2004 illustrates a line of endemic districts from the Bangladesh to the Myanmar border with a prevalence of 0–5% [5].

Studies prior to the commencement of MDA in 2004 found a bancroftian Mf prevalence of 0.61–10.27% and 0.45–1.79% in tea-estate and non-tea-estate populations, respectively [32,37–40,51]. Sub-group meta-analysis showed a significantly higher Mf prevalence in populations living in tea-estates (6.11%, 95%CI 3.49–9.41%) compared to those who did not (0.88%, 0.3–1.54) ($p = 0.000$). A more recent study found persistent microfilaraemia of 7.41% in a tea-estate following six rounds of MDA [41]. The government reports that the national infection prevalence has decreased from 1.24% in 2004 to 0.35% in 2011 [5].

The prevalence of lymphoedema and hydrocoele found in tea-estate populations was 0.12–0.72% and 1.01–8.96%, respectively [32,37,39–41,51]. One study assessed morbidity in a non-tea-estate community and found no clinical cases [40].

4.4.2. Discussion

Available data indicate that Assam is the only LF-endemic state in Northeast India. Baseline mapping and studies demonstrated very high levels of *W. bancrofti* infection amongst those living in tea-estates and a moderate prevalence in non-tea estate populations. Tea-estates are predominantly composed of workers who migrated from states such as Bengal, Bihar, Odisha, Uttar Pradesh, Madhya Pradesh, Tamil Nadu and Jharkhand as part of the British tea trade in the 19th and early 20th century. Whilst national infection prevalence has progressively declined since the commencement of the MDA program in 2004, a recent study found very high levels of persisting microfilaraemia in a tea-estate following six rounds of MDA [41]. Reports of missed MDA rounds in seven districts in 2009, as well as suboptimal drug coverage may account for the ongoing LF transmission in the region [63,74,75]. Further rounds of MDA with sufficient coverage and uptake are required.

Multiple representative studies have demonstrated an overall moderate burden of disease in the tea-estate population of Assam with a low prevalence of lymphoedema but very high prevalence of hydrocoele. Insufficient datawere available to assess the morbidity burden in the non-tea estate population. In addition to ongoing MDA, programmatic efforts should focus on assessing the morbidity burden in non-tea populations and implementing alleviation programs.

4.5. Lao PDR

4.5.1. Results

No studies on the prevalence of LF in Lao PDR were found.Grey literature indicates that *W. bancrofti* is only endemic in the southern Attapeu and Sekong Provinces of Lao PDR with 137,000 individuals at risk [65,66,72,79]. Mapping of the Attapeu's five districts in 2009 showed an antigenaemia prevalence ranging 1.9–27.4% [65]. MDA commenced in Attapeu in one district in 2008 and was expanded to all five in 2009. Only one village in Sekong Province is endemic with a prevalence of 6% [65]. Two rounds of focused MDA have been completed in this and surrounding villages.

Only one case of lymphoedema and no cases of hydrocoele have been reported in the country [66].

4.5.2. Discussion

Government data from Lao PDR suggest that *W. bancrofti* is focussed in Attapeu province (along the Cambodian border) and parts of the adjacent Sekong province. Infection prevalence was initially considered low to moderate as noted by previous reviews [1,11,14,15]. However, further baseline surveys in 2009 found very high levels of antigenaemia in Attapeu province. Since the commencement of widespread MDA, infection prevalence appears to have decreased to low to moderate levels, however no independent studies are available to validate government data.

Insufficient dataare available to assess the morbidity burden in Lao PDR. Given the infection prevalence in Attapeu and morbidity burden in neighbouring Cambodia, numerous cases would be expected. Further studies are urgently needed to validate government data and assess the morbidity burden in Lao PDR.

4.6. Malaysia

4.6.1. Results

WHO reports indicate that 116 of the 994 implementation units (subdistricts and districts) are endemic across Peninsular Malaysia, Sabah and Sarawak with 1.12 million people at risk [72,79]. Subperiodic *B. malayi* accounts for the majority of cases, with 2% caused by *W. bancrofti*. Government data suggest Mf prevalence had decreased from 1% to 0.2% in Peninsular Malaysia and 5.5% to 1.5% in Sabah and Sarawak from the 1980s until the commencement of the National MDA Program in 2004 [66,67].

Pre-MDA studies of the local population in Peninsular Malaysia, Sabah and Sarawak found a prevalence of *B. malayi* Mf of 0.26–23.85%, 20.69% and 0.90%, respectively [31,34,35,46,53].

Since 2004, Malaysia has completed five rounds of MDA in Peninsular Malaysia and seven rounds in Sabah and Sarawak. As of 2014, only five IUs were still conducting MDA rounds with the remainder commencing TAS [79]. More recent studies in Peninsular Malaysia have found a prevalence of Mf and IgG4 of 0 and 2.16% respectively [25,54].

No data on the prevalence of LF-associated morbidity in the local Malaysian population were found.

4.6.2. Discussion

Brugia malayi (and to a lesser extent *W. bancrofti*) was widely endemic across Peninsular Malaysia, Sabah and Sarawak. Government surveys reported a low to moderate baseline infection prevalence. Whilst pre-MDA studies showed greater levels of infection than government data, most were not representative. These studies likely reflected the presence of highly-endemic foci in parts of Peninsular Malaysia and Sabah, rather than a high baseline prevalence. More recent surveys suggest infection levels are declining in Malaysia, although one study was conducted in a known low-endemic area [54]. Whilst recent government data are lacking, a 2016 xenomonitoring survey across five states in Peninsular Malaysia and Sabah found no active transmission [82], suggesting a likely low level of infection and supporting Malaysia's progress toward LF elimination. Further studies are required to assess current infection prevalence and the need for ongoing MDA.

Although there are no data on the morbidity prevalence in the local Malay population, a significant burden of lymphoedema is expected given the previously highly endemic foci of *B. malayi* infection. Studies assessing the morbidity burden are needed to fill this knowledge gap.

4.7. Myanmar

4.7.1. Results

Bancroftian filariasis is endemic in 45 of the 65 districts of Myanmar with 85.5% of the population at risk [5]. No published prevalence studies on Myanmar were found. One study described in a WHO report assessed filarial antigenaemia prevalence in 1997 [73]. One hundred individuals were tested by

ICT from seventy randomly selected townships across 14 districts. The central and western dry zone was highly endemic (20–30%) with the northern, eastern and southern areas less endemic or free from filariasis. Most recent government microfilaraemia prevalence data for the western Sagaing, Magway, Rakhine and Chin regions range from 0–65% [68–70]. Prevalence in Mandalay, Kayin and Yangon regions ranges from 0–2% [68–70]. Mean national prevalence has reduced from 7.1% in 2001 to 2.7% in 2011 [5]. Myanmar commenced its MDA Program in 2001. As of 2014, the program had been scaled-up to 22 of the 24 endemic districts.

One government survey assessed self-reported morbidity in 280 000 individuals in Sagaing region in 2004 and identified 520 cases of lymphoedema (0.19%) and 827 cases of hydrocoele (0.59%) [68].

4.7.2. Discussion

Baseline surveys suggest that *W. bancrofti* were widely endemic in the low-lying parts of Myanmar with over 85% of the population at risk. They suggested very high baseline levels of infection in the central and western dry zones, consistent with that seen in Myanmar migrants in Thailand. Meanwhile, the northern, eastern and southern areas were less endemic or free from filariasis. Government data suggest declining levels of infection in Mandalay, Kayin and Yangon states since the commencement of MDA, but very high rates of persisting infection in the western states of Sagaing, Magway, Rakhine and Chin. As Myanmar continues to expand its MDA program, independent studies are required to validate government prevalence data.

The only morbidity survey found low levels of self-reported lymphoedema and moderate levels of hydrocoele in Sagaing region [68]. However, morbidity self-reporting questionnaires are not a sensitive or specific indicator of clinical disease [45,83]. The significant morbidity found in Myanmar migrants in Thailand suggests that the true morbidity prevalence is likely much higher. Representative prevalence studies are required to elucidate the morbidity burden in Myanmar.

4.8. Thailand

4.8.1. Results

Baseline government mapping in 2001 found filariasis to be endemic in two foci in Thailand with 160,000 individuals at risk [5]. *Wuchereria bancrofti* was present in five provinces along the Thai-Myanmar border, whilst *B. malayi* was endemic along the southern Thai peninsula. Studies in provinces along the Myanmar border between 1998 and 2003 found an infection prevalence of 1.01–10.20%, 13.3–26.42%, 21.89–36.79% and 53.93% by TBS, ICT, Og4C3 and IgG4, respectively [26,27, 29,49,50]. Meanwhile, studies conducted along the Thai peninsula between 2001 and 2006 reported a prevalence of *B. malayi* infection of 0–2.00% and 8.00–23.67% by TBS and IgG4 [36,43,59].

The 11 studies which assessed infection in Myanmar migrants living in Thailand found a prevalence of 0–5.83%, 0.2–13.57%, 4.0–23.98%, and 2.73–42.32% by TBS, ICT, Og4C3 and IgG4, respectively [26,28,29,42,43,48,57,58,60,61].

Thailand commenced an elimination program in 2002. Mass drug administration was completed in 2007 in all provinces except Narathiwatt, which extended rounds until 2011. Thailand commenced the process of verifying LF elimination in 2012 after all areas passed TAS. National mean data suggest infection prevalence has decreased from 0.77% in 2003 to 0.09% in 2010 [5]. No post-MDA prevalence studies on the local population were identified.

Available studies have found the prevalence of lymphoedema and hydrocoele in the local population in endemic areas was 1.2% and 0–8.15% [27,29,36]. Studies of Myanmar migrants found a prevalence of hydrocoele of 8.62–16.13% [29,48]. As of 2011, the government had 200 identified cases of lymphoedema [77].

4.8.2. Discussion

Two highly endemic LF foci previously existed in Thailand. *W. bancrofti* was present along the Thai-Myanmar border, whilst *B. malayi* was endemic along the southern Thai peninsula. Government surveys suggest that LF transmission has ceased following MDA, but no studies have independently verified this.

The influx of LF-infected Myanmar migrants into Thailand, combined with a documented ability of Thai *Culex quinquefasciatus* mosquitoes to transmit the Myanmar strain of *W. bancrofti* has raised concerns regarding the potential for re-introduction of transmission [84,85]. The Thai government has acknowledged this and expanded its MDA program to include registered migrant workers from Myanmar and Laos [57,86]. However, the considerable number of unregistered migrants still poses a threat to elimination efforts.

Whilst the government had only identified 200 cases of lymphoedema in 2011, available studies suggest a potentially moderate prevalence of lymphoedema and very high prevalence of hydrocoele in previously endemic areas. However the representativeness of these surveys is uncertain, indicating the need for further studies to establish the true disease burden in these areas.

4.9. Vietnam

4.9.1. Results

No peer-reviewed studies from Vietnam were identified. Government data suggest filariasis was endemic in six of Vietnam's eight regions during 1960–2000 [66]. However, by the start of the National Elimination Program in 2003, only the Red River delta, north-central coast and central-southern coast regions remained endemic despite no MDA [65,66]. Within these regions, 12 districts were considered endemic and six selected for MDA with a total population at-risk of 675,000. *Brugia malayi* predominates in the north with *W. bancrofti* in the south [65,66].

Baseline prevalence in endemic districts in 2002 ranged from 0 to 3.6% [65,66]. Vietnam completed its MDA program in 2011 and passed TAS in all districts in 2015. It has subsequently applied to the WHO for LF elimination confirmation [65].

A government clinical survey in 2002 in 77 districts reported 570 cases of limb morbidity and 47 cases of hydrocoele [66]. A later survey in 2012 identified 489 morbidity cases in five provinces [65].

4.9.2. Discussion

Filariasis was historically widespread in Vietnam with *Brugia malayi* predominating in the north and *W. bancrofti* in the south. However by the commencement of the MDA Program, it had become confined to the Red River delta, north-central coast and central-southern coast regions. These findings are consistent with those found in prior reviews [14–16]. It has been suggested that the reduction in infection prevalence prior to MDA was likely the result of improvements in housing and living conditions, man-made ecological changes, the use of bed-nets and individual case treatment [16,65]. These changes appear to have resulted in low baseline infection prevalence levels by the start of the MDA with the exception of Khanh Vinh and Ninh Hoa districts, where prevalence remained high. Government data suggest that since MDA, LF transmission has now ceased, although no independent studies have yet validated this.

Whilst government surveys suggest a relatively few cases of morbidity, the number of participants surveyed is unknown, and therefore prevalence estimates cannot be made. Given filariasis was historically widespread with some highly endemic foci, the true morbidity burden may be higher [16]. As Vietnam approaches LF elimination, studies are needed to validate government progress and assess the morbidity burden in the country.

4.10. Overall Prevalence Estimates for Mainland Southeast Asia

4.10.1. Meta-Analysis Results

A random effects meta-analysis of available infection and morbidity data was completed. Figures 3–7 and Figures S1–S9 show the point estimates with 95% exact binomial confidence intervals (95% CI) for each meta-analysis ordered by country and study date. Substantial heterogeneity between surveys was demonstrated by I^2 values, between 83.57% and 98.74%.

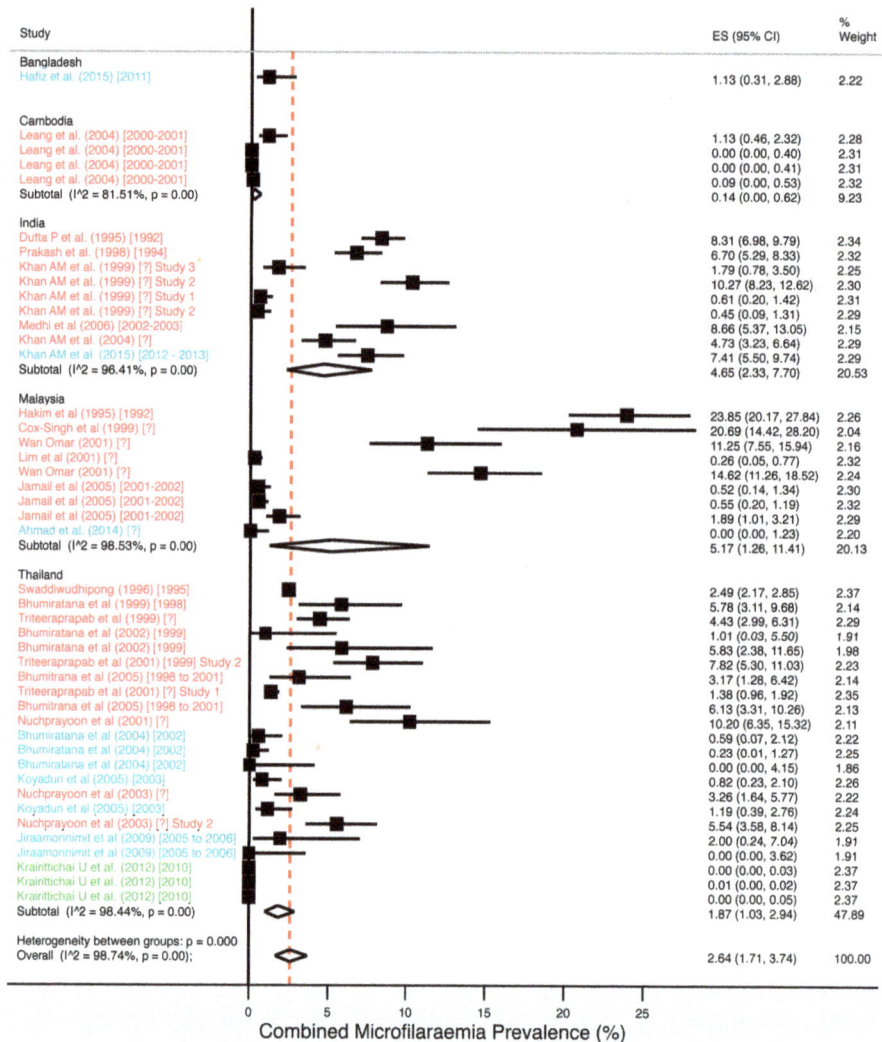

Figure 3. Percentage estimates of combined microfilaraemia prevalence by country and year. ES: prevalence estimate. Red-dashed line: overall estimate. Diamond: subgroup estimate. Horizontal line: 95% CI. Red study: pre-MDA, blue study: mid-MDA, green study: post-MDA.

For microfilaraemia, 30 studies testing 133,747 individuals estimated a pooled prevalence of *W. bancrofti* Mf of 1.77% (1.00–2.74%), *B. malayi* Mf of 0.36% (0.07–0.82%) and combined Mf of 2.64%

(1.71–3.74%). For ICT antigenaemia, 10 studies testing 7237 individuals estimated a pooled prevalence of 4.48% (1.97–7.87%). For IgG4 antibodies, 10 studies testing 14,339 individuals estimated a pooled prevalence of 7.08% (3.63–11.54%).

For combined morbidity, 16 studies testing 256,591 individuals estimated a pooled prevalence of 1.34% (0.81–1.97%). For hydrocoele, nine studies testing 4179 estimated a pooled prevalence of 3.84% (2.11–6.03%). For lymphoedema, nine studies testing 240,987 individuals estimated a pooled prevalence of 0.49% (0.24–0.80%).

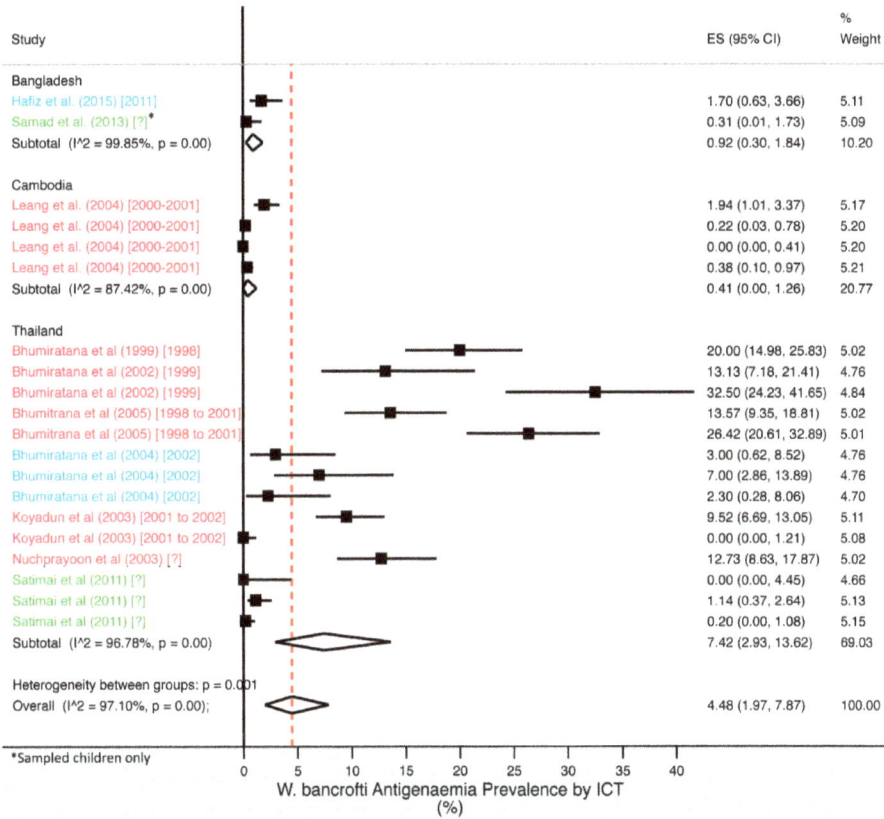

Figure 4. Percentage estimates of ICT antigenaemia prevalence by country and year. ES: prevalence estimate. Red-dotted line: overall estimate. Blue diamond: sub-group estimate. Horizontal line: 95% CI. Red study: pre-MDA, blue study: mid-MDA, green study: post-MDA.

4.10.2. Discussion

Meta-analysis showed an overall high prevalence of infection (Mf: 2.64%, antigenaemia: 4.48%) and moderate burden of morbidity (1.34%) in the region. However, pooled estimates and sub-group analyses by country are biased by the significant differences in location, time, design, diagnosis method, sampling unit and representativeness of the included studies, and should therefore be interpreted with caution. Despite this, meta-analyses show a general decline in infection prevalence with time and a higher prevalence of hydrocoele compared to lymphoedema across all countries (overall hydrocoele:lymphoedema ratio of 7.84:1).

In the context of pooled country estimates, grey literature and the quality of available data, we conclude that Lao PDR, Myanmar and Northeast India demonstrate ongoing evidence of LF transmission that will require multiple further rounds of MDA. Bangladesh, Malaysia, Thailand and Vietnam appear close to having eliminated LF, whilst Cambodia has already achieved elimination status. We estimated that the burden of morbidity is likely high in Thailand, moderate in Cambodia, Myanmar, and Northeast India, and low in Bangladesh. There was insufficient evidence to accurately estimate the disease burden in Lao PDR, Malaysia or Vietnam.

These results indicate that whilst considerable progress toward LF elimination has been made, there remains a significant filariasis burden in the region. The results will assist policy makers to advocate and budget for future MDA and morbidity control programs.

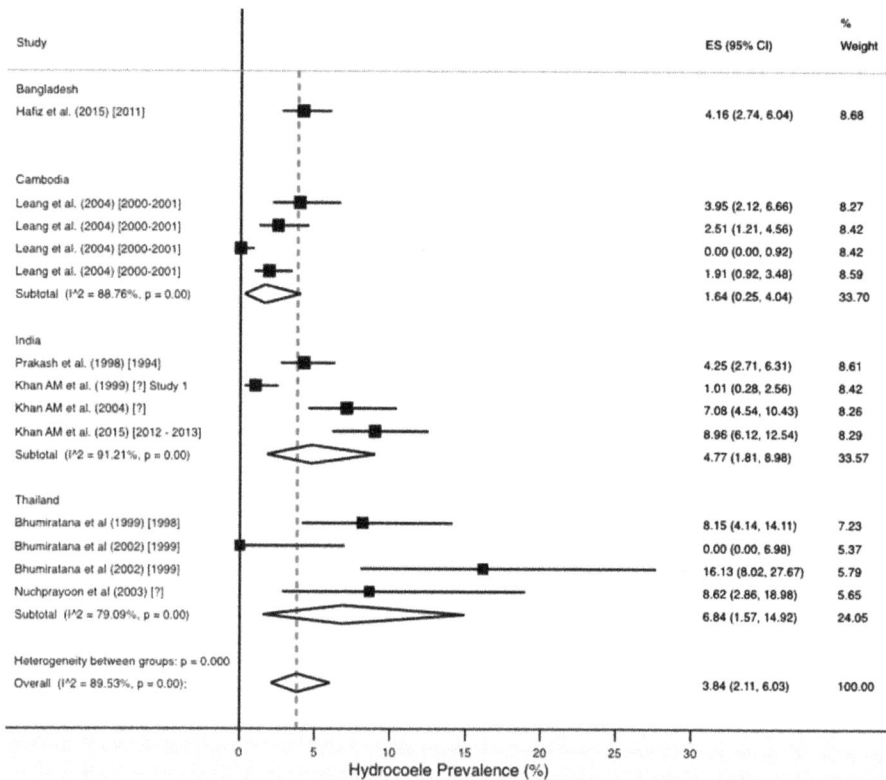

Figure 5. Percentage estimates of hydrocoele prevalence by country and year. ES: prevalence estimate. Red-dotted line: overall estimate. Diamond: sub-group estimate. Horizontal line: 95% CI.

4.11. Limitations

This systematic review was hindered by limitations at the study and review level. The overall quality of primary studies was suboptimal. Only 18% of studies used fully representative sampling methods and consensus data collection methods. Some of the studies were out-dated because one or more MDA rounds had occurred since data collection. The quality of grey literature further hindered data analysis. Available reports frequently omitted sample sizes or gave prevalence data in percentage ranges, making further analysis difficult. The uncertain methodology of government surveys further complicated grey literature assessment. Whilst national programs follow the WHO guidelines, there is often considerable variation in sampling and data collection practices in the field [22]. No published studies were available from Lao PDR, Myanmar or Vietnam to compare with government data.

Incomplete literature retrieval led to limitations at the review level. Original copies of government annual reports were obtained only from Myanmar, although use of WHO reports alleviated this deficiency to some extent. Retrieval of these data would provide a more complete picture of filariasis prevalence in these countries.

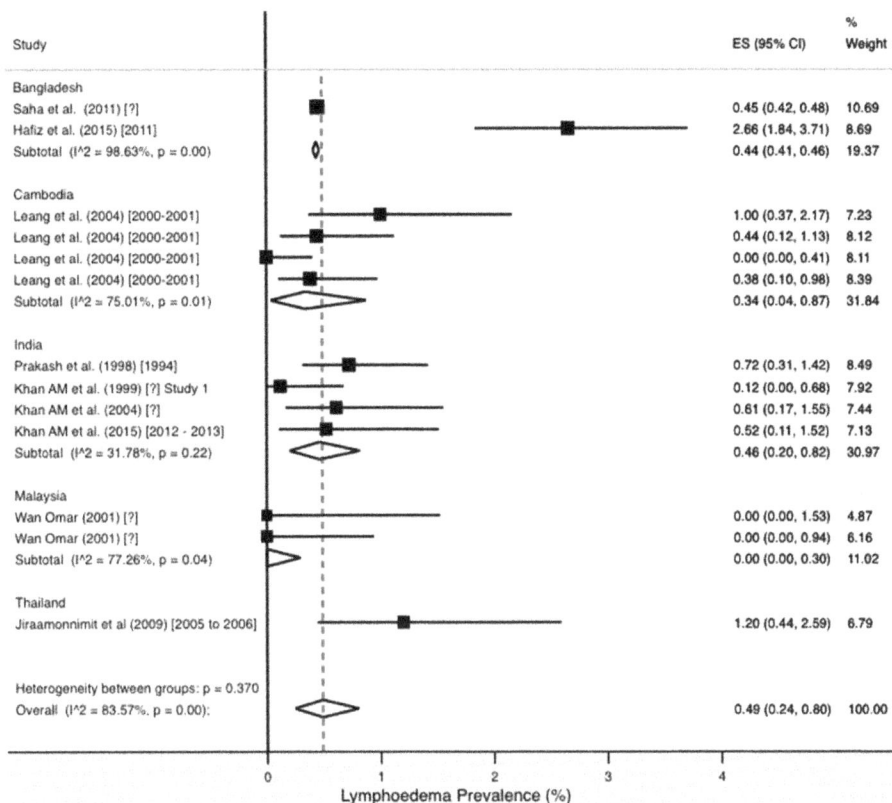

Figure 6. Percentage estimates of lymphoedema prevalence by country and year. ES: prevalence estimate. Red-dotted line: overall estimate. Diamond: sub-group estimate. Horizontal line: 95% CI.

The lack of representative and recent studies in many of the countries placed reliance on government sources for current prevalence data. Whilst sufficient information on infection was available to produce country estimates, data on the morbidity burden are notably lacking. This indicates the substantial need for further studies, with a particular focus on morbidity, to more accurately assess the current LF prevalence in the region.

It is important to note that the findings and conclusions in this paper are based solely on published prevalence data. It is therefore possible that they may not truly reflect the actual situation in these countries.

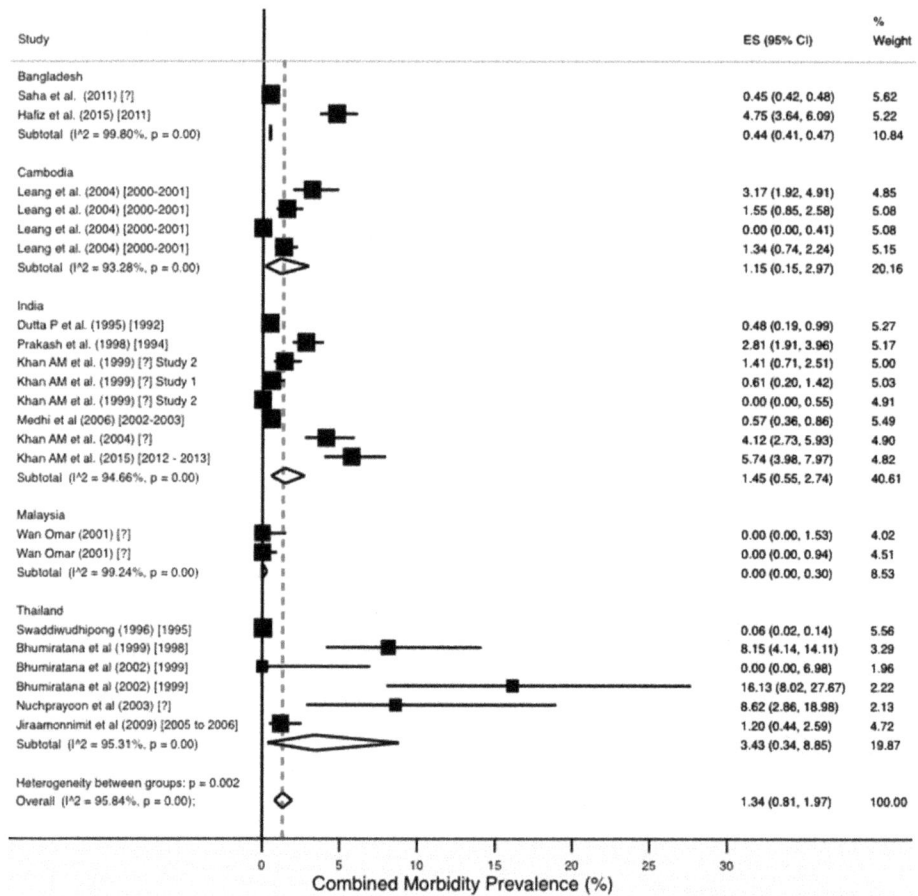

Figure 7. Percentage estimates of combined morbidity prevalence by country and year. ES: prevalence estimate. Red-dotted line: overall estimate. Diamond: sub-group estimate. Horizontal line: 95% CI.

5. Conclusions

Considerable progress has been made toward the LF elimination in mainland Southeast Asia, Bangladesh and Northeast India. Five of the eight countries reviewed are close to eliminating, or have eliminated, LF infection. The remaining three countries will require increasing support if they are to achieve LF elimination by 2020. The significant morbidity burden in the region requires increasing and urgent attention. Further studies are needed to more accurately assess the morbidity prevalence and implement desperately needed alleviation programs.

Supplementary Materials: The following are available online at www.mdpi.com/2414-6366/2/3/32/s1. Table S1: Quality Assessment of Included Peer-Reviewed Journal Articles; Table S2: Infection and Morbidity Prevalence by Country and Region in Peer-Reviewed Journals; Table S3: Infection and Morbidity Prevalence by Country and Region in Grey Literature; Figure S1: Percentage estimates of *W. bancrofti* microfilaraemia prevalence by country and year; Figure S2: Percentage estimates of *B. malayi* microfilaraemia prevalence by country and year; Figure S3: Percentage estimates of Og4C3 antigenaemia prevalence by country and year; Figure S4: Percentage estimates of IgG4 antibody prevalence by country and year; Figure S5: Percentage estimates of combined microfilaraemia prevalence in Northeast India; Figure S6: Percentage estimates of combined microfilaraemia prevalence in Thailand; Figure S7: Percentage estimates of ICT antigenaemia prevalence in Thailand; Figure S8: Percentage estimates of hydrocoele prevalence in Thailand; Figure S9: Percentage estimates of combined morbidity prevalence in Thailand. Figure S10: PRISMA checklist.

Acknowledgments: The authors would like to thank Mohamed Jamsheed (WHO SEARO), Krongthong Thimasarn (WHO Myanmar), Gawrie Galappaththy (WHO Myanmar), San San Win (WHO Myanmar), Md. Kamar Rezwan (WHO Bangladesh), Kapa Ramaiah (consultant to WHO WPRO), Ni Ni Aye (VBDC Program, Myanmar Ministry of Health) and Aya Yajima (WHO WPRO) for information, collaboration and reports. We would also like to thank James Cook University for funding this research.

Author Contributions: B.F.R.D., P.M.G. and W.J.M. designed the study. B.F.R.D. collected the data. B.F.R.D. and P.M.G. analysed the data. B.F.R.D. and P.M.G. wrote the paper with input from W.J.M. All authors reviewed the final manuscript.

Conflicts of Interest: P.M.G. was a co-investigator in Hafiz et al. 2015 and participated in the 13th and 14th Meeting of the WPR Program Review Group on NTDs and the WPR Program Managers Meeting on NTDs 2013. The paper and reports from the three meetings were included in this review.

References

1. World Health Organization. *WHO Global Programme to Eliminate Lymphatic Filariasis: Progress Report for 2000–2009 and Strategic Plan 2010–2020*; World Health Organization: Geneva, Switzerland, 2010.
2. World Health Organization. Global programme to eliminate lymphatic filariasis: Progress report, 2015. *Wkly. Epidemiol. Record* **2016**, *91*, 441–460.
3. Ramaiah, K.; Ottesen, E.A. Progress and impact of 13 years of the global programme to eliminate lymphatic filariasis on reducing the burden of filarial disease. *PLoS Negl. Trop. Dis.* **2014**, *8*, e3319. [CrossRef] [PubMed]
4. Murray, C.J.; Barber, R.M.; Foreman, K.J.; Ozgoren, A.A.; Abd-Allah, F.; Abera, S.F.; Aboyans, V.; Abraham, J.P.; Abubakar, I.; Abu-Raddad, L.J. Global, regional, and national disability-adjusted life years (DALYs) for 306 diseases and injuries and healthy life expectancy (HALE) for 188 countries, 1990–2013: Quantifying the epidemiological transition. *Lancet* **2015**, *386*, 2145–2191. [CrossRef]
5. World Health Organization: Regional Office for South-East Asia. *Towards Eliminating Lymphatic Filariasis: Progress in the South-East.Region. (2001–2011)*; World Health Organization Regional Office for South-East Asia: New Delhi, India, 2013.
6. Weil, G.J.; Jain, D.C.; Santhanam, S.; Malhotra, A.; Kumar, H.; Sethumadhavan, K.V.P.; Liftis, F.; Ghosh, T.K. A monoclonal antibody-based enzyme immunoassay for detecting parasite antigenemia in bancroftian filariasis. *J. Infect. Dis.* **1987**, *156*, 350–355. [CrossRef] [PubMed]
7. Weil, G.J.; Lammie, P.J.; Weiss, N. The ICT filariasis test: A rapid-format antigen test for diagnosis of bancroftian filariasis. *Parasitol. Today* **1997**, *13*, 401–404. [CrossRef]
8. Gass, K.; de Rochars, M.V.B.; Boakye, D.; Bradley, M.; Fischer, P.U.; Gyapong, J.; Itoh, M.; Ituaso-Conway, N.; Joseph, H.; Kyelem, D. A multicenter evaluation of diagnostic tools to define endpoints for programs to eliminate bancroftian filariasis. *PLoS Negl. Trop. Dis.* **2012**, *6*, e1479. [CrossRef] [PubMed]
9. Lammie, P.J.; Weil, G.; Noordin, R.; Kaliraj, P.; Steel, C.; Goodman, D.; Lakshmikanthan, V.B.; Ottesen, E. Recombinant antigen-based antibody assays for the diagnosis and surveillance of lymphatic filariasis—A multicenter trial. *Filaria J.* **2004**, *3*, 9. [CrossRef] [PubMed]
10. Rebollo, M.P.; Bockarie, M.J. Shrinking the lymphatic filariasis map: Update on diagnostic tools for mapping and transmission monitoring. *Parasitology* **2014**, *141*, 1912–1917. [CrossRef] [PubMed]
11. World Health Organization. *WHO Global Programme to Eliminate Lymphatic Filariasis: Practical Entomology*; World Health Organization: Geneva, Switzerland, 2013.
12. World Health Organization. *Validation of Elimination of Lymphatic Filariasis as A Public Health Problem*; World Health Organization: Geneva, Switzerland, 2017.
13. World Health Organization. *Transmission Assessment Surveys in the Global Programme to Eliminate Lymphatic Filariasis: WHO Position Statement*; World Health Organization: Geneva, Switzerland, 2012.
14. Sudomo, M.; Chayabejara, S.; Duong, S.; Hernandez, L.; Wu, W.P.; Bergquist, R. Elimination of lymphatic filariasis in Southeast Asia. *Adv. Parasitol.* **2010**, *72*, 205–233. [PubMed]
15. Michael, E.; Bundy, D.A.P.; Grenfell, B.T. Re-assessing the global prevalence and distribution of lymphatic filariasis. *Parasitology* **1996**, *112*, 409–428. [CrossRef] [PubMed]
16. Meyrowitsch, D.W.; Nguyen, D.T.; Hoang, T.H.; Nguyen, T.D.; Michael, E. A review of the present status of lymphatic filariasis in Vietnam. *Acta Trop.* **1998**, *70*, 335–347. [CrossRef]

17. Moher, D.; Liberati, A.; Tetzlaff, J.; Altman, D.G. Preferred reporting items for systematic reviews and meta-analyses: The PRISMA statement. *Ann. Intern. Med.* **2009**, *151*, 264–269. [CrossRef] [PubMed]
18. PROSPERO Registered Study Protocol. Available online: http://www.crd.york.ac.uk/PROSPERO/display_record.asp?ID=CRD42014013070#.VAihrWSSxBA (accessed on 11 December 2016).
19. World Health Organization. *Institutional Repository of Information Sharing*. Available online: http://apps.who.int/iris/ (accessed on 11 December 2016).
20. Crowe, M. *Crowe Critical Appraisal Tool (CCAT) User Guide*; Conchra House: Scotland, UK, 2013.
21. Jackson, R.; Ameratunga, S.; Broad, J.; Connor, J.; Lethaby, A.; Robb, G.; Wells, S.; Glasziou, P.; Heneghan, C. The GATE frame: Critical appraisal with pictures. *Evid. Based Nurs.* **2006**, *9*, 68–71. [CrossRef] [PubMed]
22. World Health Organization. *Monitoring and Epidemiological Assessment of the Programme to Eliminate Lymphatic Filariasis at Implementation Unit Level*; World Health Organization: Geneva, Switzerland, 2005.
23. DerSimonian, R.; Laird, N. Meta-analysis in clinical trials. *Controll. Clin. Trials* **1986**, *7*, 177–188. [CrossRef]
24. Higgins, J.; Thompson, S.G.; Deeks, J.J.; Altman, D.G. Measuring inconsistency in meta-analyses. *BMJ* **2003**, *327*, 557–560. [CrossRef] [PubMed]
25. Ahmad, A.F.; Ngui, R.; Muhammad Aidil, R.; Lim, Y.A.; Rohela, M. Current status of parasitic infections among Pangkor Island community in Peninsular Malaysia. *Trop. Biomed.* **2014**, *31*, 836–843. [PubMed]
26. Bhumiratana, A.; Koyadun, S.; Srisuphanunt, M.; Satitvipawee, P.; Limpairojn, N.; Gaewchaiyo, G. Border and imported bancroftian filariases: Baseline seroprevalence in sentinel populations exposed to infections with *Wuchereria bancrofti* and concomitant HIV at the start of diethylcarbamazine mass treatment in Thailand. *Southeast Asian J. Trop. Med. Public Health* **2005**, *36*, 390–407. [PubMed]
27. Bhumiratana, A.; Koyadun, S.; Suvannadabba, S.; Karnjanopas, K.; Rojanapremsuk, J.; Buddhirakkul, P.; Tantiwattanasup, W. Field trial of the ICT filariasis for diagnosis of *Wuchereria bancrofti* infections in an endemic population of Thailand. *Southeast Asian J. Trop. Med. Public Health* **1999**, *30*, 562–568. [PubMed]
28. Bhumiratana, A.; Siriaut, C.; Koyadun, S.; Satitvipawee, P. Evaluation of a single oral dose of diethylcarbamazine 300 mg as provocative test and simultaneous treatment in Myanmar migrant workers with *Wuchereria bancrofti* infection in Thailand. *Southeast Asian J. Trop. Med. Public Health* **2004**, *35*, 591–598. [PubMed]
29. Bhumiratana, A.; Wattanakull, B.; Koyadun, S.; Suvannadabba, S.; Rojanapremsuk, J.; Tantiwattanasup, W. Relationship between male hydrocele and infection prevalences in clustered communities with uncertain transmission of *Wuchereria bancrofti* on the Thailand-Myanmar border. *Southeast Asian J. Trop. Med. Public Health* **2002**, *33*, 7–17. [PubMed]
30. Chansiri, K.; Phantana, S. A polymerase chain reaction assay for the survey of bancroftian filariasis. *Southeast Asian J. Trop. Med. Public Health* **2002**, *33*, 504–508. [PubMed]
31. Cox-Singh, J.; Pomrehn, A.S.; Rahman, H.A.; Zakaria, R.; Miller, A.O.; Singh, B. Simple blood-spot sampling with nested polymerase chain reaction detection for epidemiology studies on Brugia malayi. *Int. J. Parasitol.* **1999**, *29*, 717–721. [CrossRef]
32. Dutta, P.; Gogoi, B.K.; Chelleng, P.K.; Bhattacharyya, D.R.; Khan, S.A.; Goswami, B.K.; Mahanta, J. Filariasis in the labour population of a tea estate in Upper Assam. *Indian J. Med. Res.* **1995**, *101*, 245–246. [PubMed]
33. Hafiz, I.; Graves, P.; Haq, R.; Flora, M.S.; Kelly-Hope, L.A. Clinical case estimates of lymphatic filariasis in an endemic district of Bangladesh after a decade of mass drug administration. *Trans. R. Soc. Trop. Med. Hyg.* **2015**, *109*, 700–709. [CrossRef] [PubMed]
34. Hakim, S.L.; Vythilingam, I.; Marzukhi, M.I.; Mak, J.W. Single-dose diethylcarbamazine in the control of periodic brugian filariasis in Peninsular Malaysia. *Trans. R. Soc. Trop. Med. Hyg.* **1995**, *89*, 686–689. [CrossRef]
35. Jamail, M.; Andrew, K.; Junaidi, D.; Krishnan, A.K.; Faizal, M.; Rahmah, N. Field validation of sensitivity and specificity of rapid test for detection of Brugia malayi infection. *Trop. Med. Int. Health* **2005**, *10*, 99–104. [CrossRef] [PubMed]
36. Jiraamonnimit, C.; Wongkamchai, S.; Boitano, J.; Nochot, H.; Loymek, S.; Chujun, S.; Yodmek, S. A cohort study on anti-filarial IgG4 and its assessment in good and uncertain MDA-compliant subjects in brugian filariasis endemic areas in southern Thailand. *J. Helminthol.* **2009**, *83*, 351–360. [CrossRef] [PubMed]
37. Khan, A.M.; Dutta, P.; Khan, S.A.; Baruah, N.K.; Sarma, C.K.; Mahanta, J. Prevalence of bancroftian filariasis in a foot-hill tea garden of upper Assam. *J. Commun. Dis.* **1999**, *31*, 145–146. [PubMed]
38. Khan, A.M.; Dutta, P.; Khan, S.A.; Baruah, N.K.; Sharma, C.K.; Mahanta, J. Bancroftian filariasis in a weaving community of lower Assam. *J. Commun. Dis.* **1999**, *31*, 61–62. [PubMed]

39. Khan, A.M.; Dutta, P.; Khan, S.A.; Mahanta, J. A focus of lymphatic filariasis in a tea garden worker community of central Assam. *J. Environ. Biol.* **2004**, *25*, 437–440. [PubMed]
40. Khan, A.M.; Dutta, P.; Khan, S.A.; Mohapatra, P.K.; Baruah, N.K.; Sharma, C.K.; Mahanta, A.J. Lymphatic filariasis in two distinct communities of upper Assam. *J. Commun. Dis.* **1999**, *31*, 101–106. [PubMed]
41. Khan, A.M.; Dutta, P.; Sarmah, C.K.; Baruah, N.K.; Das, S.; Pathak, A.K.; Sarmah, P.; Hussain, M.E.; Mahanta, J. Prevalence of lymphatic filariasis in a tea garden worker population of Dibrugarh (Assam), India after six rounds of mass drug administration. *J. Vector Borne Dis.* **2015**, *52*, 314–320. [PubMed]
42. Koyadun, S.; Bhumiratana, A. Surveillance of imported bancroftian filariasis after two-year multiple-dose diethylcarbamazine treatment. *Southeast Asian J. Trop. Med. Public Health* **2005**, *36*, 822–831. [PubMed]
43. Koyadun, S.; Bhumiratana, A.; Prikchu, P. *Wuchereria bancrofti* antigenemia clearance among Myanmar migrants after biannual mass treatments with diethylcarbamazine, 300 mg oral-dose FILADEC tablet, in Southern Thailand. *Southeast Asian J. Trop. Med. Public Health* **2003**, *34*, 758–767. [PubMed]
44. Krairittichai, U.; Pungprakiet, D.; Boonthongtho, K.; Arsayot, K. Prevalence of infectious diseases of immigrant workers receiving health examinations at Rajavithi Hospital. *J. Med. Assoc. Thail.* **2012**, *95* (Suppl. 3), S1–S6.
45. Leang, R.; Socheat, D.; Bin, B.; Bunkea, T.; Odermatt, P. Assessment of disease and infection of lymphatic filariasis in Northeastern Cambodia. *Trop. Med. Int. Health* **2004**, *9*, 1115–1120. [CrossRef] [PubMed]
46. Lim, B.H.; Rahmah, N.; Afifi, S.A.; Ramli, A.; Mehdi, R. Comparison of Brugia-ELISA and thick blood smear examination in a prevalence study of brugian filariasis in Setiu, Terengganu, Malaysia. *Med. J. Malays.* **2001**, *56*, 491–496.
47. Medhi, G.K.; Hazarika, N.C.; Shah, B.; Mahanta, J. Study of health problems and nutritional status of tea garden population of Assam. *Indian J. Med. Sci.* **2006**, *60*, 496–505. [PubMed]
48. Nuchprayoon, S.; Porksakorn, C.; Junpee, A.; Sanprasert, V.; Poovorawan, Y. Comparative assessment of an Og4C3 ELISA and an ICT filariasis test: A study of Myanmar migrants in Thailand. *Asian Pac. J. Allergy Immunol.* **2003**, *21*, 253–257. [PubMed]
49. Nuchprayoon, S.; Sanprasert, V.; Porksakorn, C.; Nuchprayoon, I. Prevalence of bancroftian filariasis on the Thai-Myanmar border. *Asian Pac. J. Allergy Immunol.* **2003**, *21*, 179–188. [PubMed]
50. Nuchprayoon, S.; Yentakam, S.; Sangprakarn, S.; Junpee, A. Endemic bancroftian filariasis in Thailand: detection by Og4C3 antigen capture ELISA and the polymerase chain reaction. *J. Med. Assoc. Thail.* **2001**, *84*, 1300–1307.
51. Prakash, A.; Mohapatra, P.K.; Das, H.K.; Sharma, R.K.; Mahanta, J. Bancroftian filariasis in Namrup tea estate, district Dibrugarh, Assam. *Indian J. Public Health* **1998**, *42*, 103–107. [PubMed]
52. Priest, J.W.; Jenks, M.H.; Moss, D.M.; Mao, B.; Buth, S.; Wannemuehler, K.; Soeung, S.C.; Lucchi, N.W.; Udhayakumar, V.; Gregory, C.J. Integration of multiplex bead assays for parasitic diseases into a national, population-based serosurvey of women 15–39 years of age in Cambodia. *PLoS Negl. Trop. Dis.* **2016**, *10*, e0004699. [CrossRef] [PubMed]
53. Rahmah, N.; Lim, B.H.; Azian, H.; Ramelah, T.S.; Rohana, A.R. Short communication: Use of a recombinant antigen-based ELISA to determine prevalence of brugian filariasis among Malaysian schoolchildren near Pasir Mas, Kelantan-Thailand border. *Trop. Med. Int. Health* **2003**, *8*, 158–163. [CrossRef] [PubMed]
54. Rahmah, N.; Nurulhasanah, O.; Norhayati, S.; Zulkarnain, I.; Norizan, M. Comparison of conventional versus real-time PCR detection of *Brugia malayi* DNA from dried blood spots from school children in a low endemic area. *Trop. Biomed.* **2010**, *27*, 54–59. [PubMed]
55. Saha, A.K.; Mohanta, M.K. Bancroftian elephantiasis in Nilphamari, Bangladesh. *Mymensingh Med. J. MMJ* **2011**, *20*, 40–44. [PubMed]
56. Samad, M.S.; Itoh, M.; Moji, K.; Hossain, M.; Mondal, D.; Alam, M.S.; Kimura, E. Enzyme-linked immunosorbent assay for the diagnosis of *Wuchereria bancrofti* infection using urine samples and its application in Bangladesh. *J. Parasitol. Res.* **2013**, *62*, 564–567. [CrossRef] [PubMed]
57. Satimai, W.; Jiraamonnimit, C.; Thammapalo, S.; Choochote, W.; Luenee, P.; Boitano, J.J.; Wongkamchai, S. The impact of a national program to eliminate lymphatic filariasis in selected Myanmar immigrant communities in Bangkok and Ranong Province, Thailand. *Southeast Asian J. Trop. Med. Public Health* **2011**, *42*, 1054–1064. [PubMed]
58. Swaddiwudhipong, W.; Tatip, Y.; Meethong, M.; Preecha, P.; Kobasa, T. Potential transmission of bancroftian filariasis in urban Thailand. *Southeast Asian J. Trop. Med. Public Health* **1996**, *27*, 847–849. [PubMed]

59. Triteeraprapab, S.; Karnjanopas, K.; Porksakorn, C.; Sai-Ngam, A.; Yentakam, S.; Loymak, S. Lymphatic filariasis caused by *Brugia malayi* in an endemic area of Narathiwat Province, southern of Thailand. *J. Med. Assoc. Thail.* **2001**, *84* (Suppl. S1), S182–S188.

60. Triteeraprapab, S.; Nuchprayoon, I.; Porksakorn, C.; Poovorawan, Y.; Scott, A.L. High prevalence of *Wuchereria bancrofti* infection among Myanmar migrants in Thailand. *Ann. Trop. Med. Parasitol.* **2001**, *95*, 535–538. [CrossRef] [PubMed]

61. Triteeraprapab, S.; Songtrus, J. High prevalence of bancroftian filariasis in Myanmar-migrant workers: A study in Mae Sot district, Tak province, Thailand. *J. Med. Assoc. Thail.* **1999**, *82*, 735–739.

62. Wan Omar, A.; Sulaiman, O.; Yusof, S.; Ismail, G.; Fatmah, M.S.; Rahmah, N.; Khairul, A.A. Epidemiological screening of lymphatic filariasis among immigrants using dipstick colloidal dye immunoassay. *Malays. J. Med. Sci.* **2001**, *8*, 19–24. [PubMed]

63. World Health Organization: Regional Office for South-East Asia. *Elimination of Lymphatic Filariasis in the South-East Asia Region: Report of the Eighth Meeting of National National Programme Managers*; WHO Regional Office for South-East Asia: New Delhi, India, 2011.

64. World Health Organization: Regional Office for South-East Asia. *Elimination of Lymphatic Filariasis in the South-East Asia Region: Report of the Fifth Meeting of National National Programme Managers*; WHO Regional Office for South-East Asia: New Delhi, India, 2006.

65. United States Agency for International Development. *FHI360/USAID. End Neglected Tropical Diseases in Asia: Final Report*; USAID: Washington, DC, USA, 2015.

66. World Health Organization: Regional Office for the Western Pacific. *First Mekong-Plus Programme Managers Workshop on Lymphatic Filariasis and Other Helminthiasis, Phnom Penh, Cambodia, 23–26 March 2009*; WHO Regional Office for the Western Pacific: Manila, Philippines, 2009.

67. World Health Organization: Regional Office for the Western Pacific. *Malaysia: Country Cooperation Strategy 2009–2013*; WHO Regional Office for the Western Pacific: Manila, Philippines, 2010.

68. Myanmar Ministry of Health. *Myanmar National Programme to Eliminate Lymphatic Filariasis: Annual Report (2005)*; Myanmar Ministry of Health: Naypyitaw, Myanmar, 2005.

69. Myanmar Ministry of Health. *Myanmar National Programme to Eliminate Lymphatic Filariasis: Annual Report (2011)*; Myanmar Ministry of Health: Naypyitaw, Myanmar, 2011.

70. Myanmar Ministry of Health. *Myanmar National Programme to Eliminate Lymphatic Filariasis: Annual Report (2012)*; Myanmar Ministry of Health: Naypyitaw, Myanmar, 2012.

71. World Health Organization: Regional Office for South-East Asia. *Regional Stategic Plan. for Elimination of Lymphatic Filariasis (2004–2007)*; WHO Regional Office for South-East Asia: New Delhi, India, 2004.

72. World Health Organization: Regional Office for the Western Pacific. *Report of the Thirteenth Meeting of the Western Pacific Regional Programme Review Group on Neglected Tropical Diseases*; WHO Regional Office for the Western Pacific: Manila, Philippines, 2013.

73. World Health Organization. *UNDP-World Bank-WHO Special Programme for Research and Training in Tropical Diseases WHO-UNICEF Joint Programme for Health Mapping World Health Organization: Division of Tropical Diseases. Research on Rapid Geographical Assessment of Bancroftian Filariasis*; World Health Organization: Geneva, Switzerland, 1998.

74. World Health Organization: Regional Office for South-East Asia. *South-East Asia Regional Programme Review Group of Elimination of Lymphatic Filariasis: Report of the Eight Meeting*; WHO Regional Office for South-East Asia: New Delhi, India, 2011.

75. World Health Organization: Regional Office for South-East Asia. *South.-East. Asia Regional Programme Review Group of Elimination of Lymphatic Filariasis: Report of the First Meeting*; WHO Regional Office for South-East Asia: New Delhi, India, 2005.

76. World Health Organization: Regional Office for South-East Asia. *South.-East. Asia Regional Programme Review Group of Elimination of Lymphatic Filariasis: Report of the Ninth Meeting*; WHO Regional Office for South-East Asia: New Delhi, India, 2012.

77. World Health Organization: Regional Office for South-East Asia. *South.-East. Asia Regional Programme Review Group of Elimination of Lymphatic Filariasis: Report of the Seventh Meeting*; WHO Regional Office for South-East Asia: New Delhi, India, 2010.

78. World Health Organization: Regional Office for South-East Asia. *South.-East. Asia Regional Programme Review Group of Elimination of Lymphatic Filariasis: Report of the Tenth Meeting*; WHO Regional Office for South-East Asia: New Delhi, India, 2013.

79. World Health Organization: Regional Office for the Western Pacific. *Report of the Fourteenth Meeting of the Western Pacific Regional Programme Review Group on Neglected Tropical Diseases*; WHO Regional Office for the Western Pacific: Manila, Philippines, 2014.

80. World Health Organization. *Strengthening the Assessment of Lymphatic Filariasis Transmission and Documenting the Achievement of Elimination*; World Health Organization: Geneva, Switzerland, 2016.

81. Cambodia Ministry of Planning. *General Population Census of Cambodia 1998: Final Results*, 2nd ed.; Cambodia Ministry of Planning: Phnom Penh, Cambodia, 2002.

82. Beng, T.S.; Ahmad, R.; Hisam, R.S.R.; Heng, S.K.; Leaburi, J.; Ismail, Z.; Sulaiman, L.H.; Soyoti, R.F.H.M.; Lim, L.H. Molecular xenomonitoring of filarial infection in Malaysian mosquitoes under the National Program for Elimination of Lymphatic Filariasis. *Southeast Asian J. Trop. Med. Public Health* **2016**, *47*, 617–624.

83. Mathieu, E.; Amann, J.; Eigege, A.; Richards, F.; Sodahlon, Y. Collecting baseline information for national morbidity alleviation programs: Different methods to estimate lymphatic filariasis morbidity prevalence. *Am. J. Trop. Med. Hyg.* **2008**, *78*, 153–158. [PubMed]

84. Triteeraprapab, S.; Kanjanopas, K.; Suwannadabba, S.; Sangprakarn, S.; Poovorawan, Y.; Scott, A.L. Transmission of the nocturnal periodic strain of *Wuchereria bancrofti* by *Culex quinquefasciatus*: Establishing the potential for urban filariasis in Thailand. *Epidemiol. Infect.* **2000**, *125*, 207–212. [CrossRef] [PubMed]

85. Bhumiratana, A.; Intarapuk, A.; Koyadun, S.; Maneekan, P.; Sorosjinda-Nunthawarasilp, P. Current bancroftian filariasis elimination on Thailand-Myanmar border: Public Health Challenges toward Postgenomic MDA Evaluation. *ISRN Trop. Med.* **2013**, *2013*. [CrossRef]

86. Toothong, T.; Tipayamongkholgul, M.; Suwannapong, N.; Suwannadabba, S. Evaluation of mass drug administration in the program to control imported lymphatic filariasis in Thailand. *BMC Public Health* **2015**, *15*, 975. [CrossRef] [PubMed]

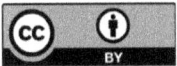

Tropical Medicine and
Infectious Disease

MDPI

Article

Concordance between Plasma and Filter Paper Sampling Techniques for the Lymphatic Filariasis Bm14 Antibody ELISA

Jesse Masson [1,*], Jan Douglass [1], Maureen Roineau [1], Khin Saw Aye [2], Kyi May Htwe [2], Jeffrey Warner [1] and Patricia M. Graves [1]

[1]   College of Public Health, Medical and Veterinary Sciences, James Cook University, Cairns, QLD 4870, Australia; jan.douglass@my.jcu.edu.au (J.D.); Maureenroineau@wanadoo.fr (M.R.); jeffrey.warner@jcu.edu.au (J.W.); patricia.graves@jcu.edu.au (P.M.G.)
[2]   Department of Medical Research, Myanmar Ministry of Health and Sports, Nay Pyi Taw, Myanmar; ksadmr@gmail.com (K.S.A.); Kyimaywin31@gmail.com (K.M.H.)
*   Correspondence: Jesse.masson@my.jcu.edu.au; Tel.: +61-434-089-108

Academic Editors: Peter Leggat and John Frean
Received: 20 February 2017; Accepted: 4 April 2017; Published: 7 April 2017

Abstract: Diagnostic testing for the antibody Bm14 is used to assess the prevalence of bancroftian and brugian filariasis in endemic populations. Using dried blood spots (DBS) collected on filter paper is ideal in resource-poor settings, but concerns have been raised about the performance of DBS samples compared to plasma or serum. In addition, two versions of the test have been used: the Bm14 CELISA (Cellabs Pty Ltd., Manly, Australia) or an in-house CDC version. Due to recent improvements in the CELISA, it is timely to validate the latest versions of the Bm14 ELISA for both plasma and DBS, especially in settings of residual infection with low antibody levels. We tested plasma and DBS samples taken simultaneously from 92 people in Myanmar, of whom 37 (40.2%) were positive in a rapid antigen test. Comparison of results from plasma and DBS samples demonstrated no significant difference in positive proportions using both the CELISA (46.7% and 44.6%) and CDC ELISA (50.0% and 47.8%). Quantitative antibody unit results from each sample type were also highly correlated, with coefficients >0.87. The results of this study demonstrate that DBS samples are a valid collection strategy and give equivalent results to plasma for Bm14 antibody ELISA testing by either test type.

Keywords: lymphatic filariasis; Bm14; filter paper; DBS; CELISA; CDC

---

1. Introduction

Screening assays used in The Global Program to Eliminate Lymphatic Filariasis (GPELF) are frequently performed in low resource settings where samples may be exposed to temperature changes during collection, storage and transport. Diagnostic tests that can utilise dried blood spots (DBS) collected on filter paper which do not require immediate cold storage have many advantages over plasma samples in rural communities where lymphatic filariasis (LF) occurs.

The parasite antibody Bm14 diagnostic ELISA is among the techniques used to identify bancroftian- and brugian-associated lymphatic filariasis (LF) [1–5] and is used alongside antigen detection tests to monitor and evaluate endemicity in populations [2,6,7]. However, concerns over the specificity and predictive values of the Bm14 ELISA have raised questions about its accuracy in detecting residual endemicity or resurgence [8,9]. Of the three species detected by the Bm14 antibody test, *Wuchereria bancrofti* and *Brugia malayi* contribute 90% and 9% of LF disease burden worldwide [10–12].

The Bm14 ELISA, commercially produced as the CELISA (Cellabs Pty Ltd., Manly, Australia), incorporates positive and negative control samples to check plate to plate consistency [13]. The kit recommends using an optical density cut-off value for defining a positive result (0.4) [13], although some studies use a lower cut-off of 0.25 [10]. The CDC Bm14 in-house version of the assay recommends use of a standard curve to generate antibody units, with sample antibody values greater or equal to the cut-off being considered positive [14]. For comparability in the current study, we used standard curves generated from the same positive serum for both CELISA and CDC versions. Both versions of the Bm14 ELISA recommend the application of either plasma or eluted DBS for antibody detection.

While there is not a true gold standard for LF positivity, previous studies have found that the Bm14 test with plasma or serum has high sensitivity compared to microfilaria microscopy, recorded at 98% for samples from people with *W. bancrofti* and 91% for *Brugia malayi* filariasis [10]. Gass et al. [9] found similar high specificity of 95% for plasma in anticoagulant ethylenediaminetetraacetic acid (EDTA). However, CELISA DBS sensitivity can range from 50.0% to 92.3% when compared with immunochromatographic testing and PCR testing, with consistently high negative predictive values (NPV) of >96.6% [10].

While the dried blood spot method would be an inexpensive and convenient alternative to plasma samples, Joseph and colleagues [8] have reported that specificity of DBS when using the CELISA may be as low as 77%, with a positive predictive value (PPV) of 60% when compared to plasma application. Knowledge gaps in the literature and the release of an improved CELISA kit by Cellabs require additional evaluation and comparison of these methods.

This study investigates whether results obtained using DBS are valid and comparable to results obtained using plasma with the CELISA and the CDC ELISA. These results will provide confidence in and promote appropriate application of the Bm14 ELISA for whichever collection method is available.

2. Materials and Methods

2.1. Study Population

Amarapura Township within the Mandalay Region of Central Myanmar was selected as a study site, as it was known from sentinel site records to have a high prevalence of LF infection. All young people aged 10–21 years were invited to participate in a cross-sectional study. Ethical approval for the study was given by the Myanmar Ministry of Health and Sports and James Cook University Research Human Ethics Committee, approval number H5261.

Individuals were screened for LF infection using the BinaxNOW® filariasis immunochromatographic test (ICT) card (Alere International Limited, Galway, Ireland). Young adults aged 18–21 years gave written consent to participate, while parents or guardians gave written consent for participants aged 10–17 years. An equal number of positive and negative participants were invited for a follow-up visit; however, some chose not to attend, resulting in a final collection of 37 ICT positives and 55 ICT negatives out of 92 total participants. The study sampling occurred shortly before the filariasis mass drug administration was offered in this township. Follow-up visits were done after the mass drug administration to ensure that positive participants took deworming drugs.

2.2. Preparation of Plasma and Blood Filter Paper Samples

Blood samples were collected by technical staff from the Myanmar Ministry of Health and Sports. A 10 mL sample of venous blood was collected from all participants and stored in cooled EDTA anticoagulant vacutainers (BD biosciences, Becton, Dickinson and Company, North Ryde, NSW, Australia). An amount of 10 µL of collected blood was transferred using a micropipette to each of the six protrusions of a filter paper disc (TropBio filter papers) and left to dry completely before storage in individual plastic bags. Remaining whole blood was kept on crushed ice and delivered to the Public Health Laboratory in Mandalay within four hours of collection. Plasma was separated from whole blood by centrifugation at $3000 \times g$ for 15 min and aliquoted into 2 mL tubes. Plasma samples were stored at $-20\ ^{\circ}\text{C}$ at the laboratory in Mandalay until transported to Yangon on dry ice and stored at $-80\ ^{\circ}\text{C}$ by the Department of Medical Research (DMR). One vial of each plasma sample was thawed, aliquoted and refrozen for transport to James Cook University in Cairns, Australia, where it was stored at −80 °C. Filter papers were sealed in plastic containers and kept in either 4 °C refrigeration or hand luggage during direct transport to Cairns, where they were stored at −80 °C.

2.3. Preparation of Eluates from DBS

DBS eluates were prepared for the application of the commercially available Bm14 kit (CELISA) [13] and the LF Bm14 CDC TMB-ELISA [14], using respective protocols. Sample diluent was prepared according to the instructions, with individual 495 μL and 245 μL sample diluent aliquots transferred into separate serum tubes for CELISA and CDC ELISA testing respectively, using a micropipette. Single blood-soaked filter paper protrusions were transferred to two separate serum tubes, one containing 495 μL of sample diluent to create 1:100 dilutions intended for CELISA application, and another containing 245 μL sample diluent to create a 1:50 dilution intended for CDC ELISA application. Each protrusion soaks exactly 10 μL of blood, with half of this volume estimated to be plasma and the remaining 5 μL containing all other blood products. Therefore, it is assumed that the 5 μL of plasma from each DBS added to 495 μL and 245 μL aliquots creates dilutions of 1:100 and 1:50 respectively. All samples were vortexed to ensure complete saturation of each disc and left to elute overnight at 4 °C before being warmed to room temperature (RT) of between 20 °C and 25 °C and vortexed again prior to testing.

2.4. Bm14 Filariasis Cellabs Enzyme Linked Immunosorbent Assay

Primary sample incubation was at 37 °C for 1 h before emptying and flooding wells with washing buffer three times, followed by a final emptying and upside down tapping of each plate to ensure wells were free of large droplets. Secondary IgG_4 conjugates were added and incubated for 45 min at 37 °C, before washing again and applying a final 15-min incubation with tetramethylbenzidine (TMB) substrate without light exposure. Plates were prepared for optical density reading through the addition of 50 μL of stopping solution per well.

2.5. Bm14 Filariasis CDC's Enzyme Linked Immunosorbent Assay

Antigen sensitising buffer (ASB) was created at 0.1 M using $NaHCO_3$ and dH_2O with a pH of 9.6 using NaOH. Working antigen solution (Atlanta, CDC) was prepared at 2 μg/mL using ASB. The binding of antigens to each well of Immulon 4HB plates (Thermofisher, Loughborough, UK) was achieved by adding 50 μL of 1:50 antigen solution to each well of a 96-well microplate before incubating at 4 °C overnight for at least 12 h. Working antigen solution was physically removed before the addition of 100 μL of PBS + 0.3% Tween (Life Technologies, Mulgrave, VIC, Australia), pH 7.2, to each well and incubated at 4 °C for 1 h.

Blanks were created by adding 50 μL of PBS with 0.05% Tween to intended blank wells. Dilutions of plasma or DBS eluates were added at 50 μL to each experimental well before incubating at room temperature on a rocker platform for 2 h. Washing steps between incubations were performed in an identical fashion to the CELISA, referred to earlier. Following the addition of horseradish peroxidase conjugated anti-human IgG_4 (mouse) (Life Technologies), made to a 1:500 dilution with PBS with 0.05% Tween, at 50 μL to each plate well, the plate was incubated at room temperature for 45 min. TMB substrate was added at 50 μL to each well and incubated at room temperature in the dark for 5 min before adding 50 μL of 1 M HCL.

2.6. Statistical Analysis

Optical density readings of each sample were measured at a dual wavelength of 450 nm/650 nm with a VersaMax™ ELISA microplate reader (Molecular Devices, Sunnyvale, CA, USA) using SoftMax Pro Software Version 6.4.1 (Molecular Devices, Sunnyvale, CA, USA) with background absorbance of sample diluent subtracted. A moderately-positive sample collected from an endemic area of Papua

New Guinea was used as a positive control, while negative controls were taken from Australian lab workers.

A standard curve was constructed using a single highly-positive sample from Papua New Guinea which was defined by an arbitrary high value of 1000 antibody units with subsequent 2-fold dilutions. A single cut-off point of >125 units was used to determine positive readings based on previous literature [5,9]. It should be noted that an optical density cut-off value of 0.4 is normally recommended by the CELISA manual. Relative sensitivity, specificity, positive predictive values (PPV), and negative predictive values (NPV), as well as paired *t*-tests, odds ratios, McNemar chi-square tests and correlations were performed using the IBM statistical software SPSS Version 23.0. Confidence intervals (CI) were reported at 95%.

3. Results

During October 2014, 377 young people residing in Amarapura Township were screened by ICT. Positive cases were age and gender matched to negative cases and 112 young people were invited to participate in a longitudinal study including provision of a blood sample. Not all participants returned for participation, leaving a final sample of 37 (40.2%) positive and 55 (59.8%) negative samples that were included in this study (Table 1).

Table 1. Positive proportions and chi-square results obtained when using the CELISA with plasma as a standard.

Standard	N Positive	% Positive (95% Confidence Interval (CI))	Comparative Test	N Positive	% Positive (95% CI)	McNemar Chi sq	P Value
CELISA Plasma 1:100	43	47 (37–57)	CELISA Dried blood spot (DBS) 1:100	41	45 (35–55)	0.5	0.7
-	-	-	CDC Plasma 1:50	46	50 (40–60)	1.3	0.5
-	-	-	CDC DBS 1:50	44	48 (38–58)	0.2	0.9

3.1. Categorical Analysis and Comparisons of Plasma and DBS Using Cellabs and CDC ELISA Assays

Holding all CELISA plasma samples tested at a 1:100 dilution as a standard, we compared how DBS application affects the proportion of positive results when using the CELISA at an identical dilution. We found no significant difference in positive proportions between plasma (47%) and DBS (45%) samples (Table 1).

The CELISA standard was also compared to the CDC version of the Bm14 ELISA to assess any similarity in positive proportions when using plasma or DBS at the CDC recommended 1:50 dilution. The proportions of samples classed as positive were not significantly different between the CELISA standard (47%) and CDC ELISA with plasma (50%) or DBS (48%), respectively (Table 1). These three comparisons suggest that high similarity in positive results is found between the CELISA and the CDC ELISA using either plasma or DBS.

To establish how the CDC ELISA is affected by the application method, plasma and DBS samples were compared using the 1:50 dilution. Positive proportions of 50% when using plasma, and 48% when using DBS were not significantly different (Table 2). This confirms that the CDC ELISA will yield similar results regardless of the sample application method.

Table 2. Positives proportions and chi-square results obtained when comparing plasma and DBS with the CDC ELISA.

Standard	N Positive	% Positive (95% CI)	Comparative Test	N Positive	% Positive (95% CI)	McNemar Chi sq	P Value
CDC Plasma 1:50	46	50 (40–60)	CDC DBS 1:50	44	48 (38–58)	1.0	0.6

3.2. Comparing the Plasma and DBS for CELISA and CDC ELISA Samples

To determine how application of plasma and filter paper affects CELISA agreement, relative sensitivity, specificity, PPV and NPV were calculated. When DBS was compared to plasma at a 1:100 dilution using the CELISA, results were high overall at 88.4% sensitivity, 93.9% specificity, 92.7% PPV, and 90.2% NPV (Table 3). These results suggest that the CELISA yields reliable agreement between plasma and DBS samples.

Table 3. Sensitivity, specificity, positive predictive value (PPV), negative predictive value (NPV) and odds ratio statistics comparisons of plasma and DBS application using the CELISA and CDC ELISA.

Standard	Comparative Test	Sensitivity (95% CI)	Specificity (95% CI)	PPV (95% CI)	NPV (95% CI)	Odds Ratio (95% CI)	P Value
CELISA Plasma 1:100	CELISA DBS 1:100	88.4% (74.9–96.1)	93.9% (83.1–98.7)	92.7% (80.8–95.5)	90.2% (80.1–95.5)	116.5 (26.15–519.4)	<0.0001
-	CDC Plasma 1:50	95.4% (84.2–99.4)	89.8% (77.8–96.6)	89.1% (78.1–95.0)	95.7% (85.0–98.8)	180.4 (33.2–981.7)	<0.0001
-	CDC DBS 1:50	95.4% (84.2–99.4)	93.9% (83.1–98.7)	93.2% (82.0–97.6)	95.8% (85.6–98.9)	314.3 (50.0–1975.4)	<0.0001

Performance of the CDC ELISA using plasma and DBS at a 1:50 dilution was also compared to the CELISA 1:100 plasma standard. Relative sensitivity was high at 95.4% for both CDC plasma and DBS samples, with specificity found at 89.8% and 93.9% respectively (Table 3). Predictive values were also high for both CDC plasma and DBS samples compared to CELISA plasma, yielding 89.1% and 93.2% respectively for PPV, and 95.7% and 95.8% respectively for NPV (Table 3). Therefore, there is good agreement between the CDC ELISA using plasma and DBS when compared to results yielded by the CELISA using plasma.

Again, we compared plasma and DBS using the CDC ELISA at the recommended dilution of 1:50, to determine how test performance and relative predictive values are affected. Sensitivity and specificity were 97.7% and 93.8% respectively, while PPV and NPV were 93.5% and 97.8% respectively (Table 4). These results suggest that the CDC ELISA performs equally well when using either plasma or DBS, as confirmed by a high odds ratio value (Table 4).

Table 4. Sensitivity, specificity, PPV, NPV and odds ratio statistics comparisons of plasma and DBS application using the CDC ELISA.

Standard	Comparative Test	Sensitivity (95% CI)	Specificity (95% CI)	PPV (95% CI)	NPV (95% CI)	Odds Ratio (95% CI)	P Value
CDC Plasma 1:50	CDC DBS1:50	97.7% (88.0–99.9)	93.8% (82.8–98.7)	93.5% (82.7–97.7)	97.8% (86.6–99.7)	645.0 (64.6–6442.6)	<0.0001

3.3. Comparing Difference in Bm14 Antibody Units between Cellabs and CDC Assays

All unit concentrations, with the addition of one to include results of zero, were converted to log values to approximate a normal distribution (Figure 1). Results were compared using geometric means. When analysing CELISA samples, the mean log value for plasma at 1.66 was significantly lower than the mean log value of 2.10 for DBS ($p < 0.0001$) (Table 5). However, the mean log values for CDC ELISA plasma and DBS samples at 2.03 and 2.07 respectively were not significantly different ($p = 0.34$) (Table 5). The data suggests a rise in estimated concentration when using DBS in comparison to plasma when using the CELISA, but not when using the CDC ELISA.

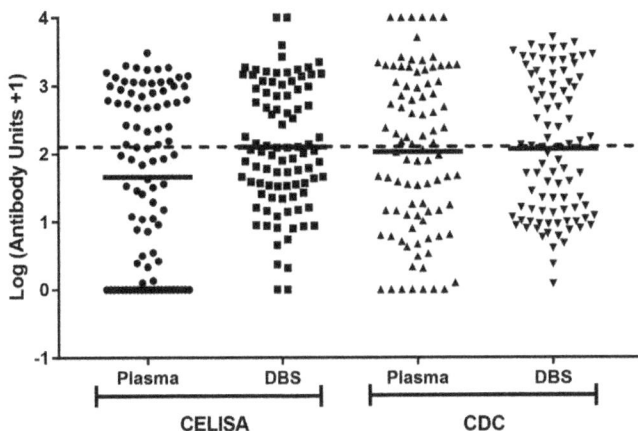

Figure 1. Filariasis Bm14 ELISA log (antibody unit concentration +1) value comparisons between plasma and DBS application of CELISA and CDC ELISA assays. Horizontal black lines refer to mean concentration of each assay, with the segmented line referring to the cut-off value at log (125 units +1). All concentrations above or equal to the defined cut-off are considered positive, while all readings below are considered negative.

Table 5. Geometric mean concentration values and *t*-test comparisons between plasma and DBS application of CELISA and CDC ELISA assays.

	Group 1			Group 2			*t*-Test		
Test	Mean log (Antibody unit +1)	Geometric mean	Test	Mean log (Antibody unit +1)	Geometric mean	N	Mean Difference	SD	*p*
CELISA Plasma	1.66	45.00	CELISA DBS	2.10	124.42	92	0.44	0.63	<0.0001
CDC Plasma	2.03	105.62	CDC DBS	2.07	115.51	92	0.04	0.39	0.34

3.4. Correlation Coefficient Analysis of Bm14 Antibody Concentrations from Plasma and Eluates from Filter Paper

The log values of Bm14 unit concentrations, with the addition of one to include results of zero, between plasma and DBS application were compared to determine correlation coefficients for both CELISA and CDC ELISA assays. Strong correlations were found at 0.87 and 0.95 for CELISA (Figure 2A) and the CDC ELISA (Figure 2B) respectively when comparing plasma and DBS samples ($p < 0.0001$). This shows that quantitative values between plasma and DBS are strongly positively associated when using the CELISA and the CDC ELISA.

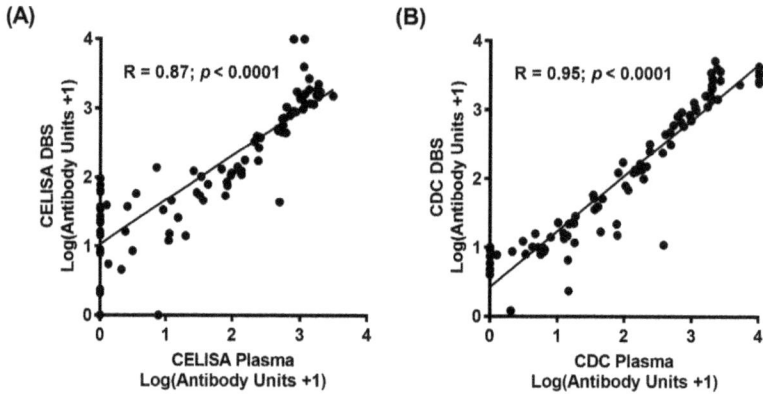

Figure 2. Filariasis Bm14 ELISA antibody unit concentration comparisons of plasma and whole blood application. (**A**) CELISA at 1:100 dilution comparisons of plasma against DBS; (**B**) CDC ELISA at 1:50 dilution comparisons of plasma against DBS.

4. Discussion

The major finding of this study is the strong agreement between plasma and DBS samples, taken from the same individuals and stored identically, when applied to either the Cellabs produced CELISA or the CDC Bm14 ELISA. In the Cellabs CELISA protocol [13], the recommended dilution is set at 1:100. According to the instructions for the in-house CDC filariasis serology assay [14], the recommended dilution is set at 1:50 dilution using serum obtained from centrifuged blood. Despite these differences in dilution optimised for the two tests, the proportions of samples classified as positive were not significantly different, with performance (relative sensitivity, specificity and predictive values) being very similar between all the tests.

High specificity and PPV values were found for comparisons of DBS against plasma using both CELISA and CDC ELISA tests. According to Joseph and Melrose [8], results obtained using the CELISA assay for DBS yielded a specificity of 77%, with 16 samples testing positive by DBS but negative by plasma, while PPV was found at 60%, suggesting that DBS sampling may result in false positives at an approximate rate of 40%. However, this work was done with an earlier version of the CELISA. Weil et al. [10] stated that blood samples with a known amount of antibody applied to DBS are not significantly different to those from serum samples under controlled conditions when using the CELISA. Our own results of 93.9% and 92.7% for specificity and PPV when comparing DBS and plasma suggest that the CELISA assay has improved in these regards.

Analysis of quantitative data showed that correlation was high between plasma and DBS for both the CELISA and CDC ELISA at >0.87. Although the mean antibody units were lower for DBS than plasma in the CDC ELISA, the difference was not significant. The significantly higher sample concentrations for DBS than plasma when using the CELISA suggests that this test gives higher background for DBS. However, the categorical results suggest no significant difference in agreement (classification of positives).If the amount of antibody present is important in future studies using DBS, it may be necessary to keep this difference in mind.

The use of DBS could facilitate more effective sample collection in endemic countries, where large-scale sampling must be undertaken with limited resources and also eliminates the risk of thawing or leaking during shipping.

Our analysis showed that both plasma and filter paper demonstrate similar results using both the CELISA and CDC ELISA. High agreement was also found when comparing the CELISA using plasma with CDC ELISA applications of either plasma or DBS. These results support the use of the

Trop. Med. Infect. Dis. **2017**, *2*, 6

Bm14 ELISA in assessing LF prevalence in the GPELF and can be used with either plasma or DBS on filter paper.

Acknowledgments: The authors would like to thank the Myanmar Ministry of Health and Sports, for study support, specifically Tint Wai. We must also thank the Vector Borne Disease Control group (Mandalay Region) for technical support and the WHO country office in Myanmar. Special thanks go to Ye Ye and Thi Thi Lwin of the Public Health Laboratory in Mandalay for sample separation and short term samples storage, and the Department of Medical Research (Lower Myanmar) for laboratory support and long-term storage of the samples. We are grateful to Luke Becker of the Australian Institute for Tropical Medicine for his assistance with training of local research assistants in all study protocols. Thanks to Graham Burgess for comments on the manuscript. We are very grateful to Kimberly Won and Jeff Priest of CDC for advice and for provision of antigen. We would like to thank Diane Dogcio Hall and Cellabs Pty Ltd., Brookvale, New South Wales, Australia for advice and donation of kits for use in Myanmar. We must also thank the Filariasis Reagent Resource Center (FR3) (http://www.filariasiscenter.org/), who provided positive controls for the ICT cards used in initial screening of the samples. And finally, Keryn Masson and Matt Hayes for their support. This study was approved by JCU HREC number H5261 and the Myanmar Department of Health.

Author Contributions: P.M.G., J.D., J.M. and J.W. conceived of and designed the experiments; J.M., M.R., K.S.A., and K.M.H. performed the experiments; J.M. and P.M.G. analysed the data; J.M., P.M.G. and J.D. wrote the paper with input from J.W.; all authors reviewed the final draft and provided input.

Conflicts of Interest: The authors declare no conflict of interest.

References

1. Simonsen, P.E.; Pedersen, E.M.; Rwegoshora, R.T.; Malecela, M.N.; Derua, Y.A.; Magesa, S.M. Lymphatic filariasis control in Tanzania: Effect of repeated mass drug administration with ivermectin and albendazole on infection and transmission. *PLoS Negl. Trop. Dis.* **2010**, *4*, e696. [CrossRef] [PubMed]
2. Hamlin, K.L.; Moss, D.M.; Priest, J.W.; Roberts, J.; Kubofcik, J.; Gass, K.; Streit, T.G.; Nutman, T.B.; Eberhard, M.L.; Lammie, P.J. Longitudinal monitoring of the development of antifilarial antibodies and acquisition of *Wuchereria bancrofti* in a highly endemic area of Haiti. *PLoS Negl. Trop. Dis.* **2012**, *6*, e1941. [CrossRef] [PubMed]
3. Shawa, S.T.; Mwase, E.T.; Pedersen, E.M.; Simonsen, P.E. Lymphatic filariasis in Luangwa District, South-East Zambia. *Parasit. Vectors* **2013**, *6*, 299. [CrossRef] [PubMed]
4. Mwakitalu, M.E.; Malecela, M.N.; Pedersen, E.M.; Mosha, F.W.; Simonsen, P.E. Urban lymphatic filariasis in the metropolis of Dar es Salaam, Tanzania. *Parasit. Vectors* **2013**, *6*, 286. [CrossRef] [PubMed]
5. Lau, C.L.; Won, K.Y.; Becker, L.; SoaresMagalhaes, R.J.; Fuimaono, S.; Melrose, W.; Lammie, P.J.; Graves, P.M. Seroprevalence and spatial epidemiology of lymphatic filariasis in American Samoa after successful mass drug administration. *PLoS Negl. Trop. Dis.* **2014**, *8*, e3297. [CrossRef] [PubMed]
6. Weil, G.J.; Kastens, W.; Susapu, M.; Laney, S.J.; Williams, S.A.; King, C.L.; Kazura, J.W.; Bockarie, M.J. The impact of repeated rounds of mass drug administration with diethylcarbamazine plus albendazole on bancroftian filariasis in Papua New Guinea. *PLoS Negl. Trop. Dis.* **2008**, *2*, e344. [CrossRef] [PubMed]
7. Harrington, H.; Asugeni, J.; Jimuru, C.; Gwalaa, J.; Ribeyro, E.; Bradbury, R.; Joseph, H.; Melrose, W.; MacLaren, D.; Speare, R. A practical strategy for responding to a case of Lymphatic filariasis post-elimination in Pacific Islands. *Parasit. Vectors* **2013**, *6*, 218. [CrossRef] [PubMed]
8. Joseph, H.M.; Melrose, W. Applicability of the filter paper technique for detection of antifilarial IgG$_4$ antibodies using the Bm14 filariasis CELISA. *J.Parasitol. Res.* **2010**, *2010*, 594687. [CrossRef] [PubMed]
9. Gass, K.; Beau de Rochars, M.V.; Boakye, D.; Bradley, M.; Fischer, P.U.; Gyapong, J.; Itoh, M.; Ituaso-Conway, N.; Joseph, H.; Kyelem, D.; et al. A multicenter evaluation of diagnostic tools to define endpoints for programs to eliminate bancroftian filariasis. *PLoS Negl. Trop. Dis.* **2012**, *6*, e1479. [CrossRef] [PubMed]
10. Weil, G.J.; Curtis, K.C.; Fischer, P.U.; Won, K.Y.; Lammie, P.J.; Joseph, H.; Melrose, W.D.; Brattig, N.W. A multicenter evaluation of a new antibody test kit for lymphatic filariasis employing recombinant *Brugia malayi* antigen Bm-14. *Acta Trop.* **2011**, *120* (Suppl. 1), S19–S22. [CrossRef] [PubMed]
11. Fenwick, A. The global burden of neglected tropical diseases. *Public Health* **2012**, *26*, 233–236. [CrossRef] [PubMed]
12. World Health Organization. Global programme to eliminate lymphatic filariasis: Progress report, 2014. *Wkly. Epidemiol. Rec.* **2015**, *90*, 489–504.

13. Cellabs Pty Ltd. *Lymphatic Filariasis Bm14 Antibody CELISA*; Cellabs Pty Ltd.: Brookvale, Queensland, Australia, 2012.

14. Centers for Disease Control. *Lymphatic Filariasis Bm14CDC HRP TMB-ELISA (Modified by JCU)*; The Centers for Disease Control: Atlanta, GA, USA, 2012.

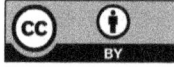

*Tropical Medicine and
Infectious Disease*

MDPI

Article

Relative Performance and Predictive Values of Plasma and Dried Blood Spots with Filter Paper Sampling Techniques and Dilutions of the Lymphatic Filariasis Og4C3 Antigen ELISA for Samples from Myanmar

Jesse Masson [1,*], Jan Douglass [1], Maureen Roineau [1], Khin Saw Aye [2], Kyi May Htwe [2], Jeffrey Warner [1] and Patricia M. Graves [1]

[1] College of Public Health, Medical and Veterinary Sciences, James Cook University, Cairns, QLD 4870, Australia; jan.douglass@my.jcu.edu.au (J.D.); Maureenroineau@wanadoo.fr (M.R.); jeffrey.warner@jcu.edu.au (J.W.); patricia.graves@jcu.edu.au (P.M.G.)
[2] Department of Medical Research, Myanmar Ministry of Health and Sports, Nay Pyi Taw, Myanmar; ksadmr@gmail.com (K.S.A.); Kyimaywin31@gmail.com (K.M.H.)
* Correspondence: Jesse.masson@my.jcu.edu.au; Tel.: +61-434-089-108

Academic Editors: Thewarach Laha and Peter A. Leggat
Received: 11 February 2017; Accepted: 4 April 2017; Published: 11 April 2017

Abstract: Diagnostic testing of blood samples for parasite antigen Og4C3 is used to assess *Wuchereria bancrofti* in endemic populations. However, the Tropbio ELISA recommends that plasma and dried blood spots (DBS) prepared using filter paper be used at different dilutions, making it uncertain whether these two methods and dilutions give similar results, especially at low levels of residual infection or resurgence during the post-program phase. We compared results obtained using samples of plasma and DBS taken simultaneously from 104 young adults in Myanmar in 2014, of whom 50 (48.1%) were positive for filariasis antigen by rapid antigen test. Results from DBS tests at recommended dilution were significantly lower than results from plasma tested at recommended dilution, with comparisons between plasma and DBS at unmatched dilutions yielding low sensitivity and negative predictive values of 60.0% and 70.6% respectively. While collection of capillary blood on DBS is cheaper and easier to perform than collecting plasma or serum, and does not need to be stored frozen, dilutions between different versions of the test must be reconciled or an adjustment factor applied.

Keywords: lymphatic filariasis; Og4C3; ELISA; filter paper; DBS; ICT; immunochromatographic test

1. Introduction

Accurate and reliable screening assays that can be performed in low-resource laboratory settings have become vital for the Global Program to Eliminate Lymphatic Filariasis (GPELF). Currently, the use of the parasite antigen Og4C3 ELISA is among several techniques used to identify infection with lymphatic filariasis (LF) in *Wuchereria bancrofti* endemic areas [1–3]. Along with rapid immunochromatographic testing (ICT), which generates positive/negative results, the Og4C3 ELISA is used in monitoring and evaluation of the mass drug administration (MDA)-led elimination programs among endemic populations, producing quantitative results based on antigen units derived from a standard curve [4–6].

The Og4C3 ELISA, originally developed under Tropbio Pty. Ltd. at James Cook University, has been commercially available since the 1990s. Since 2013, the Og4C3 ELISA has been manufactured and supplied by Cellabs Pty. Ltd., Australia. Using categorical positive/negative results generated by using a cut-off value for positivity, the test has previously demonstrated a high level of sensitivity for the detection of filarial antigen when compared with the ICT rapid test [7–9]. Typically, the Og4C3 ELISA is performed using serum or plasma, either immediately after the sample has been obtained, or more often, from frozen samples. However, the Og4C3 ELISA also offers an alternative application method through the use of dried blood spots (DBS) collected on filter paper, an inexpensive and convenient method that requires less space and less stringent refrigeration for transport and storage.

Both plasma and DBS can make an important contribution to the final stages of LF elimination and to ensuring that re-emergence of disease has not occurred, despite some differences in practicability. For example, plasma samples can be directly applied to ELISA, yielding final results within a few hours if onsite laboratory facilities are available. However, DBS may be more convenient for field work and cost-effectiveness, as laboratory conditions are not mandatory despite the required overnight elution. Limited sample variation due to fluctuations in temperature and detection of antigen even after 12 months has also been demonstrated [10].

Despite the convenience in having two methods of application, studies which have directly compared Og4C3 ELISA DBS results to those from serum or plasma have shown discordance. Reeve and Melrose [11] compared results for 354 individuals from Papua New Guinea and observed significantly higher proportions of samples classified as positive by Og4C3 ELISA for serum (48.2%) than for DBS (32.5%). They demonstrated that the DBS technique yielded high specificity (99.2%; $N = 391$) and positive predictive value (PPV) (98.8%), but that sensitivity (67.2%; $N = 354$) and negative predictive values (NPV) (77%) were low when comparing DBS to serum as the gold standard. Interestingly, Tropbio and Cellabs recommend the dilution for plasma at 1:4 [12], while filter paper is recommended at an estimated dilution of 1:13.3, suggesting that the difference in dilution could be an underlying factor for discordance.

A second study by Itoh et al. [10], compared Og4C3 results for serum and DBS using a sample of 60 people in Sri Lanka, 55% of whom were reported to be positive for microfilariae, 65% positive by Og4C3 using serum, and 63.3% positive when using DBS. While these proportions positive by DBS and serum were not significantly different, this study used serum at a 1:3 dilution, applied at 16.7 μL per well, while DBS samples at an estimated dilution of 1:5 were applied at 3.3 μL per well. The authors then employed a 5-fold upward correction to the DBS antigen unit results to correct this difference in dilution. It is not clear how the results would have aligned if both sample types had been tested at currently recommended dilutions, and not adjusted.

Given the routine use of the Og4C3 ELISA by either plasma or DBS worldwide, this study aims to validate the existing instructions regarding the different dilutions of sample collected, and to determine if DBS is appropriate and comparable to plasma at the recommended dilutions.

2. Materials and Methods

The study site was the Amarapura Township of the Mandalay Region in Central Myanmar, an area known to have a high prevalence of LF infection. Persons aged 10–21 years were invited to participate. Ethical approval for the study was obtained from the James Cook University Research Human Ethics Committee, approval number H5261, and the Myanmar Ministry of Health and Sports.

2.1. Study Population

All participants were screened for LF infection using BinaxNOW® filariasis ICT (Alere International Limited, Ireland). Participants who tested positive by ICT were age and gender matched to uninfected controls and invited to participate in the longitudinal study. Written consent was obtained from 18–21 year olds and from the parent or guardian of 10–17 year olds. Blood collection was conducted with the assistance of the Myanmar Ministry of Health and Sports.

2.2. Preparation of Plasma and DBS Samples

A 10 mL sample of venous blood was collected from each individual in cooled ethylenediaminetetraacetic acid (EDTA) anticoagulant vacutainers (BD Biosciences, Becton, Dickinson and Company, North Ryde, NSW, Australia). Ten microlitres of blood was blotted using a micropipette onto each of six protruding filter paper sections (TropBio filter papers), which were left to completely dry before being placed in individual plastic bags. The remaining whole blood was placed on crushed ice and delivered to the Public Health Laboratory in Mandalay within four hours of collection. Whole blood was spun for 15 min at $3000 \times g$ so that plasma could be aliquoted into 2 mL tubes. Plasma samples and DBS were stored short term at $-20\ ^\circ$C until transported to Yangon on dry ice for $-80\ ^\circ$C storage at the Department of Medical Research. One vial of each plasma sample was further aliquoted and refrozen before being shipped to James Cook University in Cairns, Australia, for storage at $-80\ ^\circ$C. Filter papers were sealed in plastic containers and kept in either $4\ ^\circ$C refrigeration or hand luggage during direct transport to Cairns where they were stored at $-80\ ^\circ$C.

2.3. Application of the TropBio Og4C3 Filariasis ELISA

The Og4C3 antigen was detected in plasma using the commercially available TropBio Og4C3 kits (Cellabs Pty. Ltd., Manly, Australia) at 1:4 dilution (50 μL of plasma into 150 μL of sample diluent, rather than 100 μL of plasma into 300 μL of sample diluent as recommended by the TropBio kit, to conserve samples) and at 1:16 dilution (50 μL of the 1:4 dilution into 150 μL of sample diluent). DBS samples were not tested at 1:4, since the volume of the three DBS protrusions was too large to elute in a small enough volume to test at 1:4.

The DBS dilution used three filter paper protrusions per sample, representing 30 μL of whole blood. We diluted the DBS into 200 μL of diluent. If the haematocrit was 50%, this would give a dilution of 1:13, making the assumption that the dried blood occupies no volume. Given wide individual variation in haematocrit, we are not able to specify an exact dilution factor for DBS. The filter paper insert supplied by TropBio suggests that the DBS assay is approximately 4-fold less sensitive than plasma or serum tested at recommended dilution of 1:4. Therefore the dilution is likely in the range of 1:11 to 1:16. In this study all DBS were tested as per kit recommended dilution (three spots into 200 μL). DBS were eluted overnight at $4\ ^\circ$C.

Positive control samples of serum were created at identical dilutions to ensure plate-to-plate consistency using a pool of ten known positive sera from a LF endemic area of Papua New Guinea (PNG). Negative controls from Australian lab workers were also used. Diluted samples were boiled using a water bath for 10 min before centrifuging at $2000 \times g$ for 15 min. Fifty μL of the supernatant from each diluted sample was added to each well of the plate for primary sample incubation at $37\ ^\circ$C for 1 h, with the remainder of the ELISA technique performed as described in the instructions provided with the Tropbio Og4C3 kit [12]. Following initial incubation, wells which contained DBS samples were emptied and treated with washing buffer before the addition of 50 μL of 1% hydrogen peroxide solution, made by diluting 400 μL of 30% hydrogen peroxide in 11.6 mL of prepared wash buffer, and incubated for 10 min before subsequent washing.

2.4. Statistical Analysis

A standard curve was constructed for each ELISA plate using the kit-supplied controls, assigning an arbitrary high value of 32,768 units with subsequent 4-fold dilutions. The Softmax Pro v5 software (Molecular Devices, Sunnyvale, CA, USA) was used to convert optical density readings of the test samples to units based on a four-parameter curve. A single cut off point of >32 units (representing the sixth point of the standard curve from subsequent dilutions) was used to determine positive readings. Differences in unit values, between sampling techniques and test variations, were examined using paired *t*-tests, odds ratio, chi-square and correlation analysis. All analyses were performed using the IBM statistical software SPSS Version 23.0 (IBM, Armonk, NY, USA). Sensitivity, specificity, positive predictive value (PPV), and negative predictive value (NPV) of comparisons were also analysed. Confidence intervals (CI) were reported at 95%.

3. Results

Individuals between 10 to 21 years of age, irrespective of gender, were tested by ICT using fingerprick blood collected during October 2014. For each ICT-positive participant, an age and sex matched ICT negative participant was identified. Both were invited to return for full participation in a study of physical characteristics and to give a sample of venous blood for serological testing. Not all selected individuals (cases and controls) returned for the second venous sample; therefore, a final collection of 48 positive and 56 negative samples were included in this study.

3.1. Analysis of Categorical Results Used to Compare the ICT and Og4C3 ELISA

To investigate how results classified as positive and negative varied between the ICT and the Og4C3 ELISA using plasma and DBS, categorical results were compared. Positive proportions of 46.2% obtained through the ICT were not significantly different to the proportion of 48.1% when using plasma at 1:4 dilution (Table 1). However, values became significantly different, dropping to 37.5% and 34.6% respectively, when plasma at 1:16 dilution or DBS was used (Table 1).

Table 1. Positive proportions and chi-square results of comparisons between the immunochromatographic test and the Og4C3 ELISA.

Standard	N Positive	% Positive (95% Confidence Interval (CI))	Comparative Test	N Positive	% Positive (95% CI)	McNemar Chi Sq	P Value
ICT	48	46.2 (36.9–55.7)	Plasma 1:4	50	48.1 (38.7–57.6)	0.3	$p = 0.8$
-	-	-	Plasma 1:16	39	37.5 (28.8–47.1)	6.2	$p = 0.02$
-	-	-	Dried blood spot (DBS)	36	34.6 (26.2–44.2)	8.00	$p = 0.008$

Holding the ICT as a relative standard, agreement with the Og4C3 ELISA using plasma and DBS was assessed. When ELISA using plasma at a 1:4 dilution was compared to ICT, sensitivity was 85.4% and specificity 83.9%, while PPV and NPV were 82.0% and 87.0%, respectively (Table 2). The use of a 1:16 dilution for plasma or use of DBS resulted in a decrease in sensitivity and NPV when compared to ICT, while specificity and PPV increased (Table 2). This suggests that the Og4C3 ELISA is significantly affected by dilution and application method when compared to ICT, with the 1:4 dilution yielding higher sensitivity and NPV, while the 1:16 plasma dilution or DBS yields higher specificity and PPV.

Table 2. Sensitivity, specificity, positive predictive value (PPV), negative predictive value (NPV) and odds ratio results from ICT and Og4C3 ELISA comparisons.

Standard	Comparative Test	Sensitivity (95% CI)	Specificity (95% CI)	PPV (95% CI)	NPV (95% CI)	Odds Ratio (95% CI)	P Value
ICT	Plasma 1:4	85.4% (72.2–93.9)	83.9% (71.7–92.4)	82.0% (71.2–89.3)	87.0% (77.0–93.1)	30.6 (10.5–89.4)	$p < 0.0001$
-	Plasma 1:16	77.1% (62.7–88.0)	96.4% (87.7–99.6)	94.9% (82.5–98.6)	83.1 (74.5–89.2)	90.8 (19.0–433.8)	$p < 0.0001$
-	DBS	68.8% (53.8–81.3)	94.5% (85.1–98.9)	91.7% (78.3–97.1)	77.9% (69.8–84.4)	38.9 (10.5–144.6)	$p < 0.0001$

Odds ratios were used to predict the likelihood of positive and negative results from comparative Og4C3 samples when compared to the ICT standard. Odds ratio was highest at 90.8 for comparison against plasma using a 1:16 dilution, but decreased to 30.6 when using plasma at 1:4 dilution, and to 38.9 when using DBS (Table 2). This suggests that agreement between the ICT and Og4C3 ELISA is best when using the Og4C3 with plasma at a 1:16 dilution.

3.2. Analysis of Categorical Results Used to Compare Plasma at 1:4 and 1:16 Dilutions and DBS

To assess results achieved by Og4C3 ELISA, plasma application at a 1:4 dilution was held as a standard for comparison. Again, we used chi-square tests to find a significant value of 7.5 ($p = 0.009$) when comparing plasma at 1:4 to DBS, which remained significant at 5.3 ($p = 0.04$) when plasma was compared using 1:4 and 1:16 dilutions (Table 3). Therefore, both plasma application at 1:16 and DBS give different results to plasma tested at the recommended 1:4 dilution.

Table 3. Positive proportions and chi-square results of comparisons between Og4C3 ELISA application method and dilution.

Standard	N Positive	% Positive (95% CI)	Comparative Test	N Positive	% Positive (95% CI)	McNemar Chi Sq	P Value
Plasma 1:4	50	48.1 (38.7–57.6)	DBS	36	34.6 (26.2–44.2)	7.5	$p = 0.009$
-	-	-	Plasma 1:16	39	37.5 (28.8–47.1)	5.3	$p = 0.04$

To investigate if matched dilutions might improve plasma and DBS concordance between proportions, both methods were compared using plasma at 1:16 as the new standard. The difference was not significant when comparing plasma at 1:16 and DBS, achieving a chi-square value of 0.7 (Table 4). This confirms high agreement of positive proportions when plasma and DBS are applied using similar dilutions.

Table 4. Positive proportions and chi-square results of comparisons between Og4C3 ELISA applications at 1:16 dilution.

Standard	N Positive	% Positive (95% CI)	Comparative Test	N Positive	% Positive (95% CI)	McNemar Chi Sq	P Value
Plasma 1:16	39	37.5 (28.8–47.1)	DBS	36	34.6 (26.2–44.2)	0.7	$p = 0.6$

To determine how application of plasma and DBS with recommended dilution affects final results of each test, sensitivity, specificity, PPV and NPV were calculated. Sensitivity and NPV were low at 60.0% and 70.6% when DBS was compared to plasma at 1:4 (Table 5). Higher values of 88.9% and 83.3% were recorded for specificity and PPV respectively (Table 5). Test performance remained relatively unchanged when plasma at 1:16 was compared to plasma at 1:4, with the exception of an increase in sensitivity to 66.0% over DBS when using a similar dilution (Table 5).

Table 5. Sensitivity, specificity, PPV, NPV and odds ratio results from Og4C3 method and dilution comparisons.

Standard	Comparative Test	Sensitivity (95% CI)	Specificity (95% CI)	PPV (95% CI)	NPV (95% CI)	Odds Ratio (95% CI)	P Value
Plasma 1:4	DBS	60.0% (45.2–73.6)	88.9% (77.4–95.8)	83.3% (67.2–93.6)	70.6% (58.3–81.0)	12.0 (4.3–33.3)	$p <0.0001$
-	Plasma 1:16	66.0% (51.2–78.8)	88.9% (77.4–95.8)	84.6% (69.5–94.1)	73.9% (61.5–84.0)	15.5 (5.5–43.5)	$p <0.0001$

Kappa agreement statistic was used to analyse concordance between comparisons against the 1:4 diluted plasma gold standard. Kappa values were relatively low at 0.55 and 0.49 for comparisons of plasma at 1:4 with plasma at 1:16 dilution and DBS respectively.

To assess if more closely-matched dilutions might improve positive and negative detection rates, plasma at 1:16 dilution was employed as a standard and compared against DBS. This resulted in relatively high sensitivity (79.5%), specificity (92.3%), PPV (86.1%), and NPV (88.2%), suggesting that both plasma and DBS yield highest concordance in positive and negative results when applied using similar dilutions (Table 6).

Table 6. Sensitivity, specificity, PPV, NPV and odds ratio results from Og4C3 ELISA applications of plasma at 1:16 dilution and DBS.

Standard	Comparative Test	Sensitivity (95% CI)	Specificity (95% CI)	PPV (95% CI)	NPV (95% CI)	Odds Ratio (95% CI)	P Value
Plasma 1:16	DBS	79.5% (63.5–90.7)	92.3% (83.0–97.5)	86.1% (70.5–95.3)	88.2% (78.1–94.8)	46.5 (14.0–154.2)	$p < 0.0001$

An odds ratio of 46.5 was also achieved when comparing plasma at a 1:16 dilution and DBS (Table 6) which was higher than odds ratio achieved when using plasma at 1:4 dilution as the standard (Table 5). This suggests a stronger association between plasma and DBS when dilutions are matched.

Concordance between the 1:16 diluted plasma sample and the DBS sample was also measured using kappa agreement statistic. Values were higher at 0.73 than observed with comparisons that used a 1:4 diluted gold standard. This suggests higher concordance between samples when dilutions are matched.

3.3. Analysis of Quantitative Mean Results Used to Compare Plasma at 1:4 and 1:16 Dilutions and DBS

Antigen unit values are shown for each sample type and dilution expressed as log (units+1) in Figure 1.

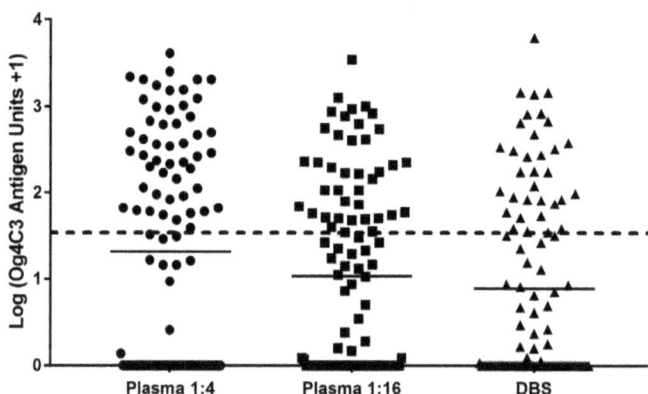

Figure 1. Filariasis Og4C3 ELISA antigen unit concentration comparisons of dilution, plasma and whole blood application. Horizontal black lines refer to mean log antigen unit concentration of each assay (Table 7). All antigen unit concentrations above the defined cut-off (log (32 antigen units + 1)), shown by the horizontal segregated line, are considered positive, while all readings below are considered negative.

Table 7. Comparison of mean Og4C3 antigen units between sample applications and dilutions.

	Group 1			Group 2			t-Test		
Test	Mean Log (Antigen Unit +1)	Geometric Mean	Test	Mean Log (Antigen Unit +1)	Geometric Mean	N	Mean Log Difference	SD	P Value
Plasma 1:4	1.32	19.75	DBS	0.89	6.81	104	0.42	0.88	$p < 0.0001$
Plasma 1:4	1.32	19.75	Plasma 1:16	1.03	9.83	104	0.28	0.74	$p < 0.001$
Plasma 1:16	1.03	9.83	DBS	0.89	6.81	104	0.14	0.67	$p = 0.03$

Analysis of log unit values + 1 was used to approximate a normal distribution for comparisons. From these units, the mean log value for plasma at 1:4 (1.32) was significantly higher than the mean log values achieved for DBS (0.89; $p < 0.0001$) (Table 7). The mean log for plasma at 1:4 was also significantly higher than for plasma at 1:16 dilution (Table 7). Despite a statistically significant p value when dilutions were similar for plasma and DBS, the mean difference was smaller than previous comparisons. These quantitative comparisons are consistent with the results described above.

3.4. Correlation Comparisons Analysis of Og4C3 Concentrations from Plasma and Eluates from DBS

To compare differences in antigen unit concentrations between tests, correlation coefficients were measured between sample types and dilutions. When comparing recommended dilutions of plasma at 1:4 against DBS, correlation was lowest at 0.7 (Figure 2A). Correlation increased to 0.8 when plasma at 1:4 and 1:16 dilutions were compared (Figure 2B), and when plasma at 1:16 and DBS were compared (Figure 2C). This suggests improved correlation is achieved through either matched sample application or dilution.

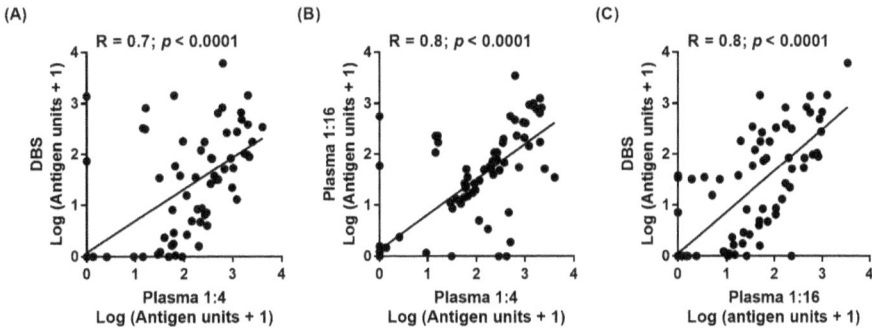

Figure 2. Filariasis Og4C3 ELISA antigen unit concentration correlation comparisons. (**A**) Plasma at recommended 1:4 dilution plotted against DBS samples. (**B**) Plasma at recommended 1:4 dilution plotted against 1:16 dilution. (**C**) Plasma at 1:16 dilution plotted against DBS samples.

4. Discussion

The major finding of this study is that the agreement of results between plasma and DBS samples is lowest when using recommended dilutions of 1:4 for plasma, and that better agreement between these tests is achieved when using plasma at 1:16 against DBS. However, significantly fewer samples are classed as positive when using the lower 1:16 dilution for plasma or using DBS.

We showed that the ICT had similar positive proportions and predictive values to the Og4C3 ELISA when using plasma at 1:4, but that sensitivity is reduced when using the 1:16 dilution. Previous literature has shown that the ICT is less sensitive than the Og4C3 ELISA at 1:4 dilution, detecting only 66.5% of known bancroftian filariasis cases with no microfilariae confirmed by microscopy [13], but that both tests yield identical detection rates when microfilariae were detectable [13–16]. Og4C3 has also been reported to detect significantly smaller titres of filarial antigen when compared to the ICT [13,17], although ICT and Og4C3 both showed an improved detection rate average of up to 25% over microfilariae detection[18]. The current study suggests that despite the higher sensitivity of Og4C3 at lower antigen dilutions, the dilution recommended for DBS application reduces the amount of antigens per sample to a titre that will not accurately yield a positive result when the disease is present.

When analysing positive proportions, results were similar at 46.15% and 48.08% for ICT and plasma at 1:4, and again at 37.50% and 34.62% for plasma at 1:16 and DBS. Positive proportion similarity between plasma and DBS has previously been discussed by Itoh and colleagues [10] as having a 97.4% concordance. However, these results were produced using a 5-fold upwards adjustment to the DBS antigen units.

Lack of concordance between plasma at 1:4 and DBS was supported by Chi-square analysis, which showed significant difference when recommended dilutions for plasma and DBS were used, but no significant difference with matched dilution comparisons. These data support the notion that it is not sample type per se but dilution factor that affects quantitative results, and lower positive proportions for plasma at 1:16 and DBS are detected when compared to ICT or plasma at 1:4 dilution.

Sensitivity and NPV was lowest when DBS was compared to plasma using recommended dilutions. This comparison also yielded an odds ratio of 12.00 and kappa of 0.49, the lowest value among each of these comparisons. These results are similar to those found by Reeve and Melrose [11], where sensitivity and NPV was 67.2% and 77.0% respectively using the dilutions recommended by the Og4C3 kit. As sensitivity and NPV increased to 79.49% and 88.24% respectively when comparing plasma at 1:16 and DBS samples, these results suggest that dilution directly affects how likely it is that the assay will detect the presence of *Wuchereria bancrofti* in someone with LF, as well as how likely it is to detect someone with a negative result when they do not have LF. These statistics were also supported by an odds ratio, which was highest at 45.50, and by the kappa agreement statistic, which was also highest at 0.73, when dilutions were matched.

There was a higher mean antigen concentration in plasma compared to DBS at recommended dilutions, but the difference in mean antigen units was greatly reduced when dilutions were more closely matched. While plasma samples were tested at 1:4 and 1:16 dilutions, equal to a 4-fold difference, geometric mean (antigen unit +1) values were 19.75 and 9.83 respectively. The difference in means is much less than 4-fold. The geometric means were 9.83 and 6.81 for plasma at 1:16 and DBS respectively. The non-linear antigen unit relationship to dilution factor may be attributed to high saturation of each ELISA well by a higher concentration of sample, which would be left with fewer spare antibodies bound to the plastic surface available for the free floating antigens to bind during the initial 1-h incubation period. It is possible that a lower concentration of sample antigen may bind fewer antibodies initially, but will not saturate the well as the higher concentration sample would, allowing a greater number of unbound antibodies on the plate to attach to free floating antigens during incubation [19,20].

Correlation was found to be highest when either dilutions or sample application methods were matched, but was low when plasma at 1:4 and DBS were compared. No previous study has compared matching low dilutions but it is not surprising that matched dilutions may result in higher agreeability between plasma and DBS. This is important as higher dilutions are less sensitive overall when compared with ICT and therefore must be used with caution.

The results of this study indicate that the currently recommended dilution for the Og4C3 ELISA using DBS is not as sensitive as for plasma, and that more than 25% of positive cases may be being missed when using DBS. Concordance between methods would improve if similar dilutions were used. Unfortunately, a 1:4 dilution is not possible with the current prescribed method of DBS preparation and amount of sample, since that would require eluting three filter paper discs in 60 μL of diluent, leaving insufficient supernatant for a single well after boiling and spinning. While high correlation can be achieved when the fold difference in antigens is matched [10], Lalitha and colleagues [21] show that correlation can drop to 0.83 when plasma and DBS are used at 1:4 and 1:20 dilutions respectively.

The outcomes of this research lead to a recommendation that further assessment be carried out to determine how both plasma and DBS perform at other matched dilutions, such as 1:8 or 1:10. Any such tests must accommodate the volume needed to fully saturate each dried blood spot, allow for boiling, precipitation and spinning, and yielding 50 μL to be applied to the well of an Og4C3 ELISA. Improved concordance between Og4C3 plasma and DBS application that also achieves a similar detection rate as the ICT would greatly support the reliability of the Og4C3 ELISA for field collection in non-laboratory locations, as DBS is a convenient method of collecting samples, requiring less in-depth training, and less storage space or refrigeration during transport.

A major limitation attributed to enzyme immunoassays, referred to as the 'hook' effect, is shown when a decrease in reactivity is seen as the concentration of free antigen or antibody increases [22–24]. As each plate will always give different readings, a reliable standard curve must be used to mitigate plate-to-plate variation and avoid error in classifications of positive or negative from test to test.

One strategy may be to perform each sample at two dilutions in order to obviate such occurrences and to ensure that antibody or antigen excess does not occur. A two-dilution application could also evaluate each individual plate by showing if any non-linearity between results has occurred.

In conclusion, the current recommended dilutions for plasma and DBS did not demonstrate adequate agreement. The data obtained shows that both plasma and DBS are capable of yielding similar results, but only when dilutions are more closely matched than is currently recommended. Definition of a single suitable dilution factor lower than 1:16 which can be applied to both DBS and plasma assays, and to compare specificity, sensitivity and predictive values between DBS and plasma upon application is required. Results achieved from antigen unit analysis using DBS assays need to be adjusted upwards to be comparable with plasma tests. We recommend that similar studies be repeated in other endemic situations, with different test predictive values, to confirm our results and to determine the adjustment factors required. In the longer term, the dilutions for the two test types need to be reconciled.

Acknowledgments: The authors would like to thank the Myanmar Ministry of Health and Sports and the Department of Medical Research (Lower Myanmar) for laboratory support and storage of the samples. We are grateful to Luke Becker of the Australian Institute for Tropical Health and Medicine and Ye Ye and Thi Thi Lwin of the Public Health Laboratory in Mandalay (Central Myanmar) for assistance with sample collection and separation. We would like to thank Diane Dogcio-Hall and Cellabs Pty. Ltd., New South Wales, Australia, for advice and discussions. We are very grateful to the NIH/NIAID Filariasis Reagent Resource Center (www.filariasiscenter.org) that provided positive controls for the ICT cards. Additional thanks must also be given to Mathew Hayes and Adam Bowen for their support and advice.

Author Contributions: P.M.G., J.D., J.M. and J.W. conceived of and designed the experiments; J.M., M.R., and K.M.H. performed the experiments; K.S.A. provided storage and lab facilities, J.M. and P.M.G. analysed the data; J.M., P.M.G. and J.D. wrote the paper with input from J.W.; all authors reviewed the final draft and provided input.

Conflicts of Interest: The authors declare no conflict of interest.

References

1. Lau, C.L.; Won, K.Y.; Becker, L.; Soares Magalhaes, R.J.; Fuimaono, S.; Melrose, W.; Lammie, P.J.; Graves, P.M. Seroprevalence and spatial epidemiology of lymphatic filariasis in American Samoa after successful mass drug administration. *PLoS Negl. Trop. Dis.* **2014**, *8*, e3297. [CrossRef] [PubMed]

2. Mwakitalu, M.E.; Malecela, M.N.; Pedersen, E.M.; Mosham, F.W.; Simonsen, P.E. Urban lymphatic filariasis in the metropolis of Dar es Salaam, Tanzania. *Parasites Vectors* **2013**, *6*, 286. [CrossRef] [PubMed]

3. Hamlin, K.L.; Moss, D.M.; Priest, J.W.; Roberts, J.; Kubofcik, J.; Gass, K.; Streit, T.G.; Nutman, T.B.; Eberhard, M.L.; Lammie, P.J. Longitudinal monitoring of the development of antifilarial antibodies and acquisition of *Wuchereria bancrofti* in a highly endemic area of Haiti. *PLoS Negl. Trop. Dis.* **2012**, *6*, e1941. [CrossRef] [PubMed]

4. Harrington, H.; Asugeni, J.; Jimuru, C.; Gwalaa, J.; Ribeyro, E.; Bradbury, R.; Streit, T.G.; Nutman, T.B.; Eberhard, M.L.; Lammie, P.J. A practical strategy for responding to a case of lymphatic filariasis post-elimination in Pacific Islands. *Parasites Vectors* **2013**, *6*, 218. [CrossRef] [PubMed]

5. Weerasooriya, M.V.; Gunawardena, N.K.; Itoh, M.; Qiu, X.G.; Kimura, E. Prevalence and intensity of *Wuchereria bancrofti* antigenaemia in Sri Lanka by Og4C3 ELISA using filter paper-absorbed whole blood. *Trans. R. Soc. Trop. Med. Hyg.* **2002**, *96*, 41–45. [CrossRef]

6. World Health Organization. *Lymphatic Filariasis: A Manual for National Elimination Programmes*; WHO Press: Geneva, Switzerland, 2011; pp. 7–8.

7. Gass, K.; Beau de Rochars, M.V.; Boakye, D.; Bradley, M.; Fischer, P.U.; Gyapong, J.; Itoh, M.; Ituaso-Conway, N.; Joseph, H.; Kyelem, D.; et al. A multicenter evaluation of diagnostic tools to define endpoints for programs to eliminate bancroftian filariasis. *PLoS Negl. Trop. Dis.* **2012**, *6*, e1479. [CrossRef] [PubMed]

8. Rocha, A.; Braga, C.; Belém, M.; Carrera, A.; Aguiar-Santos, A.; Oliveira, P.; Texeira, M.G.; Furtado, A. Comparison of tests for the detection of circulating filarial antigen (Og4C3-ELISA and AD12-ICT) and ultrasound in diagnosis of lymphatic filariasis in individuals with microfilariae. *Mem. Inst. Oswaldo Cruz* **2009**, *104*, 621–625. [CrossRef] [PubMed]

9.   Gounoue-Kamkumo, R.; Nana-Djeunga, H.C.; Bopda, J.; Akame, J.; Tarini, A.; Kamgno, J. Loss of sensitivity of immunochromatographic test (ICT) for lymphatic filariasis diagnosis in low prevalence settings: Consequence in the monitoring and evaluation procedures. *BMC Infect. Dis.* **2015**, *15*, 579. [CrossRef] [PubMed]

10.   Itoh, M.; Gunawardena, N.K.; Qiu, X.G.; Weerasooriya, M.V.; Kimura, E. The use of whole blood absorbed on filter paper to detect *Wuchereria bancrofti* circulating antigen. *Trans. R. Soc. Trop. Med. Hyg.* **1998**, *92*, 513–515. [CrossRef]

11.   Reeve, D.; Melrose, W. Evaluation of the Og34C filter paper technique in lymphatic filariasis prevalence studies. *Lymphology* **2014**, *47*, 65–72. [PubMed]

12.   Tropbio Pty. Ltd. *ELISA Kit for Detecting and Quantifying Wuchereria bancrofti Antigen*; Cellabs Pty. Ltd.: Brookvale, NSW, Australia, 2014.

13.   Nuchprayoon, S.; Porksakorn, C.; Junpee, A.; Sanprasere, V.; Poovorawan, Y. Comparative assessment of an Og4C3 ELISA and an ICT filariasis test: A study of Myanmar migrants in Thailand. *Asian Pac. J. Allergy Immunol.* **2003**, *21*, 253–257. [PubMed]

14.   Freedman, D.O.; de Almeida, A.; Miranda, J.; Plier, D.A.; Braga, C. Field trial of a rapid card test for *Wuchereria bancrofti*. *Lancet* **1997**, *350*, 1681. [CrossRef]

15.   Simonsen, P.E.; Dunyo, S.K. Comparative evaluation of three new tools for diagnosis of bancroftian filariasis based on detection of specific circulating antigens. *Trans. R. Soc. Trop. Med. Hyg.* **1999**, *93*, 278–282. [CrossRef]

16.   Nuchprayoon, S.; Sanprasert, V.; Porksakorn, C.; Nuchprayoon, I. Prevalence of bancroftian filariasis on the Thai-Myanmar border. *Asian Pac. J. Allergy Immunol.* **2003**, *21*, 179–188. [PubMed]

17.   Nguyen, N.L.; Plichart, C.; Esterre, P. Assessment of immunochromatographic test for rapid lymphatic filariasis diagnosis. *Parasite* **1999**, *6*, 355–358. [CrossRef] [PubMed]

18.   Melrose, W.; Pisters, P.; Turner, P.; Kombati, Z.; Selve, B.P.; Hii, J.; Speare, R. Prevalence of filarial antigenaemia in Papua New Guinea: Results of surveys by the School of Public Health and Tropical Medicine, James Cook University, Townsville, Australia. *P. N. G. Med. J.* **2000**, *43*, 161–165. [PubMed]

19.   Butler, J.E.; McGivern, P.L.; Swanson, P. Amplification of the enzyme-linked immunosorbent assay (ELISA) in the detection of class-specific antibodies. *J. Immunol. Methods* **1978**, *20*, 365–383. [CrossRef]

20.   Winzor, D.J. Allowance for antibody bivalence in the characterization of interactions by ELISA. *J. Mol. Recognit.* **2011**, *24*, 139–148. [CrossRef] [PubMed]

21.   Lalitha, P.; Ravichandran, M.; Suba, S.; Kaliraj, P.; Narayanan, R.B.; Jayaraman, K. Quantitative assessment of circulating antigens in human lymphatic filariasis: A field evaluation of monoclonal antibody-based ELISA using blood collected on filter strips. *Trop. Med. Int. Health* **1998**, *3*, 41–45. [CrossRef] [PubMed]

22.   Pesce, A.J.; Michael, J.G. Artifacts and limitations of enzyme immunoassays. *J. Immunol. Methods* **1992**, *150*, 111–119. [CrossRef]

23.   Rodbard, D.; Feldman, Y.; Jaffe, M.L.; Miles, L.E. Kinetics of two-site immunoradiometric (sandwich) assays—II. Studies on the nature of the 'high-dose hook-effect'. *Immunochemistry* **1978**, *15*, 77–82. [CrossRef]

24.   Ryall, R.G.; Story, C.J.; Turner, D.R. Reappraisal of the causes of the 'hook-effect' in two-site immunoradiometric assays. *Anal. Biochem.* **1982**, *27*, 308–315. [CrossRef]

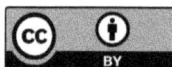

Tropical Medicine and Infectious Disease

MDPI

Article

Lymphatic Filariasis Increases Tissue Compressibility and Extracellular Fluid in Lower Limbs of Asymptomatic Young People in Central Myanmar

Janet Douglass [1,*], Patricia Graves [2], Daniel Lindsay [1], Luke Becker [2], Maureen Roineau [2], Jesse Masson [2], Ni Ni Aye [3], San San Win [4], Tint Wai [3], Yi Yi Win [3] and Susan Gordon [1,5]

[1] Division of Tropical Health and Medicine, James Cook University, Townsville 4811, Australia; daniel.lindsay1@jcu.edu.au (D.L.); sue.gordon@flinders.edu.au (S.G.)
[2] Division of Tropical Health and Medicine, James Cook University, Cairns 4870, Australia; patricia.graves@jcu.edu.au (P.G.); luke.becker@jcu.edu.au (L.B.); maureenroineau@wanadoo.fr (M.R.); jesse.masson@my.jcu.edu.au (J.M.)
[3] Department of Health, Myanmar Ministry of Health and Sports, Nay Pyi Taw 15011, Myanmar; shwewaethu@gmail.com (N.N.A.); mr.tintwaitun2013@gmail.com (T.W.); yywin2008@gmail.com (Y.Y.W.)
[4] World Health Organization, Country Office, Yangon 11201, Myanmar; wins@who.int
[5] College of Nursing & Health Sciences, Flinders University, Bedford Park 5042, Australia
* Correspondence: jan.douglass@my.jcu.edu.au; Tel.: +61-419-848-589

Received: 15 August 2017; Accepted: 17 September 2017; Published: 27 September 2017

Abstract: When normal lymphatic function is hampered, imperceptible subcutaneous edema can develop and progress to overt lymphedema. Low-cost reliable devices for objective assessment of lymphedema are well accepted in clinical practice and research on breast-cancer related lymphedema but are untested in populations with lymphatic filariasis (LF). This is a cross-sectional analysis of baseline data in a longitudinal study on asymptomatic, LF antigen-positive and -negative young people in Myanmar. Rapid field screening was used to identify antigen-positive cases and a group of antigen-negative controls of similar age and gender were invited to continue in the study. Tissue compressibility was assessed with three tissue tonometers, and free fluids were assessed using bio-impedance spectroscopy (BIS). Infection status was confirmed by Og4C3 antigen assay. At baseline ($n = 98$), antigen-positive cases had clinically relevant increases in tissue compressibility at the calf using a digital Indurometer (11.1%, $p = 0.021$), and in whole-leg free fluid using BIS (9.2%, $p = 0.053$). Regression analysis for moderating factors (age, gender, hydration) reinforced the between-infection group differences. Results demonstrate that sub-clinical changes associated with infection can be detected in asymptomatic cases. Further exploration of these low-cost devices in clinical and research settings on filariasis-related lymphedema are warranted.

Keywords: neglected tropical disease; lower extremity; lymphatic filariasis; tissue tonometry; bio-impedance spectroscopy; lymphedema

1. Introduction

Lymphatic filariasis (LF) is a parasitic disease in which thread-like worms inhabit the human lymphatic system, where they can impair normal lymphatic pumping. Classified as a neglected tropical disease and affecting many of the world's poorest populations, LF can lead to lymphedema, a progressively debilitating swelling of the skin and subcutaneous tissue in any body part, most frequently the legs [1]. Normal lymphatic pumping actively removes circulating proteins and fluid from the tissue spaces, maintaining a slightly negative interstitial pressure. When lymphatic capacity is impaired, extracellular fluid (ECF) and circulating proteins begin to accumulate in the interstitial spaces [2]. If normal lymphatic function is not restored, this initially covert edema gradually becomes overt, and the affected body part visibly enlarges. Over time, the protein-rich fluid is replaced with fat and fibrous tissue, and normal limb contours are lost. The outdated eponym 'elephantiasis' was inspired by the appearance of a grossly enlarged limb in late-stage lymphedema where the skin is thick, discolored, and formed into folds. In developed countries, lymphedema is frequently caused by surgical damage when lymph nodes are removed or irradiated during cancer treatment. Much of what is known about initiation and progression of lymphedema comes from research on breast cancer-related lymphedema (BCRL) of the arm [3].

A wide spectrum of devices and methods is used to objectively evaluate lymphedema depending on the setting. At the highly resourced end of the spectrum, nuclear imaging and other sophisticated technologies are often used to assess BCRL of the arm. Tissue tonometry to quantify tissue compressibility and portable bio-impedance spectroscopy (BIS) to track fluctuations in free fluid are also used and are relatively inexpensive. Using BIS, it has been shown that covert pathologic change due to lymphatic damage during breast cancer treatment can be detected, and that early intervention in this latent stage can prevent the onset of overt disease [4]. At the low-resourced end of the spectrum, assessment of LF related-lymphedema (LFRL) of the leg usually relies on classification of visible and palpable soft tissue changes [5], where subjectivity may lead to inconsistent classification. There is no differentiation or assessment of covert change, so subtle but important alterations in tissue composition may be missed.

In LF, mosquitoes pick up the microfilariae during a blood meal. The larvae develop to third stage within the mosquito before being transmitted by a subsequent bite. Transmission is relatively inefficient with a low risk of infection per bite, and after transmission there is a lag between being infected and the development of adult worms. This means that most children with LF will remain asymptomatic until young adulthood, which affords a long, latent period in which to implement preventive strategies [6]. Primary prevention in the Global Program to Eliminate LF (GPELF) is preventive chemotherapy, which is delivered annually via mass drug administration (MDA) in endemic regions [7]. This will eventually prevent any new cases of morbidity as infection rates fall too low to sustain transmission. However, preventive chemotherapy conveys no real benefit to advanced cases, most of whom will no longer be antigenemic, but will require life-long health care. In between the asymptomatic cases that will never progress to overt disease and the advanced cases that have irreversible lymphedema, there are many cases of latent and early stage lymphedema. There is some evidence that MDA may reverse very early tissue changes in LFRL [8], but without standardized assessment or diagnostic criteria for Stage 0, or devices sensitive enough to detect small changes in tissue composition, it is not clear at what stage or which individuals will remain at risk of disease progression. Reliable, sensitive, low-cost devices to provide objective assessment of LFRL are needed [9].

A pilot study in Papua New Guinea (PNG) found the skin over the posterior thigh was 20% more compressible in asymptomatic young people who had tested positive for LF antigen compared to antigen-negative peers, using a mechanical tonometer [10]. Subsequently, three tissue tonometers and a portable BIS device have demonstrated intra-operator reliability in assessing tissue composition in the lower limbs of young Australian and Myanmar populations without any history or risk of lymphedema [11]. It is not yet known if covert lymphedema can be detected by tissue tonometry or BIS in these populations.

There is no agreed standard for assessment of Stage 0 lymphedema, and diagnostic criteria for clinical onset are not well defined [3]. One study on BCRL used a 3% change in BIS values to trigger preventive treatment [4], and clinical lymphologists may use a percentage change in limb girth or volume to track lymphedema change, with a variation of more than 10% considered clinically relevant [12]. Variations in body composition will influence measurements with these devices as muscle holds more free fluid than fat, fat is more compressible than muscle, and the ECF in the subcutaneous compartment fluctuates slightly depending on overall body hydration. Individual characteristics that influence body composition should be considered when assessing superficial tissues of the lower limb, including expected changes associated with growth from child to young adult and gender-based differences in muscle and fat distribution. Habitual patterns of muscle use should also be considered, and significant between-leg differences in healthy young Australian and Myanmar people have been reported when using these devices [13].

This cross-sectional study on young people residing in an LF endemic region in Central Myanmar investigated whether tissue tonometry and BIS measures were altered in asymptomatic cases who tested positive for *Wuchereria bancrofti* antigen. The results will assist researchers and clinicians to objectively quantify changes occurring in early LFRL and may contribute to formal recognition and intervention for Stage 0 lymphedema of the leg.

2. Materials and Methods

2.1. Study Site Selection, Participant Recruitment, and Screening

Sentinel site records kept by the Vector Borne Disease Control (VBDC) Centre in Mandalay identified Amarapura Township as a densely populated area with a high prevalence of LF. It was also close enough to laboratory services for blood sample processing. A study site was set up in the Administration Centre in the village of Nge Toe and baseline data were collected over a two-week period in October 2014. The study was conducted in accordance with the Declaration of Helsinki and the protocol was approved by the Myanmar Ministry of Health (MoH) and James Cook University Human Research Ethics Committee (approval number H5261).

A sample size of 32 in each group was predicted to detect a 10% difference between groups with 80% power, based on a mean mid-calf value of 2.5 with SD of 0.7 using the digital Indurometer [13,14]. A convenience sample of local young people aged 10–21 years was invited to be screened for LF antigen and to participate in a longitudinal study on early detection of LFRL. Participant information sheets and informed consent forms were provided in Burmese. Staff of the VBDC and Amarapura Township Hospital, the World Health Organization (WHO) technical officer for Myanmar (SSW), and locally-trained research assistants explained all procedures to the participants, determined their eligibility to participate, and obtained informed consent. Written consent was given by young adults aged 18–21 and by a parent or guardian for minors aged 10–17. A further verbal assent for each procedure was obtained from all participants prior to performing that procedure. Participant inclusion and exclusion criteria are shown in Figure 1.

Inclusion criteria	Exclusion criteria
• Aged 10 – 21 years at screening • Residing in Amarapura Township • Able to give informed consent (18 – 21 year olds) • Accompanied by an adult relative able to give informed consent (10 – 17 years olds)	• Any clinical sign of lymphedema • Acute injury to the lower limb(s) • Past surgery to the trunk or lower limb(s) • Heart disease • Pacemaker or other implanted device • Pregnancy • Unable to give informed consent

Figure 1. Participant inclusion and exclusion criteria.

2.2. Screening and Baseline Data Collection

A rapid field test for the presence of LF antigen was performed using an immunochromatographic test (ICT) card (Binax Now, Alere, Waltham, MA, USA). This involved placing a 100 μL draw of blood from a fingerprick onto a test strip. The sample was allowed to flow for 10 min and the result appeared as one or two lines across the test strip. One line is a control and if this line was not visible then the test was void and if possible, repeated. Appearance of the second line indicated the presence of circulating *W. bancrofti* antigen that is produced by adult worms. The young people who tested positive by ICT (cases), and a sample of the negative participants of the same age and gender (controls), were invited to return and participate in the longitudinal study. A James Cook University (JCU) technical staff member (LB) trained the local research assistants in correct use of the ICT card and selected participants invited for follow-up.

Participants returned during the following fortnight for the blood draw and device measures. Local research assistants conducted a short interview to elicit information on current health status, prescription or traditional medications, surgical history, family history of lymphedema, time since the last drink (as a proxy for hydration), and if they had consumed preventive chemotherapy during the previous annual MDA. Leg dominance was determined by asking the question 'Which foot do you use to kick a ball?' Height was measured using a chart marked on a wooden post in centimeters and a set square, and weight in kilograms was recorded using digital scales purchased locally. Device measures were conducted in a small side office or screened off area and an adult relative was asked to be present during the measurement of minors.

2.2.1. Device Measures

Three tissue tonometers were used to assess tissue compressibility. The Indurometer (SA Biomedical Engineering, Adelaide, Australia) is a hand-held electro-mechanical device with a 1 cm diameter plunger/indenter extending through a 7 cm diameter reference plate and a built-in force sensor. The reference plate is aligned to the surface of the skin while the device is pressed evenly into the tissue. A beep is emitted once the equivalent to 200 g of force has been applied, and the degree of displacement is displayed in 0.01 increments on a light-emitting diode (LED) screen. An image of the Indurometer is shown in Figure S1. The mechanical Tonometer (SA Biomedical Engineering, Adelaide, Australia) is a similar device, in which a 1 cm diameter plunger extends beyond a 7 cm diameter reference plate. This purely mechanical device uses a 200 g mass to drive the indenter into the underlying tissue, and the degree of displacement is shown on an analogue scale. Both of these devices record the displacement of the indenter in relation to the reference plate as an indication of compliance (compressibility) of the underlying skin and tissue. The values provided by these devices are not absolute measures and can be considered as arbitrary units used to compare measures of tissue compressibility [15]. A third device, the SkinFibroMeter (Delfin Technologies, Kuopio, Finland), uses a smaller reference plate with a 1.25 mm length fixed indenter and built-in force sensors. The reference plate is pressed evenly onto the skin and the device emits a beep when the equivalent of 50 g has been applied. The device is applied five times and the average resistance in newtons is displayed on a digital screen. A tape measure and washable skin marker were used to locate and mark the midpoint of each thigh (front and back) and the back of each calf, and all tonometry measures were taken at these marks.

Extracellular and intracellular fluid loads were assessed using bio-impedance spectroscopy (BIS), which measures the resistance to multifrequency, low-level electrical currents. The difference between resistance in the intracellular (Ri) and extracellular (Re) fluid compartments was represented as a ratio Ri:Re. As the intracellular fluid (ICF) compartment is tightly regulated, any changes in the ratio usually represent changes in the extracellular fluid (ECF). Whole-leg BIS measures were recorded for each leg with the SFB7 (Impedimed, Australia) using self-adhesive electrodes applied to the skin according to manufacturer's instructions for lower limb measures.

A detailed description of data collection methods was published in a reliability study on these devices in Australia and Myanmar [11]. All devices were operated by the principal researcher (JD), who was blinded to the infection status of the participants. Tonometry scores were recorded on data collection sheets by a research assistant, and BIS data was downloaded to an Excel file (Microsoft Office 365, version 1706).

2.2.2. Blood Collection and Processing/Storage

Blood samples were collected by local research assistants, who were trained in specific blood collection and handling protocols by the JCU technician (LB). A 10 mL draw of venous blood was collected from each participant into cooled ethylenediaminetetraacetic acid (EDTA) anticoagulant vacutainers (BD Biosciences, North Ryde, Australia). The antigen test was repeated using 100 uL of the venous blood pipetted onto an ICT card, and the remaining blood was kept on ice until delivery to the Public Health Laboratory in Mandalay. Separation of plasma and red blood cells was performed using a centrifuge for 15 min at 3000 rpm; the plasma was transferred into 2-mL cryotubes by pipette in duplicate (4 mL per person) and stored at $-20\,^\circ$C. Once all baseline data had been collected, the plasma was transferred on dry ice to the Department of Medical Research in Yangon for long-term storage at $-80\,^\circ$C in a monitored freezer connected to a back-up generator and with daily monitoring. There were no thaws during plasma transportation or storage. One set of the cryotubes was aliquoted and used to conduct ELISA assay for the presence of Og4C3, an antigen marker for *W. bancrofti*, using the recommend 1:4 dilution for plasma as per the manufacturer (Cellabs, Sydney, Australia) kit instructions [16]. Samples were classified as positive if the antigen units, estimated using the standard curve of controls provided with the kit, exceeded 32 units. Detailed methods for the ELISA assays were previously published in a study on diagnostic testing for LF antigen [16].

2.3. Data Analysis

LF antigen-positive cases were defined as those who were positive by either antigen test (ICT or Og4C3). Body mass index (BMI) was calculated as kg/m^2, but adult values cannot be used for children; therefore, WHO growth charts and definitions were used to identify underweight participants, who were defined as being more than two standard deviations below the median BMI for their age [17]. Chi-squared tests, Fisher's exact tests, and independent samples *t*-tests were used to compare antigen-positive and -negative group characteristics at baseline for known moderating factors. Paired sample *t*-tests were used to compare device measures of dominant and non-dominant legs. Statistical analysis was conducted in SPSS version 23 (IBM Corp), and significance was set at 0.05 with a 95% confidence interval. Clinically-relevant difference for tonometry measures was set at >10% and for BIS measures it was set at >3%. Stepwise regression was performed for dominant and non-dominant legs separately to determine the level of variance in device measures associated with infection status (univariate) and other potential moderating factors (multivariate).

3. Results

3.1. Participants

Screening for LF found 60 antigen-positive cases among 316 volunteers, and 114 young people (57 cases and 57 controls of the same age and gender) were invited to continue in the longitudinal study (see Figure 2). Ten people either could not be found or refused to return, and 104 participants were available for baseline blood draw and physical measures. Data from six participants were excluded from the final analysis; four were found at a later measure to have been outside the target age range at baseline, one had a prosthetic leg, and another had a heart condition, neither of which had been disclosed at the screening interview. The final study population was comprised of 46 antigen-positive cases detected by ICT plus a further four cases identified as antigen positive by Og4C3 ELISA ($n = 50$). There were 48 antigen-negative (control) cases.

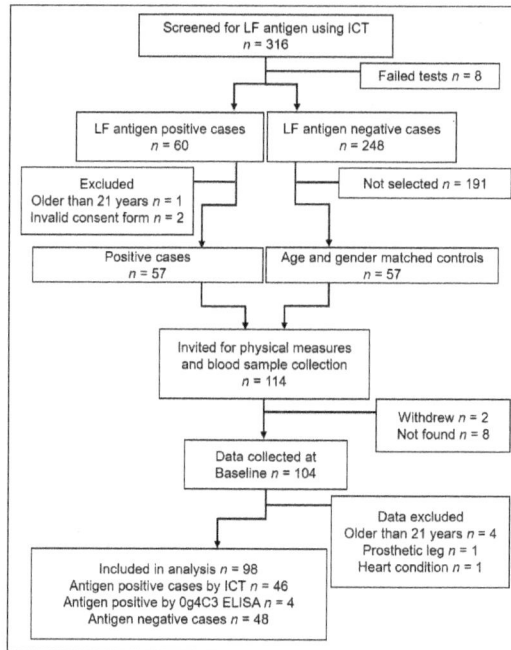

Figure 2. Flow of participants through recruitment, screening, and baseline data collection.

3.1.1. Participant Characteristics

All participants (n = 98) were aged between 10 and 21 years (mean 15.3 SD 3.4) and there were 55 females and 43 males. The mean height, weight, and BMI were 152.0 cm (SD 12.0, range 118.8–174.0), 42.3 kg (SD 11.5, range 17.5–82.7), and 18.0 kg/m^2 (SD 3.0, range 12.4–29.7), respectively. The cohort was 95.9% right leg dominant and 13.3% (n = 13) were considered underweight. Almost half (44.9%) of the participants were working in weaving workshops, 27.6% were students, 8.2% were street vendors, 2.0% were construction workers, and the remaining 17.3% worked in other occupations or did not disclose their occupation. None had a history of lymphedema in their immediate family, previous surgery or medical implants, and all were in good health. Two participants were taking prescription medications and one was using traditional medicine. One participant felt unwell on the day scheduled for taking the measures and was asked to return when feeling better. Comparing antigen-positive and antigen-negative groups, there were no significant between-group differences for any physical attribute or moderating factor. Participant characteristics at baseline are shown in Table 1.

Table 1. Group characteristics of antigen-positive and antigen-negative participants (positive by either immunochromatographic test (ICT) or Og4C3) at baseline.

	LF Antigen-Positive Cases	LF Antigen-Negative Controls	Mean Diff (95% CI)	*p=*
	n = 50	*n* = 48		
Age in years—mean (SD)	15.20 (3.38)	15.48 (3.46)	0.28 (−1.09, 1.07)	0.691 [a]
Gender				
Female *n* (%)	27 (54%)	28 (58%)		0.410 [b]
Male *n* (%)	23 (46%)	20 (42%)		0.410 [b]
Height in cm—mean (SD)	151.80 (12.56)	152.20 (11.52)	0.399 (−4.44, 5.24)	0.870 [a]
Weight in kg—mean (SD)	42.27 (12.81)	42.30 (10.12)	0.028 (−4.617, 4.670)	0.990 [a]
BMI in kg/m^2—mean (SD)	18.05 (3.46)	18.03 (2.65)	−0.012 (−1.239, 1.216)	0.985 [a]
Body composition *n* = (%)				0.976 [c]
Median weight	41 (82%)	40 (83%)		
Underweight > −2SD	7 (14%)	6 (13%)		
Overweight > +1SD	2 (4%)	2 (4%)		
Dominant leg right/left	47/3	47/1		0.324 [b]
Occupation *n* = (%)				0.395 [c]
Student	14 (28%)	13 (27%)		
Working/other	32/4 (72%)	34/1 (73%)		
Drank liquid *n* = 97				0.590 [c]
<60 min	13 (26%)	12 (26%)		
>60 min	37 (74%)	35 (74%) (1 NA)		
Consumed 2013 MDA *n* (%)	17 (34%)	22 (46%)		0.383 [c]

LF = lymphatic filariasis; BMI = body mass index; SD = standard deviation; [a] independent samples *t*-test; [b] Fishers exact test; [c] Pearson chi-square; NA = participant was not asked.

3.2. Moderating Factors Associated with Device Measures

3.2.1. Effect of Infection on Device Measures

In the antigen-positive group, tissue compressibility was higher at all measuring points, and there was more free fluid in both legs compared to that of the antigen negative group. Independent *t*-tests found that, at mid-calf on the non-dominant side, the increase in Indurometer measures was both clinically (11.1%) and statistically significant (*p* = 0.021). In addition, whole leg BIS measures found clinically-relevant (>3%) increases in free fluid in both legs (dominant leg, 4.9% (*p* = 0.220), non-dominant leg, 9.2% (*p* = 0.053)). Mean values and between-group differences for the Indurometer and BIS measures are shown in Table 2. Neither the mechanical Tonometer nor SkinFibroMeter found any clinically relevant or statistically significant differences between infection groups, with many differences too small to be evident at two decimal places. The only between-group difference of interest with these two devices was increased tissue compressibility with the Tonometer at the non-dominant calf (4.8% softer, *p* = 0.296). Mean values and between-group differences for all devices including the Tonometer and SkinFibroMeter are given in Table S1.

Table 2. Between-infection group differences for Indurometer and BIS measures, size, and direction of variation.

Measurement Point Indurometer	Positive $n = 50$ Mean (SD)	Negative $n = 48$ Mean (SD)	Mean Difference (%)	Direction in Positive Cases	$p=$
Dominant anterior thigh	4.80 (0.76)	4.72 (0.69)	0.05 (1.1%)	Softer	0.731
Non-dominant anterior thigh	5.10 (0.88)	5.00 (0.69)	0.10 (1.9%)	Softer	0.546
Dominant posterior thigh	4.13 (0.93)	4.06 (0.87)	0.07 (1.7%)	Softer	0.701
Non-dominant posterior thigh	3.88 (0.83)	3.86 (0.95)	0.02 (0.4%)	Softer	0.933
Dominant calf	2.91 (0.57)	2.70 (0.68)	0.21 (7.8%)	Softer	0.096
Non-dominant calf	2.73 (0.65)	2.46 (0.65)	0.27 (11.1%) *,#	Softer	0.021
BIS					
Dominant leg $n = 47/45$	2.44 (0.46)	2.56 (0.45)	0.12 (4.9%) #	More fluid	0.220
Non-dominant leg $n = 46/44$	2.62 (0.56)	2.86 (0.59)	0.24 (9.2%) #	More fluid	0.053

SD = standard deviation; * Significant between-group difference $p \leq 0.05$; # clinically relevant between-group difference.

3.2.2. Effect of Infection Status, Age, Gender, Body Composition, and Hydration on Device Measures

Regression was first performed with infection status (antigen positivity) alone, and then stepwise regression was used to add moderating factors. Being antigen positive was significantly associated with increased compressibility in the non-dominant calf when using the Indurometer (Table 3, step 1) which is consistent with the *t*-test results given above in Table 2. Using multivariate regression, after adjustment for other factors (gender, age, underweight, and hydration), increased compressibility remained significantly associated with being antigen positive (in the non-dominant calf) using the Indurometer, and was also significant in the dominant calf using the same device. When considering all factors, being antigen positive was significantly associated with increased fluid in the non-dominant leg using BIS (Table 3, step 2).

In the stepwise regression, being female was significantly associated with higher tissue compressibility using all three tonometers. The largest gender-related effect using the Indurometer was in calf measures where there is a relatively thin fat layer over the muscles, making small differences in fat and muscle composition more likely to be detected (dominant leg B (SE) = 0.639 (0.117), $p < 0.000$) (see Table 3). The least effect of gender was found over the anterior thighs where the relatively thicker fat layer reduces the influence of the underlying muscle tone and a small difference between the sexes is not likely to register as much change. Using BIS, being female was significantly associated with less free fluid in both legs, and this is consistent with females having relatively smaller muscle/higher fat mass (less fluid) than males of the same age. The largest coefficient was in the non-dominant leg (B (SE) = 0.485 (0.103), $p < 0.001$) (see Table 3).

Being less well hydrated, defined as not having a drink within one hour of measures, was associated with lower tissue compressibility. This was significant at the non-dominant calf (B (SE) = -0.239 (0.110), $p = 0.032$). Being older was significantly associated with a small increase in free fluid in both legs, consistent with normal growth increase in muscle mass. Being underweight was significantly associated with a small increase in free fluid in the non-dominant leg (BIS) which may be associated with reduced fat mass or an increased capillary filtrate due to proteinemia.

In summary, when accounting for known moderating factors of age, gender, BMI, and hydration, there was a highly significant association between antigen positivity and increased Indurometer measures at the non-dominant calf ($p = 0.007$). At the dominant calf, the same association was also significant ($p = 0.038$). When these factors are taken into account for BIS measures, there was a clinically relevant and significant increase in free fluid (Table 2) in the non-dominant leg ($p = 0.038$). All associations between moderating factors and device measures are given in Table S2.

Table 3. Stepwise regression for moderating factors associated with variation in Indurometer and bio-impedance spectroscopy (BIS) measures.

	Indurometer				BIS	
	Higher Values = Increased Tissue Compressibility				Lower Values = Increased ECF	
	Posterior Thigh B (SE)		Calf B (SE)		Whole Leg B (SE)	
Factor	Dominant	Non−dominant	Dominant	Non−dominant	Dominant	Non−dominant
Step 1 $R^2=$	*0.002*	*0.000*	*0.029*	*0.054*	*0.017*	*0.042*
Antigen Positive	0.070 (0.182)	0.015 (0.180)	0.212 (0.126)	0.272 (0.116) *	−0.117 (0.095)	−0.238 (0.122)
Step 2 $R^2=$	*0.189*	*0.187*	*0.283*	*0.269*	*0.283*	*0.398*
Antigen Positive	0.093 (0.168)	0.049 (0.166)	0.234 (0.111) *	0.286 (0.104) **	−0.108 (0.083)	−0.210 (0.099) *
Gender = Female	0.751 (0.178) **	0.679 (0.175) **	0.639 (0.117) **	0.492 (0.110) **	0.230 (0.087) **	0.485 (0.103) **
Older age	0.022 (0.025)	0.041 (0.025)	0.010 (0.017)	0.024 (0.016)	−0.051 (0.012) **	−0.061 (0.015) **
Underweight	0.136 (0.250)	0.277 (0.247)	−0.052 (0.165)	−0.094 (0.155)	−0.237 (0.120)	−0.302 (0.142) *
Less Recent Hydration	−0.338 (0.177)	−0.223 (0.174)	−0.139 (0.117)	−0.239 (0.110) *	0.107 (0.085)	0.124 (0.101)

ECF = extracellular fluid; SE = standard error; * $p < 0.05$; ** $p < 0.01$.

3.3. Patterns of Tissue Compressibility and Free Fluid in Dominant and Non-Dominant Legs

There was a consistent pattern of tissue compressibility at the measurement sites that held true for all devices and all subgroups by age, gender, or infection status. The most compressible tissue was located at the (relatively) fatty anterior thigh, the least compressible tissue was over the dense tendomuscular junction at mid-calf, and values for the posterior thigh fell between the two. When comparing dominant and non-dominant legs, a consistent pattern of between-leg differences was seen and can be attributed to expected muscle activity during a kick. The skin was less compressible (more muscle tone) over the front of the 'dominant' kicking thigh and over the back of the 'non-dominant' thigh and calf muscles that propel the body forward during the kick. Using BIS, there was more free fluid (more muscle mass or less fat) in the dominant leg compared to the non-dominant leg (9.6%); this difference was both clinically relevant (>3%) and statistically significant ($p < 0.01$) using paired samples t-tests. Mean values and between-leg differences for the Indurometer and BIS are given in Table 4. Mean values and between-leg differences for all devices including the Tonometer and SkinFibroMeter and are given in Table S3.

Table 4. Mean values and between-leg differences using the Indurometer and BIS.

	Indurometer ($n = 98$)			BIS ($n = 90$)
	Anterior Thigh	**Posterior Thigh**	**Calf**	**Whole Leg**
Dominant leg mean (SD)	4.74 (0.72)	4.10 (0.90)	2.81 (0.63)	2.50 (0.46)
Non−dominant leg mean (SD)	5.05 (0.79)	3.87 (0.89)	2.60 (0.59)	2.74 (0.59)
Mean difference (SD)	−0.31 (0.31)	0.23 (0.23)	0.21 (0.21)	−0.24 (0.32)
95% CI of the difference	−0.41, −0.21	0.11, 0.35	0.13, 0.28	−0.31, −0.17
% difference	6.5% **	5.6% **	7.5% **	9.6% **,#
Direction (dominant leg)	Harder	Softer	Softer	More fluid

SD = standard deviation; ** Significant between-leg difference $p \leq 0.01$; # Clinically relevant between-leg difference (tonometry > 10%, BIS > 3%).

The overall pattern of between-leg differences (dominant vs. non-dominant), as demonstrated by kicking a ball, was maintained in the antigen-positive cases, but the degree of difference was altered. Figure 3 is a radar graph showing the percentage of between-leg differences in Indurometer and BIS values for the whole cohort and by infection group. In the infected group, between-thigh differences in tissue compressibility were exaggerated (closer to the outer ring in the radar chart) but only slightly, with similar percentage differences for positive (7%), negative (6.1%), and whole cohort groups (6.5%). The between-infection group differences were more pronounced at the calf where the mean between-calf difference in the positive cases (6.5%) was much smaller (closer to the middle) than that of the negative cases (9.7%) or whole cohort (7.5%). Similarly, as well as an overall increase in free fluid, BIS results indicated that positive cases had smaller between-leg differences compared to those of their negative counterparts (7.5% vs. 11.7%). Although not statistically significant, these reduced between-leg differences in the distal legs of the antigen-positive cases suggest a covert edema overlying and masking normal between-leg variations in muscle tone and mass.

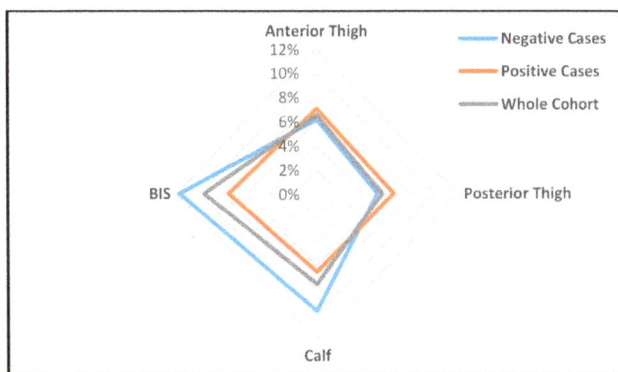

Figure 3. Percentage between-leg differences using the Indurometer and BIS in the LF antigen-negative cases, LF antigen-positive cases, and whole cohort. Data points which are closer to the outer ring indicate greater between-leg differences.

4. Discussion

In this study, tissue compressibility and free fluid loads were higher in asymptomatic young people infected with LF compared to their uninfected peers. Both groups displayed normal patterns of within-leg tissue compressibility; i.e., tissue was most compressible over the anterior thigh and least compressible at the calf, and between-leg differences were consistent with kicking a ball. However, when stratified by infection status, the size and direction of between-leg differences in the positive cases were consistent with a covert accumulation of subcutaneous fluid in the lower leg. Usually, LFRL appears distally and progresses proximally, so detectable tissue changes may occur earlier at the calf than at the thigh. The relatively thin layer of skin and tissue over the muscle of the calf may also render early tissue changes more evident than in fattier parts of the leg. Accordingly, the association with LF antigenemia and Indurometer measures was statistically significant at mid-calf, and large enough on the non-dominant side to also be clinically relevant. This early appearance of lymphatic dysfunction in the non-dominant leg is consistent with reports on BCRL, which show an increased risk of arm lymphedema if the operated side is also the non-dominant arm [18]. This tendency for fluid to accumulate more readily on the non-dominant side could be the result of differences in muscular activity that naturally promotes lymph flow and may be greater or more frequent on the dominant side.

For all devices, the significant associations between higher tissue compressibility and lower free fluid in females reflect expected variation in muscle to fat ratios between the sexes. Other moderating factors such as hydration, although not as universal as gender, did have significant associations with measures at the calf, but this could be reduced by administering a standardized drink during the assessment protocol. Increased free fluid associated with age and being underweight can be attributed to a year-by-year increase in muscle mass, or a systemic reduction in fat mass, respectively.

Results in the Myanmar study reinforce earlier findings from PNG [10], where clinically significant between-infection group differences were found in physical leg measurements. However, some differences in observations between studies were noted. In particular, in young PNG people, increased tissue compressibility was found in the posterior thighs of the infected group using the mechanical Tonometer. In the Myanmar cohort, the between-infection group differences were found using the digital Indurometer at the calf. There may be several reasons for this discrepancy. The PNG cohort had a higher proportion of females (64% vs. 54%) than the Myanmar cohort and a higher mean BMI (19.7 vs. 18.05). In addition, age, gender and hydration were not considered in that analysis. In the current study, the Tonometer did return slightly softer measures in the dominant posterior thigh and non-dominant calf in the Myanmar group, but in this cohort, the differences were not significant. (Table S1). In PNG, no MDA had been available prior to the study, after which treatment was offered to all participants; in Myanmar, MDA had been offered in 2013 and earlier, although less than half of the participants reported taking it. Taken together, these two studies provide the first empirical evidence that there are covert but measurable increases in tissue compressibility and free fluid associated with LF antigenemia, although the optimal site for assessment may differ for different populations. The advance in the current study over that done in PNG was the availability of newer, digital devices and inclusion of age, gender, BMI, and hydration in multivariate regression, which confirmed an independent effect of infection.

The proportion of all infected individuals that will progress to LFRL, while considered to be relatively small, is not well understood. It appears to depend on multiple factors including genetics, geography, exposure to infection, and worm species, and it was not possible in this cross-sectional study to determine which of the positive cases may be at risk of progression to advanced disease, if any. The fact that mean between-infection group differences can be objectively measured suggests that there is an insidious effect of LF antigenemia on skin and subcutaneous tissues in the lower limb, and this is consistent with the current understanding of the pathogenesis of lymphedema [19,20]. Follow-up on this Myanmar cohort may provide some insight into individual variation among antigen-positive persons to define who is most at risk.

The Indurometer gave the clearest indication that tonometry can be used to detect covert lymphatic change in the lower limb. While the Tonometer and SkinFibroMeter may not have detected latent changes in asymptomatic cases in this cohort, their use in assessment of established leg lymphedema from all causes warrants further study. When using these devices to track changes in the same person over time, moderating factors such as age and gender will be immaterial, hydration can be controlled for by administering a drink prior to measurement, and any change in BMI can be considered when interpreting the results, as is already the practice in BCRL. Indurometry and BIS measures may be useful in monitoring clinical progression in people at risk of lower limb lymphedema and may provide an inexpensive means to objectively measure lymphedema in LF populations.

The presence and direction of clinically-relevant changes in the antigen-positive cases in Myanmar support the hypothesis that LF can induce covert changes in the subcutaneous tissues of the lower limbs. This contributes to the case for formal recognition of a Stage 0 in the classification of LF-related lymphedema. The disparity in resources between BCRL and LFRL settings should not be a barrier to transferring reliable and effective protocols for early detection and intervention in lymphedema to LF populations.

Supplementary Materials: The following are available online at www.mdpi.com/2414-6366/2/4/50/s1, Figure S1: Indurometer, SA Biomedical Engineering; Table S1: Between-infection group differences (independent samples *t*-test) for (a) Digital Indurometer, (b) Mechanical Tonometer, (c) SkinFibroMeter and (d) BIS measures, size and direction of variation; Table S2: Stepwise regression for moderating factors associated with variation in (a) Digital Indurometer, (b) Mechanical Tonometer, (c) SkinFibroMeter and (d) BIS measures; Table S3: Mean values and between-leg differences (paired samples *t*-test) for (a) Digital Indurometer, (b) Mechanical Tonometer, (c) SkinFibroMeter and (d) BIS measures.

Acknowledgments: This study formed part of the doctoral research project of Janet Douglass and received no formal institutional or grant funding and no funds were received for the cost of open access publication. All data collection activates were funded by private donors who contributed through crowdfunding. Grateful acknowledgement is given to the following individuals and organizations:

- Louise Kelly-Hope, Centre for Neglected Tropical Diseases, Liverpool School of Tropical Medicine for early advice on the study design and country selection.
- Myanmar Ministry of Health and Sports, for permission to conduct the study, translation of participant information documents and data collection support.
- Vector Borne Disease Control, Mandalay, for access to sentinel site records and providing research assistants.
- Public Health Laboratory and Staff, Mandalay, for blood separation and short-term storage of plasma.
- Department of Medical Research and Staff, Yangon, for long term storage of plasma and processing of Og4C3 ELISAQ assays.
- Impedimed Australia, for loan of an SFB7 back-up unit and donation of electrodes.
- Delfin Finland, for loan of a SkinFibroMeter.
- JCU Physiotherapy, for use of a Tonometer and Indurometer.

- Cellabs Australia, for Og4C3 reagents.
- Pentagon Freight, for provision of international freight services.
- Singapore International Airlines, for discounted airfares.
- Kyaw San Tun, Mandalay, for interpretation and transport services.

Author Contributions: J.D., S.G. and P.G. conceived and designed the experiments; J.D., L.B. and M.R. performed the experiments; N.N.A., S.S.W., Y.Y.W. and T.W. provided in-country advice and data collection; J.D., D.L. and J.M. analyzed the data; J.D. wrote the manuscript with editorial input from all co-authors.

Conflicts of Interest: The authors declare no conflict of interest.

References

1. World Health Organization. Wha50.29 elimination of lymphatic filariasis as a public health problem. In *World Health Assembly Resolutions and Decisions*, 3rd ed.; Ninth Plenary Meeting, 13 May 1997—Committee A, Third Report; Hbk, R., Ed.; World Health Organization: Geneva, Switzerland, 1997; Volume III.

2. Guyton, A.C.; Hall, J.E. *Textbook of Medical Physiology*, 11th ed.; Elselvier Inc.: Philadelphia, PA, USA, 2006.

3. International Society of Lymphology. The diagnosis and treatment of peripheral lymphedema: 2016 consensus document of the international society of lymphology. *Lymphology* **2016**, *49*, 170–184.

4. Stout Gergich, N.L.; Pfalzer, L.A.; McGarvey, C.; Springer, B.; Gerber, L.H.; Soballe, P. Preoperative assessment enables the early diagnosis and successful treatment of lymphedema. *Cancer* **2008**, *112*, 2809–2819. [CrossRef] [PubMed]

5. Dreyer, G.; Addiss, D.; Dreyer, P.; Noroes, J. *Basic Lymphoedema Management, Treatment and Prevention Problems Associated with Lymphatic Filariasis*; Hollis Publishing Company: Hollis, NH, USA, 2002.

6. Shenoy, R.K. Clinical and pathological aspects of filarial lymphedema and its management. *Korean J. Parasitol.* **2008**, *46*, 119–125. [CrossRef] [PubMed]

7. World Health Organization. *Progress Report 2000–2009 and Strategic Plan 2010–2020 of the Global Programme to Eliminate Lymphatic Filariasis: Halfway towards Eliminating Lymphatic Filariasis*; WHO: Geneva, Switzerland, 2010.

8. Addiss, D.G. Mass treatment of filariasis in New Guinea. *N. Engl. J. Med.* **2003**, *348*, 1179–1181. [PubMed]

9. Douglass, J.; Graves, P.; Gordon, S. Self-care for management of secondary lymphedema: A systematic review. *PLoS Negl. Trop. Dis.* **2016**, *10*, e0004740. [CrossRef] [PubMed]

10. Gordon, S.; Melrose, W.; Warner, J.; Buttner, P.; Ward, L. Lymphatic filariasis: A method to identify subclinical lower limb change in PNG adolescents. *PLoS Negl. Trop. Dis.* **2011**, *5*, e1242. [CrossRef] [PubMed]

11. Douglass, J.; Graves, P.; Gordon, S. Intrarater reliability of tonometry and bioimpedance spectroscopy to measure tissue compressibility and extracellular fluid in the legs of healthy young people in Australia and Myanmar. *Lymphat. Res. Biol.* **2017**, *15*, 57–63. [CrossRef] [PubMed]

12. Lawenda, B.D.; Mondry, T.E.; Johnstone, P.A.S. Lymphedema: A primer on the identification and management of a chronic condition in oncologic treatment. *CA Cancer J. Clin.* **2009**, *59*, 8–24. [CrossRef] [PubMed]

13. Douglass, J.; Graves, P.; Gordon, S. Moderating factors in tissue tonometry and bio-impedance spectroscopy measures in the lower extremity of healthy young people in Australia and Myanmar. *Lym. Res. Biol.* **2017**. in submit.

14. Biomath. Available online: http://biomath.info/power/ttestnoninf.htm (accessed on 14 August 2017).

15. Pallotta, O.; McEwen, M.; Tilley, S.; Wonders, T.; Waters, M.; Piller, N. A new way to assess superficial changes to lymphoedema. *J. Lymphoedema* **2011**, *6*, 34–40.

16. Masson, J.; Douglass, J.; Roineau, M.; Aye, K.; Htwe, K.; Warner, J.; Graves, P. Relative performance and predictive values of plasma and dried blood spots with filter paper sampling techniques and dilutions of the lymphatic filariasis Og4c3 antigen ELISA for samples from Myanmar. *Trop. Med. Infect. Dis.* **2017**, *2*, 7. [CrossRef]

17. Onis, M.D.; Onyango, A.W.; Borghi, E.; Siyam, A.; Nishida, C.; Siekmann, J. Development of a WHO growth reference for school-aged children and adolescents. *Bull. World Health Organ.* **2007**, *85*, 660–667. [CrossRef] [PubMed]

18. Hayes, S.C.; Janda, M.; Cornish, B.; Battistutta, D.; Newman, B. Lymphedema after breast cancer: Incidence, risk factors, and effect on upper body function. *J. Clin. Oncol.* **2008**, *26*, 3536–3542. [CrossRef] [PubMed]

19. Nutman, T.B. Insights into the pathogenesis of disease in human lymphatic filariasis. *Lymphat. Res. Biol.* **2013**, *11*, 144–148. [CrossRef] [PubMed]
20. Carlson, J.A. Lymphedema and subclinical lymphostasis (microlymphedema) facilitate cutaneous infection, inflammatory dermatoses, and neoplasia: A locus minoris resistentiae. *Clin. Dermatol.* **2014**, *32*, 599–615. [CrossRef] [PubMed]

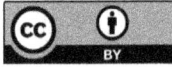

*Tropical Medicine and
Infectious Disease*

MDPI

Review

Soil-Transmitted Helminths in Tropical Australia and Asia

Catherine A. Gordon [1,*], Johanna Kurscheid [2], Malcolm K. Jones [3], Darren J. Gray [2] and
Donald P. McManus [1]

[1]   QIMR Berghofer Medical Research Institute, Molecular Parasitology Laboratory, Queensland 4006, Australia;
      Don.McManus@qimrberghofer.edu.au
[2]   Australian National University, Department of Global Health, Research School of Population Health,
      Australian Capital Territory 2601, Australia; Johanna.Kurscheid@anu.edu.au (J.K.);
      darren.gray@anu.edu.au (D.J.G.)
[3]   School of Veterinary Science, University of Queensland, Brisbane, QLD 4067, Australia; m.jones@uq.edu.au
*   Correspondence: Catherine.Gordon@qimrberghofer.edu.au; Tel.: +61-7-3845-3069

Received: 29 August 2017; Accepted: 17 October 2017; Published: 23 October 2017

Abstract: Soil-transmitted helminths (STH) infect 2 billion people worldwide including significant numbers in South-East Asia (SEA). In Australia, STH are of less concern; however, indigenous communities are endemic for STH, including *Strongyloides stercoralis*, as well as for serious clinical infections due to other helminths such as *Toxocara* spp. The zoonotic hookworm *Ancylostoma ceylanicum* is also present in Australia and SEA, and may contribute to human infections particularly among pet owners. High human immigration rates to Australia from SEA, which is highly endemic for STH *Strongyloides* and *Toxocara*, has resulted in a high prevalence of these helminthic infections in immigrant communities, particularly since such individuals are not screened for worm infections upon entry. In this review, we consider the current state of STH infections in Australia and SEA.

Keywords: soil-transmitted helminths; *Trichuris trichiura*; *Ascaris lumbricoides*; hookworm; *Ancylostoma ceylanicum*; *Strongyloides stercoralis*; South East Asia; Australia

1. Introduction

Soil-transmitted helminths (STH) are estimated to infect 2 billion people worldwide. Many of these infections occur in South-East Asia (SEA) [1,2]. Species included in the term STH are the human hookworm species *Ancylostoma duodenale* and *Necator americanus*, the human roundworm *Ascaris lumbricoides*, and the human whipworm *Trichuris trichiura* [3]. Hookworm and *Trichuris* have zoonotic counterparts (*A. caninum, A. ceylanicum, T. suis,* and *T. vulpis*) [4–14]. *A. lumbricoides* itself is a zoonosis as the previously-identified pig roundworm, *A. suum*, has been found through molecular characterisation to be nearly identical to *A. lumbricoides*, and instead represents a haplotype of *A. lumbricoides* [6,15]. *Toxocara canis* and *Strongyloides stercoralis* are additional important nematode species of dogs that can also infect humans and are included in this review. *Strongyloides* is estimated to infect 30–100 million people [16,17], while the seroprevalence (2–5% in urban areas, 14.2–37% in rural areas) of *Toxocara* in developed countries indicates that the number of people at risk of infection may be in the millions [18]. While *Toxocara* and *Strongyloides* have low prevalences in Australia, our closest neighbours in SEA, as well as many countries from which refugees and immigrants originate, are highly endemic for these parasites. These helminths are also considered neglected tropical diseases (NTD) due to their occurrence in low socio-economic regions and have thus not received as much attention as other diseases occurring in developed countries. Primarily, these helminthic infections are endemic in tropical and subtropical areas due to the requirements for warm moist soil for egg or larval development.

Another potential reason for their status as NTDs is the chronic rather than acute nature of the infections they cause. Symptoms are similar between the causative species and are generally non-specific; namely nausea and/or vomiting, diarrhoea, abdominal pain, and fever. In adults the impact can be seen as lower ability to work. As such, the impact of these parasites should be examined by considering the disability adjusted life years (DALYs) to measure disease burden. According to the WHO definition, one DALY is one year of life quality lost compared to a healthy individual, and the sum of these DALYs across a population is a measurement of the gap between current health status and an ideal health situation [19].

As of 2010 there were an estimated 438.9 million people infected globally with hookworm, 819.0 million with *A. lumbricoides,* and 464.4 million with *T. trichiura* [20]. It was calculated that STH contributed to 4.98 million years lived with disability (YLDs), with 65% attributed to hookworm, 22% to *A. lumbricoides,* and 13% to *T. trichiura* [20]. The DALYs for intestinal helminths (including only *A. lumbricoides, T. trichiura,* and hookworm) have been reduced from 170 per 100,000 (94–290) in 1990 to 75 per 100,000 (43–128) in 2010 and 69.4 per 100,000 (43.3–106.4) in 2013 [21,22]. DALYs are not considered a good measurement of the burden of disease for *S. stercoralis* since the majority of infections cause limited clinical symptoms; the most common complaint and symptom is stomachache. Poor diagnostics for *S. stercoralis* also result in the true prevalence being underestimated [23].

Infection with hookworm or hyper-infection with *S. stercoralis* can result in anaemia, and hookworm can also present with cutaneous rash from larval migration. *Ascaris, Strongyloides* and hookworm larvae migrate to the lungs to be coughed up and swallowed, thus entering the gut where they mature. Lung-stage infection by *Ascaris* can cause pneumonia, called Loeffler's pneumonia, while disseminated *Strongyloides* can also cause pneumonia and pulmonary haemorrhage; hookworm-associated pneumonia, 'eosinophilic pneumonia', is a rare manifestation [24–26]. *Toxocara* infections can result in a range of symptoms depending on where the larvae migrate. The migrating larvae themselves, much like in *Strongyloides* and hookworm infections, can result in a rash, or larval tracks, due to inflammation. In the eye, *Toxocara* can cause partial or total retinal detachment leading to blindness and may result in neurological symptoms if the larvae are present in the brain [18,27].

Strongyloides stercoralis, which is endemic in aboriginal communities of Australia, can be a serious roundworm infection with severe health implications due to autoinfection and dissemination. Infection in immunocompromised individuals is particularly serious, and can be fatal. Autoinfection with *S. stercoralis* occurs when the larvae produced by the adult worms cause reinfection without ever having to leave the body. In such instances there is no immune response against the migrating larvae and this can lead to hyperinfection and dissemination. Continuous reinfection with *S. stercoralis* through autoinfection can also lead to persistent infections lasting many years (Figure 1). Infections in immigrants in Australia have been found more than 20 years after moving away from an endemic area (Table 1). Disseminated strongyloidiasis occurs when the parasite is distributed throughout the body and is more commonly seen in people with impaired immune systems [28]. It can lead to abdominal pain and swelling, pulmonary and neurological complications and meningitis, depending on where the parasite is located, as well as septicaemia, a leading cause of death in *S. stercoralis* infection [28,29]. Septicaemia occurs due to migration of larvae through the gastrointestinal wall. While generally considered as a human parasite, *S. stercoralis* has also been found in non-human primates and dogs [30–32]. There are also haplotypes identified for this species, and grouping of haplotypes from humans with haplotypes from canids and indicates potential zoonotic transmission [33,34]. Sequencing of isolates found in dogs and humans in Cambodia found two haplotypes of *S. stercoralis* in dogs, one of which was indistinguishable from that found in humans, again indicating the potential for zoonotic transmission [30]. Dogs are an important reservoir for zoonotic infections in terms of transmission as they live in close contact with humans, increasing the likelihood of transmission when compared with other potential zoonotic hosts such as non-human primates, which have a far more limited association with humans. Australia has a high pet ownership, particularly dogs and cats, with many also living inside homes, thus providing clear potential for transmission [35].

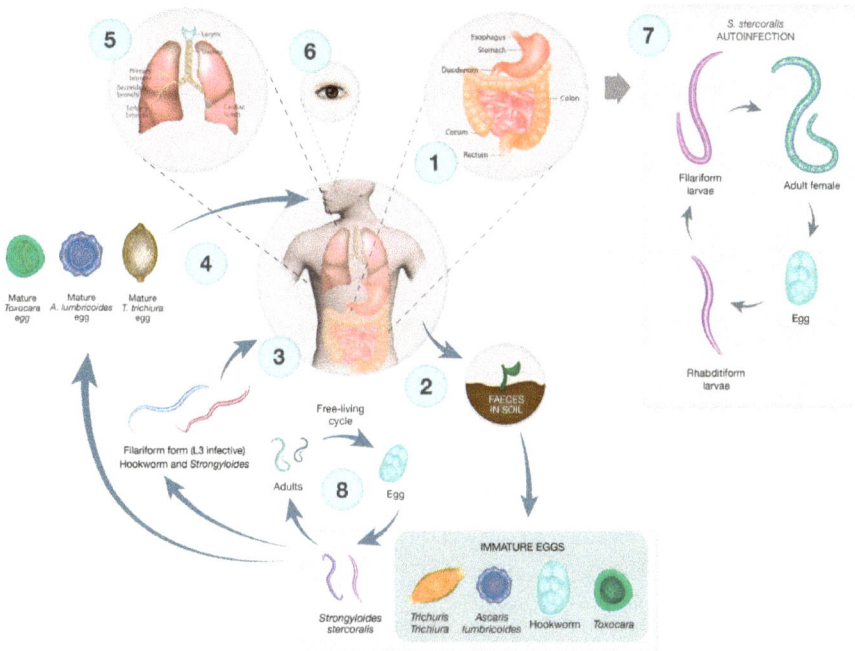

Figure 1. Lifecycles of soil-transmitted helminths (STH), *S. sterocoralis*, and *Toxocara*. **1.** Adult worms reside in the gastrointestinal tract (GIT). Hookworm, *A. lumbricoides*, and *S. stercoralis* adults reside in the small intestine while *T. trichiura* adults reside in the cecum and ascending colon. Female worms produce eggs which are passed in the stool of an infected person. **2.** *T. trichiura*, *Toxocara*, and *A. lumbricoides* eggs mature in soil but do not hatch. Hookworm eggs hatch in soil and mature into L3 hookworm larvae. *S. stercoralis* eggs hatch into rhabditiform larvae in the gut, which are then excreted via the faeces. Rhabditiform larvae then mature into infective filariform larvae or free-living adults. **3.** Infectious L3 filariform larvae of hookworm and *S. stercoralis* penetrate the skin directly, enter the circulation and migrate to the GIT after passing into the lumen of the lungs. **4.** Mature eggs of *Toxocara*, *A. lumbricoides*, and *T. trichiura* are swallowed by the host. The eggs hatch, releasing larvae in the GIT. *T. trichiura* larvae hatch in the small intestine and mature into adults while *Toxocara* and *A. lumbricoides* larvae penetrate the gut. *Toxocara* larvae are carried by the circulation to a variety of tissue types while *A. lumbricoides* larvae are carried to the lungs. **5.** Hookworm and *A. lumbricoides* larvae penetrate the alveolar walls and ascend the bronchial tree to the throat and are swallowed. Once they reach the small intestine the larvae mature into adults. *S. stercoralis* can also follow bronchial migration, or they can penetrate straight to the GIT. **6.** *Toxocara* larvae can be carried to any tissue type. As humans are dead-end hosts the larvae do not undergo further development once they reach these sites, they can cause local reactions, known as the disease toxocariasis. Ocular toxocariasis, where the larvae penetrate the eye, can result in blindness. **7.** *S. stercoralis* can also undergo autoinfection, where the rhabditiform larvae become infective filarial form larvae in the small intestine and penetrate the gut or perianal region. The filariform larvae can then disseminate to throughout the body. **8.** *Strongyloides* rhabditiform larvae develop into free-living adults that produce eggs from which rhabditidorm larvae hatch. Rhabditiform larvae then develop into infectious filariform larvae and penetrate a human host. The free-living cycle exists for one generation cycle only.

Trop. Med. Infect. Dis. **2017**, *2*, 56

Table 1. Prevalence of soil-transmitted helminths diagnosed in immigrants, refugees, ADF[#] personnel, and returned travellers in Australia since 2000.

Years Sampled	Reference	Status	Country of Origin	Parasite Species	Prevalence	Diagnostics
2000, 2002	[36]	Immigrant	East Africa / Cambodia	S. stercoralis / T. trichiura / S. stercoralis / Hookworm spp.	11% (n = 124) / 4% (n = 124) / 42% (n = 230) / 1.96% (n = 230)	Faecal samples (method unclear) / Serology (method unclear)
7–20 years after resettlement	[37]	Immigrant	Laos	S. stercoralis	24.21% (n = 95)	Faecal microscopy / Strongyloides serology
2–52 years after resettlement 1998–2005	[38] *	Immigrant	Fiji (1), SEA (5), China (1), Sri Lanka (1), India (2), Seychelles (2), Ethiopia (2), Russia (1), Italy (1), Greece (1)	S. stercoralis	100% (n = 17) *	Faecal microscopy / Strongyloides serology
1998–2005	[38]*	Returned travellers	Papua New Guinea (1), Vanuatu (1), SEA (7), Africa (2)	S. stercoralis	100% (n = 11) *	Faecal microscopy / Strongyloides serology
2004	[39]	Returned ADF[#] member	Solomon Islands	A. ceylanicum	100% (n = 1)	Harada-Mori culture, direct faecal smear
Served 1962–1975 2010	[40]	ADF veterans	Vietnam	S. stercoralis	11.6% (n = 249)	Faecal microscopy / ELISA
2006–2007	[41]	RAMSI personnel ***	Solomon Islands	S. stercoralis	100% (n = 14) *	Faecal microscopy, Serology (ELISA)

Table 1. *Cont.*

Years Sampled	Reference	Status	Country of Origin	Parasite Species	Prevalence	Diagnostics
2002–2012	[42]	Residents Northern Territory	Australia	*T. trichiura*	0.65% (n = 63,668) **	Wet mount microscopy, Concentration method
2002–2011	[43]	Residents Northern Territory	Australia	Hookworm	0.17% (n = 64,691) **	Wet mount microscopy, Concentration method
2004–2008	[44]	Immigrants	Burma	*S. stercoralis*	26% (n = 156)	Serology
2002	[45]	Immigrants	Cambodia	*S. stercoralis*	36% (n = 234) *	ELISA, faecal microscopy
2010–2011	[46]	Residents Northern Territory	Australia	*S. stercoralis*	16.5% (n = 124) pre-treatment 12% (n = 30) post-treatment	Serology (NIE ELISA, NIE-DBS-ELISA)
2000–2006	[29]	Residents	Australia	*S. stercoralis*	100% (n = 18) *	Faecal microscopy, serology
1994–1996	[47]	Residents	Australia	*T. canis* *S. stercoralis* *S. stercoralis*	21% (n = 29) 28% (n = 29) 19% (n = 314)	Serology Serology Formol-ether
	[48]	Immigrant	Laos	*S. stercoralis*	Single patient	Larvae in sputum
2010–2011	[49]	Immigrants Residents Residents	Australia	*N. americanus* *A. ceylanicum* *A. duodenale*	(n = 5/227) **** (n = 2/227) (n = 4/227)	PCR Sequencing

Australian Defence Force (ADF); * retrospective review of positive cases; ** faecal samples; *** Regional Assistance Mission to Solomon Islands; **** faecal samples from individuals with a documented history of gastrointestinal disorders.

Recent molecular analysis of hookworm species has been important for speciation and shows a different epidemiological pattern than previously thought, including a much higher prevalence of *A. ceylanicum*, which had been considered to be only a rare infection in humans [4,11,50–53]. This is due in part to the morphological similarity of eggs and larval stages between hookworm species leading to misdiagnosis, and partly due to initial erroneous assumptions of their epidemiology [53]. While dogs are thought to be the primary source of zoonotic *A. ceylanicum*, there is evidence that human–human transmission can occur [11]. Two haplotypes have been identified, with the zoonotic haplotype also identified in cats [11,54]. This has public health implications, since dogs and cats will act as reservoir hosts and will thus need to be taken into consideration for control. Dogs are also the main host for *A. caninum*, which can cause gastric enteritis in humans, and *Toxocara canis* which can cause serious eye disease often resulting in blindness, as well as neurological symptoms depending on where the parasite migrates to in the body. *T. cati*, found in cats, can also cause similar pathology.

We review the STH, *Strongyloides* and *Toxocara* in SEA and Australia, considering their lifecycles; prevalence in SE Asia and Australia; diagnosis; and treatment and control. In addition, their zoonotic potential will be further explored.

2. Lifecycles

The lifecycles of the STH are shown in Figure 1, illustrating key differences in infection strategy and migration pathways. Adults of all STH species and *S. stercoralis* live in the gastrointestinal tract (GIT) and produce eggs that are excreted into the environment via the stool. STH and *S. stercoralis* require moist, warm soil to develop, largely restricting these parasites to tropical areas. Hookworm eggs hatch in the faecal mass and moult from L1 to infective L3 larvae. The L3 larvae then migrate onto vegetation, penetrate the skin, are carried via the blood to the lungs where they undergo tracheal migration, pass through to the small intestine, mature into adults and attach to the gut wall [55]. For both *T. trichiura* and *A. lumbricoides*, eggs are passed unembryonated and mature to an infectious stage after 15 days. The now infectious eggs are ingested, often due to poor hygiene and contaminated food, and hatch in the small intestine. Larvae of *T. trichiura* then mature in the small intestine into adults [56]. *A. lumbricoides* larvae penetrate the gut and undergo tracheal migration similar to hookworm larvae, and develop into mature adults once in the small intestine (Figure 1) [57].

The lifecycle of *S. stercoralis* is more complicated than other STH since it has a free-living stage in addition to the parasitic lifecycle [58]. Adults in the gut produce eggs that hatch into first-stage larvae, which have a distinctive oesophageal appearance that gives rise to the descriptive term 'rhabditiform larva'. This first stage larva will moult to become either free-living, a dioecious adult or an infectious larva, the filariform larva. Free-living adults produce eggs that hatch as rhabditiform larvae that moult twice to become 3rd stage filariform larvae. Filariform larvae then penetrate the skin, much like hookworm L3 larvae, and migrate to the gut – this can be via the lungs and they are coughed up as occurs in the hookworm lifecycle, or direct travel to the gut. Autoinfection occurs when eggs from adult parasites hatch into rhabditiform larvae that become filariform larvae while still in the gut. The filariform larvae can complete the lifecycle in the gut, or disseminate, migrating to other organs and tissues (Figure 1). The free-living cycle for *S. stercoralis* only persists for one generation, not indefinitely as in *Parastrongyloides sp.* [59,60].

Humans are accidental hosts of *Toxocara* spp. and become infected by ingesting eggs in contaminated soil [61]. The eggs hatch in the gut and the larvae penetrate the gut and are carried by the blood to different organs where they can promote a local reaction, which is the cause of toxocariasis. Visceral and ocular migrans are the most common presentations. There is also a suggested link between seropositivity for toxocariasis and epilepsy [62].

3. STH and *Strongyloides* in SEA

STH infections are common in SEA, where approximately one-third of global STH cases occur, with active, stable transmission occurring in all countries of the region [63–65] (Figure 2). Risk factors for infection include poverty, lack of access to clean water and toilets, as well as unhygienic practices such as not washing hands [64].

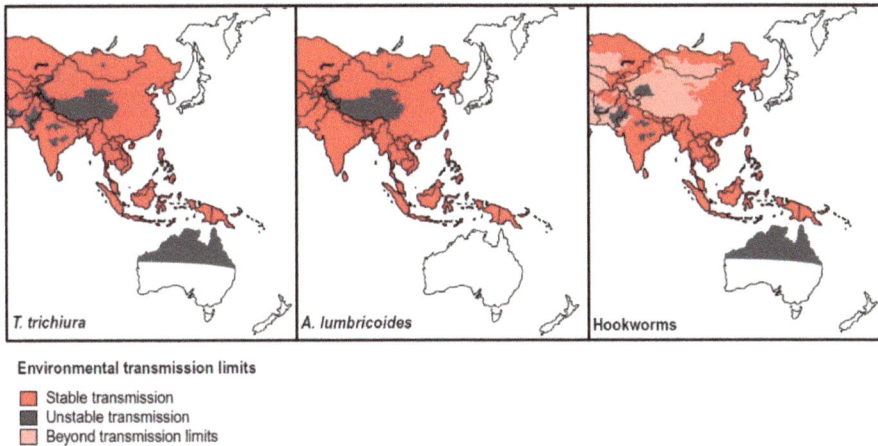

Figure 2. Distribution of STH in South-East Asia and Australia, modified from Brooker et al., [64].

T. trichiura, A. lumbricoides and hookworm are the most prevalent STH and infected individuals are often found with co-infections. Polyparasitism with STH is very common in SEA, mainly due to the shared geographical locations in tropical areas, where these worms are endemic. Additionally, the infection pathways of the STH are similar (Figure 1). Polyparasitism with STH is more likely than mono-infection in endemic areas, where co-infection with other helminths and protozoan parasites is also very high [66–71]. Because STH endemicity is quite low in Australia, data for polyparasitism is limited, although it may occur in remote Aboriginal communities [42].

Co-infections with parasites have been identified with increased disease status, and synergism between parasite infections. Infection intensity of helminths in co-infections also seems to differ, with hookworm infection intensity significantly increased with multiple infections [72]. Maternal infection with STH may also increase susceptibility of the unborn child to infection with STH, but it is unclear if this is due to shared environmental factors [73,74]. Co-infections may necessitate combination chemotherapy depending on drug efficacy for the infecting species.

The precise global prevalence of *Strongyloides* is unknown although it is estimated to infect 30–100 million people worldwide [75]. There are also issues with diagnosis because serology can return negative results, particularly in early infections, and may not pick up disseminated cases [16]. Eggs are rarely seen in the stool; rather the rhabditiform larvae are present instead, although often in low numbers. Both copro-culture, which can be laborious, and direct smears, can be used to identify larvae [76]. Other methods include the formalin ethyl acetate sedimentation method, which has low sensitivity, immunodiagnostics, and molecular methods [77]. Molecular methods, specifically PCR, have been used to sensitively diagnose *Strongyloides* [78,79]. *Strongyloides* is endemic in SEA and there are a number of reports from countries in the region using an array of different diagnostic techniques [80–83]. A comprehensive review is available of its global distribution based on community, hospital, and refugee and immigrant surveys [84] (Figure 3). Depending on the diagnostic method used, the prevalence of *S. stercoralis* given in Figure 3 may be an underestimate due to the low sensitivity of many of the procedures used, and the low number of larvae that are excreted, even in heavy infections [77,79,84].

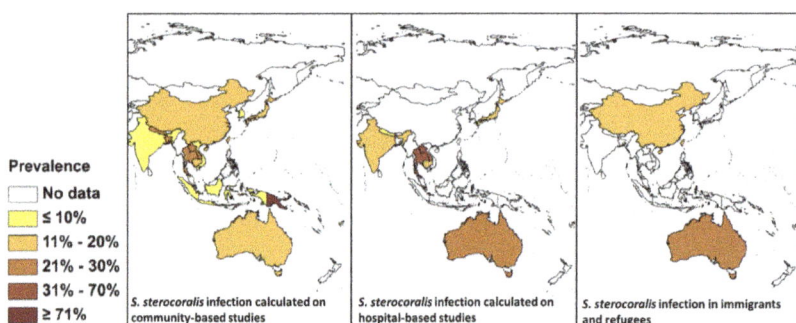

Figure 3. Prevalence of *S. stercoralis* in Asia and Australia based on community-based studies, hospital-based studies, and prevalence in immigrants and refugees. Modified from Schäret al., [84].

4. STH and *Strongyloides* in Australia

Australia has a low number of STH cases, largely because these worm infections can be readily controlled by good hygiene, access to safe, clean water, and the use of toilets. The overall prevalence of hookworm and *T. trichiura* in the Australian Northern Territory is quite low at 0.17% and 0.65%, respectively (Table 1), based on hospital data collected between 2002 and 2012 [42,43]. These cases were primarily detected in people admitted to hospital for reasons other than hookworm or *Trichuris* infection; thus the true prevalence may be much higher, and may follow a more focal intensity that would not be accounted for by recording state-wide or country-wide prevalence. For both species the prevalence has been reduced; with *T. trichiura*, there was a drop from 123.1 cases per 100,000 in 2002 to 35.8 cases per 100,000 in 2012 [42]. The zoonotic STHs, particularly *A. caninum* and *A. ceylanicum*, are of importance in Australia since they are found in domestic and wild canids (Table 2) [85,86]. Intestinal parasites of pigs in Australia also include *T. suis* and *A. suum*, which can infect humans, although the extent of human disease is unclear [4,87].

In 1918, hookworm was considered such a serious problem in North Queensland that a five-year campaign to eradicate the disease was instigated and although considered successful, hookworm infection continued to be a problem in Aboriginal communities [53,88]. The majority of published papers on STH in Australia are relatively old, with very few published in the last 10 years. Prociv and Luke [88] provide a solid review of the early history of hookworm infections in Australia. *Ascaris* spp. infection has never been very prevalent despite the requisite tropical climate and moist soil existing in Australia [89].

S. stercoralis appears to be more prevalent in Australia than the other STH, or at least, there are more published data available (Table 1) (Figure 2). The parasite is endemic in tropical regions of Australia including Queensland, the Northern Territory, Western Australia, as well as Northern NSW. It is primarily found among Aboriginal people living in remote communities, with a prevalence of >60% recorded (Table 1) [90–94]. This worm has persisted due to lack of attention to the disease it causes, despite the potential for high morbidity and mortality in immunosuppressed individuals [94]. Its true prevalence is unknown in Australia, and probably globally. As reported by Speare *et al* – "if you don't look, you won't find" [94]. As a human-only parasite, it can be readily treated with ivermectin and eliminated from the community. A retrospective study examined indigenous Australians in Central Australia who were positive for *S. stercoralis* infection and who may also have been positive for human T cell lymphotropic virus type I (HTLV-I). This virus invades adult T cells, thereby reducing the effectiveness of the immune system [29]. Of these subjects, eleven (n = 18) were tested for HTLV-I, of which seven were positive. Of those who tested positive for HTLV-I, four were never treated for *Strongyloides*, and of those who were treated, many were not treated at initial diagnosis and infection status was not checked on subsequent visits [29]. Of these eighteen patients, fifteen died from sepsis.

Table 2. Reported prevalences of *A. ceylanicum* human and animal infections in studies conducted in Australia and Asia since 2000.

Ref	Year	Country *	Human/Animal	Prevalence % (Total no.)	Species	Diagnostic
[95]	-	Taiwan	Human	Single patient	*A. ceylanicum*	Morphology
[69]	2009	Laos	Human	17.6% (n = 17) 82.4% (n = 17)	*A. ceylanicum* *N. americanus*	Nested PCR
[96]	2012	Cambodia	Human	51.6% (n = 124) 51.6% (n = 124) 3.2% (n = 124)	*A. ceylanicum* *N. americanus* *A. duodenale*	Microscopy, PCR
			Dog	94.4% (n = 90) 8.9% (n = 90) 1.1% (n = 90)	*A. ceylanicum* *A. caninum* *N. americanus*	Microscopy, PCR
[49] #	2010–2011	Australia	Human	0.88% (n = 227) 1.76% (n = 227) 1.76% (n = 227)	*A. ceylanicum* *A. duodenale* *N. americanus* [a]	PCR
[97]	-	China	Dog Cat Human	3 (n = 254) 5 (n = 102) 14 (n = 14)	*A. ceylanicum*	PCR sequencing
[98]	-	Malaysia	Dog	52% (n = 224) 48% (n = 224)	*A. ceylanicum* *A. caninum*	FECT, PCR
[99]	2007–2010	Malaysia	Cat	29.5% (n = 543)	*A. ceylanicum*	Microscopy
[100]	2009–2011	Malaysia	Human	87.2 (n = 47) 23.4 (n = 47)	*N. americanus* *A. ceylanicum*	Microscopy, PCR
[101]	2013	Malaysia (Chinese)	Human	Single patient	*A. ceylanicum*	Microscopy
[11]	2009–2011	Malaysia	Human	12.8% (n = 634) 76.6% (n = 634) 10.6% (n = 634)	*A. ceylanicum* *N. americanus* Both species	Microscopy, PCR
			Cats and dogs	52% (n = 105) 46% (n = 105)	*A. caninum* *A. ceylanicum*	Microscopy, PCR
[102]	-	Myanmar	Human	72.72% (n = 11) 27.27% (n = 11)	*N. americanus* *A. ceylanicum*	PCR sequencing
[103]	2004–2005	Australia	Dog	6.5% (n = 92) 70.7% (n = 92) 4.3% (n = 92) 2.2% (n = 92)	*A. ceylanicum* *A. caninum* *A. caninum + A. ceylanicum* *A. caninum + U. stenocephala*	Microscopy, PCR-RFLP
			Cat	30% (n = 10)	*A. caninum*	

Table 2. *Cont.*

Ref	Year	Country *	Human/Animal	Prevalence % (Total no.)	Species	Diagnostic
[12]	2011–2013	Thailand	Human	60% (n = 10) 30% (n = 10) 10% (n = 10)	*N. americanus* *A. ceylanicum* *A. duodenale*	PCR sequencing
[86]	>2007	Australia	Wild dog	100% (n = 26) 11.5% (n = 26)	*A. caninum* *A. ceylanicum + A. caninum*	Microscopy, PCR
			Dog scat	65.31% (n = 89) 71.43% (n = 89) 38.78% (n = 89)	*A. ceylanicum* *A. caninum* *A. caninum + A. ceylanicum*	
[39]	2004	Australia (Solomon Islands)	Human	Single patient	*A. ceylanicum*	Microscopy
[51]	2004–2005	Thailand	Dog	77% (n = 229) 9% (n = 229) 14% (n = 229)	*A. ceylanicum* *A. caninum* Both species	PCR
			Human	71.43% (n = 204) 28.57% (n = 204)	*N. americanus* *A. ceylanicum*	
[104]	2008	India	Dog	50.46% (n = 325) 51.92% (n = 104) 33.65% (n = 104) 15.38% (n = 104)	Hookworm spp. *A. caninum* *A. ceylanicum* *A. caninum + A. ceylanicum*	Microscopy, PCR-RFLP
[105]	2000	India	Dog	36% (n = 101) 38% (n = 101)	*A. caninum* *A. caninum + A. braziliense*	Microscopy, PCR-RFLP + sequencing
[85]	2011	Australia	Dog	96.4% (n = 84) 16.67% (n = 84) 14.0% (n = 84)	*A. caninum* *A. ceylanicum* *A. caninum + A. ceylanicum*	Microscopy, PCR
[106]	2013–2014	Malaysia	Dog Soil samples Cat	29.6% (n = 227) 6.6% (n = 227) 14.3% (n = 126) 2.4% (n = 126) 29.6% (n = 152) 6.6% (n = 152)	*A. ceylanicum* *A. caninum* *A. ceylanicum* *A. caninum* *A. ceylanicum* *A. caninum*	FECT, PCR
[107]	2015	Japan (Lao)	Human	Single patient	*A. ceylanicum*	Microscopy, PCR

Table 2. *Cont.*

Ref	Year	Country *	Human/Animal	Prevalence % (Total no.)	Species	Diagnostic
[108]	2013–2015	India	Human	100% (n = 143) 16.8% (n = 143) 8.4% (n = 143)	N. americanus A. caninum A. duodenale	PCR-RFLP
			Dog	27.9% 76.4%	A. ceylanicum A. caninum	
			Soil samples	60.2% (n = 78) 29.4% (n = 78) 16.6% (n = 78) 1.4% (n = 78)	A. ceylanicum A. caninum A. duodenale N. americanus	
[109]	2014	Thailand	Dog Cat	33.0% (n = 197) 58.46% (n = 180)	A. ceylanicum	Microscopy, PCR
[110]	2014	France (Myanmar)	Human	Single patient	A. ceylanicum	Microscopy, PCR
[111]	2014	Vietnam	Dog	54.3% (n = 94) 33% (n = 94) 12.7% (n = 94)	A. ceylanicum A. caninum Both species	PCR-RFLP, PCR (cox1)
[112]	2014	China	Cat	40.8% (n = 112) 59.2% (n = 112) 20.4% (n = 112)	A. ceylanicum A. caninum Both species	Microscopy, PCR
[113]	-	India	Human	95% 15% 5%	N. americanus A. duodenale A. ceylanicum	PCR-RFLP
[114]	2005	Thailand	Human	92% 4% 2% 2%	N. americanus A. ceylanicum A. duodenale N. americanus + A. ceylanicum	KK, PCR
[115]	2008	Lao	Human	5.91% 2.46% 1.48% 0.49%	N. americanus A. duodenale A. caninum A. ceylanicum	KK, PCR
[99]	2007–2010	Malaysia	Feral cats	29.5% (n = 251)	A. ceylanicum	Microscopy of adults (staining paracarmine)
[116]	-	Lao	Feral cats	69% (n = 55)	A. ceylanicum	Microscopy of adults (staining Mayers carmine)
[117]	-	Taiwan	Human	Single patient	A. ceylanicum	Method unclear. Adult identification.

* Origin of infection in brackets if not the same as the country of detection; # faecal samples from individuals with a documented history of gastrointestinal disorders; a individuals infected with N. americanus were refugees from Sierra Leone and Sudan, likely to be acquired in those countries.

A complication of disseminated strongyloidiasis is secondary bacterial infection that can become systemic, and has likely contributed to mortality in at least four cases. Further studies have found high prevalence of HTLV-I in Aboriginal communities (33.6% n = 889), which may lead to more cases of hyperinfection with *S. stercoralis* in the future [118,119]. Along with immune suppression due to infection with HIV or HTLV-I, and immunosuppression due to organ transplantation, treatment with steroid drugs suppresses the inflammatory response and can also result in hyperinfection [29,119–124]. There is a clear need to increase knowledge of physicians in endemic areas, perhaps as part of a database for NTDs. Speare et al [93] advocated that *S. stercoralis* be added to the national notifiable diseases surveillance system in Australia to help combat this sadly neglected disease. Notification would bring with it greater oversight and available information to physicians, which would help lead to better management of cases, including the provision of effective treatment. To date this has not occurred and, indeed, there are no helminth diseases on the list; malaria is the sole parasite infection listed.

5. Immigration Screening in Australia

Outside remote communities, it is primarily in immigrants from developing nations and returning travellers that STH cases occur in Australia (Table 1) (Figure 2). Current health screening for immigrants does not include testing for parasites and focuses on notifiable diseases such as tuberculosis and HIV/AIDS. Since STH infections are not notifiable, it is possible that there are autochthonous and returned traveller cases occurring in Australia that are not identified or reported.

Cross-sectional surveys have been performed on recent (1997–2000) and long-term immigrants to Australia in the East African and Cambodian communities in 2000 and 2002, and long-term immigrants from Cambodia [36] (Table 1). *S. stercoralis* and *T. trichiura* were identified in the East African cohort, with only *S. stercoralis* present in the Cambodian cohort. Despite having been in Australia for some years and subject to immigration screening, the high prevalence recorded, particularly in the Cambodian cohort (42%, Table 1), indicates a need to include NTDs such as STH in pre-immigration screening. *Entamoeba histolytica, Hymenolepis nana, Schistosoma* spp. (East African cohort), and *Dientamoeba fragilis* were also identified [36]. Far from being an isolated occurrence, there is a history of STH found in resettled immigrants (Table 1). An earlier study on immigrants from Laos, who had been resettled in Australia for at least 12 years prior to the survey, found *S. stercoralis* in 24% of participants (23/95) [37]. *Strongyloides* is the most commonly reported helminth infection in immigrants (Table 1). Generally *S. stercoralis* infections are asymptomatic. More severe complications from infection include eosinophilic pneumonia, malnutrition, and disseminated strongyloidiasis.

While screening for helminth and protozoan parasites does not occur upon entry to Australia, the government does provide reimbursement for GPs who perform heath assessments within 12 months of arrival [125]. There are also state-funded refugee services in most states and territories [126–130]. In theory, these services could include parasitological identification. As of June 2016, 28.5% of Australians were born overseas, with five of the top 10 countries of birth in SEA (China, India, the Philippines, Vietnam, Malaysia) [131], countries with high STH endemicity. A global distribution map for STH [64] shows stable transmission occurring in SEA and Africa, origins of many immigrants coming to Australia (Figures 2 and 3).

6. Returned Service Personnel

Another cohort for Australian STH infections are Australian army veterans, including older veterans who served in STH-endemic areas from World War II onwards (Table 2) [39–41,132]. *Strongyloides* is the most commonly identified helminth infection in this cohort, possibly the only STH actually considered. In Vietnam veterans, 11.6% had positive serology in 2013 for *Strongyloides*, despite serving between 1962 and 1975 [40]. This shows that the adult worms can persist for many years, as highlighted earlier for immigrants who had been long-term residents in Australia still testing positive for this disease.

7. Diagnostics

Microscopy

Stool-based microscopy remains the most common diagnostic method for STH, including in Australia, with the formol ethyl acetate sedimentation technique most commonly employed [133,134]. For *S. stercoralis*, serology is recommended, due to low and irregular numbers of larvae excreted in the stool even in heavy infections, with stool microscopy used to rule out other infections [133,135]. Diagnosis of STH in Australia is largely done on a case-by-case basis rather than by case detection. Case detection, involving diagnostic sweeps of a community, is more likely to occur as part of a research program in endemic countries. The diagnostic method used will vary. Case-by-case studies are likely to use more sensitive, albeit more laborious, diagnostics than prevalence surveys, which examine a large number or individuals and usually necessitating faster, cheaper diagnostics such as the Kato-Katz (KK) method.

In Asia, a number of different diagnostics have been employed, often as part of specific research projects or for assessing government control programs. The main diagnostic employed is the KK method, a tool also used for diagnosis of schistosomiasis and STH in the Philippines and China. The KK procedure is cheap and easy to perform, particularly under field conditions, which are the reasons it is generally used in large-scale studies. However, the KK is known to lack sensitivity, particularly in low prevalence/intensity infections, and particularly for *Strongyloides* [136–138]. Additionally, hookworm eggs hatch rapidly after stool deposition, with the result that KK slides need to be prepared and examined quickly before eggs lyse [139,140]. FLOTAC is another microscopic, albeit more recent, technique that has been used in STH diagnostics, and has a higher sensitivity than the KK procedure [136,137,141–144]. The main disadvantage of FLOTAC is the length of time it takes to implement, with a single FLOTAC taking around 30 minutes to produce a result [145]. Other methods include the Baermann technique, which is based on the movement of larvae out of stool, the formalin-ether concentration technique (FECT), and coproculture [136]. *Strongyloides* has low sensitivity on stool examination so either multiple stool samples need to be examined or serology undertaken, which is the recommended diagnostic approach [77]. Other methods such as PCR, agar plate culture, and Baermann sedimentation can also be performed on stool samples, and have a higher sensitivity than microscopy [77]. Both agar plate and the Baermann technique can be time consuming. While PCR is more expensive than microscopy, agar plate, or Baermann, it achieves higher sensitivity than all of these techniques [78].

8. Immunodiagnostics

As indicated, serology is often used in Australia for diagnosis of *S. stercoralis* [133], with microscopy employed for the other STH. In general, this holds true for Asia as well. For hookworms, which as discussed earlier, have fragile eggs, immunodiagnostics can be a more sensitive detection method than faecal microscopy. However, lack of specificity, cross-reactivity, and the inability to distinguish between past and current infections are limitations of many immunodiagnostic tests. The most common immunodiagnostic methods used for STH detection are enzyme-linked immunosorbent assays (ELISAs), western blots, and ELISPOT [14,146,147]. Dipstick assays are rapid diagnostics that usually detect antibodies in blood to a target parasite. A dipstick developed for *S. stercoralis*, which is no longer available, had a similar sensitivity (91%) to the ELISA assays it was compared to and a specificity of 97.7% [148]. While serology is recommended for strongyloidiasis due to the poor sensitivity of stool examination, serology can also miss heavy infections as demonstrated by a recent fatal case from Israel of hyperinfection with *S. stercoralis* that was ELISA-negative [23]. An assortment of immunodiagnostics are available for *Strongyloides*, which have a range of sensitivities and specificities [149].

Dried blood spot (DBS) testing occurs by blotting blood samples onto filter paper. Samples can be collected and stored for later analysis, allowing for large numbers of samples to be collected but without requiring large amounts of storage space, and allows relative ease of collection because only a drop from a fingerprick is required. Dried blood spots have been used for molecular diagnostic tests, but can also be used for immunodiagnostics [46]. Most recently, the application of DBS was utilised in serology to diagnose *S. stercoralis* in a remote community in Northern Australia [46].

9. Molecular Diagnostics

There is a range of molecular diagnostic tests available that offer higher sensitivity than microscopy-based diagnostics, albeit with a higher price tag, and these have been reviewed elsewhere [150]. The main benefit of molecular methods is the ability to multiplex assays, that is, identify multiple species using a single assay. However, as well as being more costly than microscopy techniques, they also require specialised equipment. An exception is loop-mediated isothermal amplification (LAMP), which can be performed in the field due to much reduced equipment requirements [151,152]. However LAMP does not allow for multiplexing and to date, of the STH, has only been used to detect hookworm infections [152].

Molecular methods with multiplexing capabilities include conventional polymerase chain reaction (cPCR), real-time PCR (qPCR), multiparallel and tandem qPCR, and digital droplet PCR (ddPCR). Both cPCR and ddPCR are endpoint PCRs, which rely on designing primers that produce amplicons of different lengths to distinguish individual parasite species. ddPCR also uses fluorescent dyes, while real-time PCR reactions utilise fluorescent probes to distinguish between amplicons; the use of taqman probes can increase the sensitivity and specificity of an assay. Of these methods only ddPCR has yet to be used to diagnose STH infections, although it has been utilised for other parasites such as *Schistosoma* spp., detecting cell-free DNA (cfDNA) in a range of body fluids (stool, serum, urine, saliva) [153,154]. The assay provides absolute quantification and can detect very low levels of target DNA; it is also more sensitive than qPCR. While currently only providing for two channels, it is possible to multiplex the reactions for four targets by utilising different size amplicons, much as for a conventional PCR multiplex, because targets can be separated based on size. While schistosomes are blood parasites, and are thus in contact with host blood and tissues, the STH live in the gut and the potential for detection of parasite cfDNA in body fluids such as blood, urine, and saliva would likely be reduced. However, since hookworm is a blood feeder it does gain access to the host blood stream and it is possible that hookworm cfDNA would be detectable in sera. Likewise, the larvae of hookworm and *Ascaris* penetrate the alveolae of the lungs to be coughed up and swallowed, thereby reaching the gut. It is therefore possible that a saliva or sputum sample would yield cfDNA or the larvae themselves. Regardless, the use of ddPCR on stool samples will readily amplify target parasite genes with very high sensitivity. Because it confers absolute quantification and by partitioning the PCR mix (containing master mix, primers, and DNA) into ~20,000 droplets pre-amplification, it effectively means that each sample has ~20,000 technical replicates. Therefore there is no need to run samples in duplicate or triplicate for ddPCR as there is for qPCR. This can save on costs, although in practice the cost of ddPCR and qPCR is similar.

10. Costs of Diagnostics

The cost of a single KK slide, excluding personnel costs and stool collection costs, is US$0.30 [155]. The total cost for single and duplicate KK slides have been estimated to be $US1.73 and US$2.06, respectively, while the FLOTAC costs $2.35 [145]. In comparison, a multiplex qPCR costs $7.68. For qPCR the major costs result from DNA extraction as the qPCR assay itself costs $1.68 per sample in triplicate. A multiparallel qPCR has been costed at $1 per sample, excluding DNA extraction costs [156].

11. Treatment and Mass Drug Administration (MDA) of STH Infections

Mass drug administration (MDA) is a hallmark of many control programs aimed at controlling STH infections. The benzimidazoles (albendazole and mebendazole) are the most commonly used drugs for STH infection in humans, and are recommended for MDA. In the Philippines there is an annual deworming program among school-aged children. In 2003 the prevalence of STH in pre-school children was 66%, after which the Philippines Department of Health introduced the national school deworming program, The Integrated Helminth Control Program (IHCP) [157], with albendazole or mebendazole being recommended for use. The program has been successful in reducing overall prevalence at least in some areas, although MDA coverage can vary. Chemotherapy does not prevent re-infection, and once out of the school program there is no mandated MDA for STH treatment in adults. Fear of birth defects has also been recorded as a reason for refusing STH treatment by pregnant women in the Philippines [158]. School-based MDA has a compliance of >75% while community wide MDAs tend toward low compliance (25–65%) [158,159]. In some cases this is due to poor community involvement, but also because of concerns with possible side effects of the drugs. In the IHCP school deworming program, there was an increase in STH in at least one city (46.05% in 2007 to 56.60% in 2011), and the overall prevalence remained high at 45% as of 2011 [160]. Assuming 100% coverage, the problem of STH will still exist, since re-infection can occur very quickly after treatment, and STH eggs/larvae can live in the environment for several weeks to months, remaining viable for infection. Another issue is drug efficacy. While most available drugs for STH are highly efficacious for *A. lumbricoides*, there are varying efficacies for hookworm, *Strongyloides* spp. and *Trichuris* spp. Efficacy varies depending on the drug given, whether the drug is given as a single or multiple dose, and the amount given. Most programs of MDA rely on a single dose, being easier and not relying on individuals returning for treatment on multiple days. Drug efficacy for hookworm species can be difficult to untangle, as many studies do not speciate the infecting worms. There are documented differences in drug efficacy between *A. duodenale* and *N. americanus,* with mebendazole less effective against *N. americanus*, and pyrantel pamoate less effective against *A. duodenale* [161]. For all STH, drug efficacy likely varies on a regional level depending on parasite populations and treatment programs, particularly those involving MDA.

A World Health Organization (WHO) report [162] showed a range of efficacies against STH for mebendazole, albendazole, pyrantel, levamisole, and ivermectin. For *A. lumbricoides*, efficacy was up to 100% for all drugs except ivermectin. For hookworm the highest efficacy, in terms of cure rate (CR), was achieved with levamisole (66%–100%), and for *T. trichiura* with mebendazole (45%–100%). In the same report comparing differing single doses of albendazole and mebendazole (recommended by the WHO for STH control and treatment) with multiple doses of mebendazole, multiple doses resulted in a higher CR for both hookworm and *Trichuris* spp., albeit the median CR was still around 80% [162]. However, the WHO also recommends periodic worming with albendazole or mebendazole where prevalence is >20% [163]. The aim of the WHO with regards to STH control is to carry out preventative worming in endemic countries with a prevalence of >20%. However if drug efficacy is low, particularly for hookworm and *Trichuris* spp., this approach is unlikely to decrease prevalence in the long term.

Of relevance to treatment of STH cases in Australia and SEA, a study on immigrant populations (in Canada) found an overall reduction in intestinal parasites (STH and *Giardia*) 6 years after resettlement and treatment with thiabendazole, from 63.7% down to 21.9%; however the prevalence of *S. stercoralis* remained relatively high with a reduction from 15% to 11% [37,164]. However, since that report, ivermectin has been designated the drug of choice for *Strongyloides* spp. infection because this has a high efficacy given singly as a 200 mcg/kg dose (96% CR) or as a split 400 mcg/kg dose (98% CR) [165]. This highlights the need for combined chemotherapy when treating individuals infected with more than one species of STH.

Cure rates may be lower than reported due to insensitive diagnostics used in many drug efficacy trials, primarily stool microscopy, and variation in CR given by the same drug regimens in different trials may be due to the methods used to assess treatment success or failure. The sensitivity of diagnosis varies considerably with the more traditional microscopic diagnostics, such as the Kato-Katz procedure, lacking the sensitivity of more recently developed techniques such as real-time PCR-based diagnostics. Serological diagnosis measuring antibodies should not be used to assess CR since they will detect antibodies from previous infections for several months post-treatment, assuming 100% efficacy. Antigen-based tests are more specific but many detected antigens tend to break down quickly in the body.

In an interesting development, the bacterium *Bacillus subtilis* has been engineered to express the anthelmintic protein Cry5B, which proved lethal to *Caenorhabditis elegans* and experimental *A. ceylanicum* hookworm infections in hamsters [166]. This approach could be used by modifying 'good' bacteria that are safe for human ingestion. There are numerous probiotics on the market, of which the most common bacterial species are *Lactobacillus acidophilus*, *L. casei*, *Bifidobacterium lactis*, *B. bifidum*, and *Bacillus subtilis*.

Resistance to anthelmintics continues to be a concern. Currently, resistance has been reported for the human helminth, *Onchocerca volvulus* against ivermectin [167]. *N. americanus* eggs heterozygous for a β-tubulin mutation associated with resistance to benzimidazoles (albendazole, mebendazole) in *A. caninum* were recovered from a small number of individuals (n = 28) in Haiti [168]; homozygous eggs were not identified, but may be present. This raises the possibility of emerging benzimidazole resistance in human hookworm infections, as it has in veterinary hookworm. Drug resistance is common in helminths of veterinary importance where resistance has been reported against not only benzimidazoles but also levamisole, avermectins, and milbemycins (which include ivermectin) [169,170]. Resistance has not been reported for any of the zoonotic helminths. With the increase of MDA programs in STH-endemic areas, there is increasing evolutionary pressure on parasite populations, which may lead to resistance. To rigorously assess resistance, however, sensitive diagnostics will be required, and research needs to be undertaken in the search for alleles conferring resistance. Wolstenholme *et al* [170] have provided an excellent overview of drug resistance in veterinary helminths, while Vercruysse *et al* [171] consider the potential of resistance to currently-available drugs developing in human helminths.

12. Control Programs

STH reinfections can largely be controlled with appropriate hygiene, including washing hands after defecation, and using a toilet, as augmentation to treatment. There are several programs operating in Asia that seek to combat STH infection by using educational interventions. These include the 'Magic Glasses' program in China [172,173], which has now been extended to the Philippines, and the WASH (water, sanitation, and hygiene) program, which aims to provide clean water, toilets, and promoting good hygiene practices, implemented, for example, in Timor-Leste [174,175]. Helminth infection is of lesser concern in developed countries, where toilets and clean running water are available. While STH chemotherapy is effective, it does not prevent re-infections that can happen very quickly after treatment [176]. The aim of currently applied interventions is to prevent re-infection, and thus reduce the overall prevalence and eventually eliminate STH from a community.

The Magic Glasses program targets school aged children in China to reduce prevalence of STH and to increase knowledge of STH parasites to reduce re-infections occurring [172]. The focal point of the intervention is a cartoon, produced along with other teaching aids, to teach children about STH and what they can do personally and in their homes to prevent infection, including washing hands after defecation, only using a toilet, covering food, and wearing shoes. In some schools, water tanks were provided outside toilets to facilitate handwashing. Parasite prevalence and intensity levels were assessed pre-intervention and a year later post-intervention; knowledge was also tested at these times using a questionnaire and quiz. The project was highly successful in reducing re-infection and increasing knowledge in Hunan province [172], and has been further trialled in Yunnan province. It is ongoing in the Philippines, where a new video was created to match local popular cartoons, culture and language. The program has the potential to be modified for many different cultures and areas, including Australia.

WASH for WORMS has been implemented in Timor-Leste as part of a trial where intervention villages had WASH implemented alongside mass drug administration (MDA) using albendazole, while control villages only received MDA [174,175]. Intervention villages were provided with access to clean water, the building of latrines and improving hygiene, particularly handwashing. Results of this intervention and the Magic Glasses trial in Yunnan and the Philippines are currently being formulated.

In both these types of interventions community involvement was crucial. With the Magic Glasses, one of the key components was to increase STH knowledge, focusing on school children whereas the WASH program was community-wide. Targeting only children, or any one group, may not significantly impact transmission in a community, but educational interventions in schools can be delivered by teachers, with the children and teachers taking the lessons learnt back to their families, thereby increasing community knowledge and practice [177]. Paradoxically, children often have the highest helminth infection prevalence in a community [178].

13. Zoonotic Roundworms

Zoonotic Hookworms

Ancylostoma duodenale and *N. americanus* are responsible for the majority of human hookworm infections. However, there are two prominent zoonotic hookworm species, *A. ceylanicum* and *A. caninum,* which can also infect humans. *A. ceylanicum,* particularly, is gaining prominence since many cases originally identified as *A. duodenale* may actually be due to *A. ceylanicum* [51]. Both *A. caninum* and *A. ceylanicum* are found in dogs, and *A. ceylanicum* infects cats (Table 2). *A. caninum* has been identified in cats, although this is uncommon (Table 2). While human infections with *A. ceylanicum* do occur, there is some discussion around whether infection with this species produces hookworm disease and morbidity (Table 1) [50,179]. Table 1 shows recent cases of *A. ceylanicum* infection in humans and animals since 2000. Conlan *et al* [179] provide a review of the historical perspective of *A. ceylanicum.* Infection with *A. ceylanicum* was confirmed by molecular methods using PCR, PCR-RFLP, sequencing, or microscopy. In Australia there have been only two recent studies, including one case study of a returned peacekeeper, identifying human infection with *A. ceylanicum.* Studies in dogs have shown that this species is present in Australia, but to a much lesser degree than *A. caninum.* In the Asia-Pacific, the main hookworm species identified is *N. americanus* (81.8%), while 18.18% harboured *A. ceylanicum,* including one individual who harboured both species [132]. An equal prevalence of *A. ceylanicum* and *N. americanus* was found in Cambodia (51.6%) [96,132]. Prevalence of hookworm in animals in Asia is also high, with dual infections of *A. ceylanicum* and *A. caninum* also occurring (Table 2). Certainly, therefore, the presence of *A. ceylanicum* in animals in Asia and Australia poses a risk to human health.

Pets or companion animals are increasingly popular and a potential source of zoonotic hookworms. Observing good hygiene practices, wearing footwear, and regular worming of pets will help prevent transmission of zoonotic hookworms to humans. However, studies on pets and their owners in Europe, which presents a similar socio-economic situation as Australia where handwashing practices, access to clean water and toilets, are similar, have shown that pet owners do not always wash their hands after handling their pets [180]. Only 15% of dog owners and 8% of cat owners stated that they always washed their hands. The same studies have also found *Toxocara* eggs on the fur of the study animals (both cats and dogs) [180–184]. Cats pose a particular risk for egg contamination because cat litter trays reside inside the house and are cleaned by the owner, while dog owners may also be required to pick up after their animals as well.

The rate of pet ownership in Australia is very high. As of 2016, an estimated 62% of households had at least one pet, with dogs the most popular (39%) followed by cats (29%) [35]. Handwashing among Australia children was examined, with only 41% reported to always or mostly wash their hands after playing with animals, indicating that this is an issue in Australia as with comparable countries in Europe [185]. Pet ownership data are also available for China (25% dogs, 10% cats), South Korea (20% dogs, 6% cats), Japan (7% dogs, 14% cats) and Hong Kong (14% dogs, 10% cats) [35].

There have been few human infections in Australia and Asia identified as *A. caninum,* with the two most recent reports of human infection with this species both coming from Asia (Laos and India)

(Table 2). In Australia, *A. caninum* has historically been associated with eosinophilic enteritis [186–192], although there are limited reports on this condition since the mid-1990s.

14. Toxocara

Toxocariasis is caused by the migration of *Toxocara* larvae to various tissues, causing visceral larva migrans. Traditionally the species involved are *T. canis* and *T. cati* nematodes of dogs and cats respectively, with the latter most likely to be involved in human disease [193]. Other *Toxocara* species may also cause infection such as *T. malaysiensis*, which is found in Malaysia, Vietnam, and China, although its potential to infect humans at this point is unknown [193–195]. *Toxocara malaysiensis* also infects cats. Stray dogs and cats are a primary source of infection in developing countries, while high pet ownership in developed countries means that pets are the main source of infection there. Soil samples taken from playgrounds in Malaysia found that 95.7% of samples tested had *Toxocara* eggs, and 88.3% had hookworm, showing very high contamination of the local soil with parasite eggs infectious to humans [196].

The most serious result of infection with *Toxocara* is ocular toxocariasis, which can lead to blindness. Humans are dead-end hosts; the parasite larvae migrate to many tissues, and while they do not develop further they can cause granulomas and inflammation in the tissues they reside in [197].

In Australia *T. canis* has long been known to exist with high prevalence found in dogs and in environmental samples [198,199]. There are very few reports of recent surveys of animals, environmental samples, or humans in Australia. In the 1990s the *T. canis* prevalence in the general population of Australia was 5.7% while in Aboriginal communities it ranged from 11.1%–43% [47]. Historical infections reported included serological examination of patients with ocular symptoms in Victoria (3.86% n = 621) [200]; 7% (n = 660) seroprevalence was recorded in healthy blood donors from the Australia Capital Territory [201]. More recently 21% (n = 29) prevalence was reported in a remote Aboriginal community in the Northern Territory [47].

15. *Ascaris suum*

It was originally thought that *A. suum* infected humans only rarely, but molecular tools have shown that the two species (*A. lumbricoides* and *A. suum*), which are morphologically identical, may in fact be one species and *A. suum* represents a haplotype of *A. lumbricoides*. It has been recognised that the haplotype, *A. suum*, can cause human infections; and has also been found in non-human primates [15,202]. A study in Japan sequenced the ITS1 region of *Ascaris* derived from humans and pigs, finding that 3 of 9 isolates derived from humans were identical to those derived from pigs [6]. A phylogeny study performed in China utilising the mitochondrial genes *cox1* and *nad1*, and found a high level of gene flow between human- and pig-derived *Ascaris*, as well as indicating the presence of 20 haplotypes based on the *cox1* gene and 26 based on the *nad1* [203]. There is also evidence from China of hybrid forms of *Ascaris* [204]. In India PCR-RFLP was performed on dog stools identifying the presence of *A. lumbricoides* eggs [205].

A. suum has been identified in pigs in Australia; however, limited molecular work has been done to characterise the genotypes. Due to control measures in pigs it is estimated that only 3% of pigs in Australia harbour *Ascaris* [206]. There is also limited information on *A. suum* human infections in Australia. Two cases of *Ascaris* infection in Tasmania were thought to be *A. suum* based on morphology of mouthparts, and based on history of contact with pigs; no molecular tools were utilised [207].

Worldwide, 800 million people are estimated to be infected with *Ascaris*. A number of prevalence studies have been done in developing countries using both microscopy, primarily KK, and molecular techniques [66,208–210]. Speciation, or the presence of haplotypes, is rarely looked for in prevalence studies; it is therefore difficult to calculate the number of *Ascaris* infections due to pig-derived worms.

16. *Trichuris suis* and *T. vulpis*

Pigs and canines are the primary hosts of *T. suis* and *T. vulpis*, respectively. Human infections with both species have been recorded, as have hybrids of *T. suis* and the human species *T. trichiura* [5,9,10,13]. In Thailand, both dogs and humans harbour *T. vulpis* and *T. trichiura*, indicating the likelihood of zoonotic transmission occurring for both species [5]. However, dogs in India appear to only carry *T. trichiura*, while further human infections with *T. vulpis* have occurred in North America and Africa [13,205,211].

Genetic analysis of *Trichuris* species in humans, pigs, and non-human primates indicates that there may be several genotypes of *Trichuris* circulating in humans and animals [212–214]. Sequencing of pig and human derived *Trichuris* indicates that they are separate species [215], unlike *A. suum* discussed above, which is considered to be the same species as *A. lumbricoides*. Experimental infections of humans with *T. suis* documented the previously undocumented symptoms of infection which included flatulence, diarrhoea, and upper abdominal pain, although these symptoms regressed over time, after repeated exposure to eggs, to subclinical symptoms [216].

17. Helminth Therapy

While not all STH have as severe consequences as *Strongyloides*, it is clear that treatment of STH is needed in infected individuals. However, it has also been suggested that intestinal worms may actually be beneficial to human health, particularly to bowel health and diseases of hypersensitivity. This is usually described as part of the hygiene hypothesis, linking 'cleaner' living conditions with higher levels of allergic disease, and now extended to inflammatory disorders such as inflammatory bowel disease (IBD) [217]. Helminth parasites are known to modulate the host immune system and it is thought that by doing so for self-benefit, this may cause a bystander effect on other immune-related diseases [218,219].

There have been clinical trials with hookworm and *Trichuris* for treatment of a range of syndromes, including coeliac disease, asthma, allergies, and psoriasis [220]. Hookworm and *Trichuris* eggs are available online through companies such as Wormswell [221], which provides *N. americanus* eggs, and Tanawisa, which provides *T. suis* (porcine *Trichuris* species) (TSO) [222] eggs. The link between asthma regulation and helminths has been studied for some time, although concrete significance in trials has yet to eventuate, and exact mechanisms of action are unclear [223]. Recent trials for asthma, where individuals were experimentally infected with hookworm, indicated some improvement between groups with hookworm and those without, but the results were not significant [220]. A study in Uganda showed maternal hookworm infections decreased the risk of childhood eczema [224]. Australian studies of hookworm therapy largely focus on coeliac disease, which has had mixed results with null or positive associations; any causal link between allergies and parasite infection has not been shown [225,226]. Gut microbiota may also play a role, although it is still unclear how parasites and the microbiota interact with each other [227]. While *T. suis* is primarily a parasite of pigs, it can establish patent infections in humans [9,10,228] and treatment with TSO has been linked to improvement of psoriasis [229].

So, whereas STH and *Strongyloides* are generally thought to be detrimental to health, the presence of a few worms might be beneficial, although more research needs to be performed to confirm this. Because of the risk of self-infection with helminth eggs, most current work aimed at clinical trials is focused on the isolation of particular components in worm secretions that provide beneficial protection or immune modulation of IBD diseases [230,231].

18. Discussion and Conclusion

While STH infections are generally low in Australia, they are still endemic and of significant health importance in remote Aboriginal communities, particularly *S. stercoralis*, which can be fatal in immunocompromised people. Limited data are available for hyperinfection and mortality due to strongyloidiasis in the Asia-Pacific area, but in Australia, infection has led to fatalities, which, in such a resource-rich country, is alarming and unacceptable. Part of the problem may be due to a general lack of awareness of worm infections, which have a low prevalence in the country as a whole. A physician in an urban area may never see, diagnose or treat a helminthiasis case [93,94]. In Aboriginal communities, where the prevalence of strongyloidiasis can be quite high (0.25%–59.5%) [90–92,94,232,233], the very high cost of healthcare delivery limits available services, and physicians may only be resident for a short time so that knowledge about STH and *S. stercoralis*, in particular, may not be being passed on or recorded in the hospital system. Adding STH, particularly especially *S. stercoralis*, to the national notifiable disease system would help increase knowledge and provide access to more information about the appropriate handling of these parasitic worm infections.

High prevalence of STH in refugees and immigrants from endemic areas, particularly the Asia-Pacific, where the majority of immigrants to Australia now originate, highlights a need for better and more comprehensive health screenings of these groups that include parasite diagnosis and treatment. This holds true for army veterans and current members who have served, or are serving, in STH-endemic areas, including long-term follow-ups in case of poor drug efficacy or ongoing autoinfection in the case of *S. stercoralis*. The Asia-Pacific area has particularly high endemicity for STH and, with so much movement between Asia-Pacific and Australia, better understanding and treatment of STH infections are key from a public health perspective.

Author Contributions: CAG wrote the first draft of the manuscript, CAG, DPM, MJ, JK, and DJG contributed to editing and rewrites. All authors have read and approved the final paper.

Conflicts of Interest: The authors declare no conflict of interest.

List of Abbreviations

STH	soil transmitted helminths
SEA	South-East Asia
DNA	deoxyribonucleic acid
qPCR	quantitative real-time polymerase chain reaction
cPCR	conventional polymerase chain reaction
ddPCR	digital droplet polymerase chain reaction
RFLP-PCR	restriction fragment length polymorphism polymerase chain reaction
Cox 1	cytochrome oxidase 1
LAMP	Loop-mediated isothermal amplification
GIT	gastrointestinal tract
WASH	water, sanitation, and hygiene
MDA	mass drug administration
NTDs	neglected tropical diseases
DALYs	disability adjusted life years
YLDs	years lived with disability
HTLV-I	human T cell lymphotropic virus type I
CR	cure rate
IHCP	the integrated helminth control program
WHO	World Health Organization
IBD	inflammatory bowel disease
KK	Kato-Katz
ELISA	enzyme linked immunosorbent assay
DBS	dried blood spot
TOS	*Trichuris suis* eggs

References

1. Bethony, J.; Brooker, S.; Alboico, M.; Geirger, S.M.; Loukas, A.; Diemart, D.; Hotez, P.J. Soil-transmitted helminth infections: Ascariasis, trichuriasis, and hookworm. *Lancet* **2006**, *367*, 1521–1532. [CrossRef]
2. Utzinger, J.; Keiser, J. Schistosomiasis and soil-transmitted helminthiasis: Common drugs for treatment and control. *Expert Opin. Pharmacother.* **2004**, *5*, 263–285. [CrossRef] [PubMed]
3. WHO; UNICEF. *Prevention and Control of Schistosomiasis and Soil-Transmitted Helminthiasis*; WHO: Geneva, Switzerland, 2004.
4. Gordon, C.A.; McManus, D.P.; Jones, M.K.; Gray, D.J.; Gobert, G.N. The increase of exotic zoonotic helminth infections: The impact of urbanization, climate change and globalization. *Adv. Parasitol.* **2016**, *91*, 311–397. [PubMed]
5. Areekul, P.; Putaporntip, C.; Pattanawong, U.; Sitthicharoenchai, P.; Jongwutiwes, S. *Trichuris vulpis* and *T. trichiura* infections among schoolchildren of a rural community in northwestern Thailand: The possible role of dogs in disease transmission. *Asian Biomed.* **2010**, *4*, 49–60.
6. Arizono, N.; Yoshimura, Y.; Tohzaka, N.; Yamada, M.; Tegoshi, T.; Onishi, K.; Uchikawa, R. Ascariasis in Japan: Is pig-derived *Ascaris* infecting humans? *Jpn. J. Infect. Dis.* **2010**, *63*, 447–448. [PubMed]
7. Betson, M.; Nejsum, P.; Bendall, R.P.; Deb, R.M.; Stothard, J.R. Molecular epidemiology of ascariasis: A global perspective on the transmission dynamics of *Ascaris* in people and pigs. *J. Infect. Dis.* **2014**, *210*, 932–941. [CrossRef] [PubMed]
8. Dutto, M.; Petrosillo, N. Hybrid *ascaris suum/lumbricoides* (ascarididae) infestation in a pig farmer: A rare case of zoonotic ascariasis. *Cent. Eur. J. Public Health* **2013**, *21*, 224–226. [PubMed]
9. Cutillas, C.; Callejon, R.; de Rojas, M.; Tewes, B.; Ubeda, J.M.; Ariza, C.; Guevara, D.C. *Trichuris suis* and *Trichuris trichiura* are different nematode species. *Acta Trop.* **2009**, *111*, 299–307. [CrossRef] [PubMed]
10. Nissen, S.; Al-Jubury, A.; Hansen, T.V.; Olsen, A.; Christensen, H.; Thamsborg, S.M.; Nejsum, P. Genetic analysis of *Trichuris suis* and *Trichuris trichiura* recovered from humans and pigs in a sympatric setting in Uganda. *Vet. Parasitol.* **2012**, *188*, 68–77. [CrossRef] [PubMed]
11. Ngui, R.; Lim, Y.A.; Traub, R.; Mahmud, R.; Mistam, M.S. Epidemiological and genetic data supporting the transmission of *Ancylostoma ceylanicum* among human and domestic animals. *PLoS Negl. Trop. Dis.* **2012**, *6*, e1522. [CrossRef] [PubMed]
12. Phosuk, I.; Intapan, P.M.; Thanchomnang, T.; Sanpool, O.; Janwan, P.; Laummaunwai, P.; Aamnart, W.; Morakote, N.; Maleewong, W. Molecular detection of *Ancylostoma duodenale*, *Ancylostoma ceylanicum*, and *Necator americanus* in humans in northeastern and southern Thailand. *Korean J. Parasitol.* **2013**, *51*, 747–749. [CrossRef] [PubMed]
13. George, S.; Geldhof, P.; Albonico, M.; Ame, S.M.; Bethony, J.M.; Engels, D.; Mekonnen, Z.; Montresor, A.; Hem, S.; Tchuem-Tchuente, L.A.; et al. The molecular speciation of soil-transmitted helminth eggs collected from school children across six endemic countries. *Trans. R. Soc. Trop. Med. Hyg.* **2017**. [CrossRef] [PubMed]
14. Bahgat, M.A.; El Gindy, A.E.; Mahmoud, L.A.; Hegab, M.H.; Shahin, A.M. Evaluation of the role of *Ancylostoma caninum* in humans as a cause of acute and recurrent abdominal pain. *J. Egypt. Soc. Parasitol.* **1999**, *29*, 873–882. [PubMed]
15. Leles, D.; Gardner, S.L.; Reinhard, K.; Iniguez, A.; Araujo, A. Are *Ascaris lumbricoides* and *Ascaris suum* a single species? *Parasit. Vectors* **2012**, *5*, 42. [CrossRef] [PubMed]
16. Siddiqui, A.A.; Berk, S.L. Diagnosis of *Strongyloides stercoralis* infection. *Clin. Infect. Dis.* **2001**, *33*, 1040–1047. [CrossRef] [PubMed]
17. Genta, R.M. Global prevalence of strongyloidiasis: Critical review with epidemiologic insights into the prevention of disseminated disease. *Rev. Infect. Dis.* **1989**, *11*, 755–767. [CrossRef] [PubMed]
18. Magnaval, J.-F.; Glickman, L.T.; Dorchies, P.; Morassin, B. Highlights of human toxocariasis. *Korean J. Parasitol.* **2001**, *39*, 1–11. [CrossRef] [PubMed]
19. WHO. Metrics: Disability-Adjusted Life Year (DALY). Available online: http://www.who.int/healthinfo/global_burden_disease/metrics_daly/en/ (accessed on 6 July 2017).
20. Pullan, R.L.; Smith, J.L.; Jasrasaria, R.; Brooker, S.J. Global numbers of infection and disease burden of soil transmitted helminth infections in 2010. *Parasit. Vectors* **2014**, *7*, 37. [CrossRef] [PubMed]
21. Murray, C.J.; Vos, T.; Lozano, R.; Naghavi, M.; Flaxman, A.D.; Michaud, C.; Ezzati, M.; Shibuya, K.; Salomon, J.A.; Abdalla, S.; et al. Disability-adjusted life years (DALYs) for 291 diseases and injuries in 21

regions, 1990–2010: A systematic analysis for the Global Burden of Disease Study 2010. *Lancet* **2012**, *380*, 2197–2223. [CrossRef]

22. Murray, C.J.; Barber, R.M.; Foreman, K.J.; Ozgoren, A.A.; Abd-Allah, F.; Abera, S.F.; Aboyans, V.; Abraham, J.P.; Abubakar, I.; Abu-Raddad, L.J.; et al. Global, regional, and national disability-adjusted life years (DALYs) for 306 diseases and injuries and healthy life expectancy (HALE) for 188 countries, 1990–2013: Quantifying the epidemiological transition. *Lancet* **2015**. [CrossRef]

23. Osiro, S.; Hamula, C.; Glaser, A.; Rana, M.; Dunn, D. A case of *Strongyloides* hyperinfection syndrome in the setting of persistent eosinophilia but negative serology. *Diagn. Microbiol. Infect. Dis.* **2017**, *88*, 168–170. [CrossRef] [PubMed]

24. Ramamoorthy, K.G. Anaesthesia and *Ascaris* pneumonia (Loeffler's syndrome). *Indian J. Anaesth.* **2015**, *59*, 125–126. [CrossRef] [PubMed]

25. Cataño, J.C.; Pinzón, M.A. *Strongyloides* Pneumonia. *Am. J. Trop. Med. Hyg.* **2012**, *87*, 195. [CrossRef] [PubMed]

26. Cheepsattayakorn, A.; Cheepsattayakorn, R. Parasitic pneumonia and lung involvement. *BioMed Res. Int.* **2014**, *2014*, 18. [CrossRef] [PubMed]

27. Fan, C.K.; Holland, C.V.; Loxton, K.; Barghouth, U. Cerebral toxocariasis: Silent progression to neurodegenerative disorders? *Clin. Microbiol. Rev.* **2015**, *28*, 663–686. [CrossRef] [PubMed]

28. Keiser, P.B.; Nutman, T.B. *Strongyloides stercoralis* in the immunocompromised population. *Clin. Microbiol. Rev.* **2004**, *17*, 208–217. [CrossRef] [PubMed]

29. Einsiedel, L.; Fernandes, L. *Strongyloides stercoralis*: A cause of morbidity and mortality for indigenous people in Central Australia. *Intern. Med. J.* **2008**, *38*, 697–703. [CrossRef] [PubMed]

30. Jaleta, T.G.; Zhou, S.; Bemm, F.M.; Schar, F.; Khieu, V.; Muth, S.; Odermatt, P.; Lok, J.B.; Streit, A. Different but overlapping populations of *Strongyloides stercoralis* in dogs and humans - dogs as a possible source for zoonotic strongyloidiasis. *PLoS Negl. Trop. Dis.* **2017**, *11*, e0005752. [CrossRef] [PubMed]

31. Kouassi, R.Y.; McGraw, S.W.; Yao, P.K.; Abou-Bacar, A.; Brunet, J.; Pesson, B.; Bonfoh, B.; N'Goran, E.K.; Candolfi, E. Diversity and prevalence of gastrointestinal parasites in seven non-human primates of the Tai National Park, Cote d'Ivoire. *Parasite* **2015**, *22*, 1. [CrossRef] [PubMed]

32. Thanchomnang, T.; Intapan, P.M.; Sanpool, O.; Rodpai, R.; Tourtip, S.; Yahom, S.; Kullawat, J.; Radomyos, P.; Thammasiri, C.; Maleewong, W. First molecular identification and genetic diversity of *Strongyloides stercoralis* and *Strongyloides fuelleborni* in human communities having contact with long-tailed macaques in Thailand. *Parasitol. Res.* **2017**, *116*, 1917–1923. [CrossRef] [PubMed]

33. Bergquist, R.; Yang, G.J.; Knopp, S.; Utzinger, J.; Tanner, M. Surveillance and response: Tools and approaches for the elimination stage of neglected tropical diseases. *Acta Trop.* **2015**, *141*, 229–234. [CrossRef] [PubMed]

34. Nagayasu, E.; Aung, M.; Hortiwakul, T.; Hino, A.; Tanaka, T.; Higashiarakawa, M.; Olia, A.; Taniguchi, T.; Win, S.M.T.; Ohashi, I.; et al. A possible origin population of pathogenic intestinal nematodes, *Strongyloides stercoralis*, unveiled by molecular phylogeny. *Sci. Rep.* **2017**, *7*, 4844. [CrossRef] [PubMed]

35. *Pet Ownership Statistics*; Animal Medicines Australia: Barton ACT, Australia, 2016.

36. Caruana, S.R.; Kelly, H.A.; Ngeow, J.Y.; Ryan, N.J.; Bennett, C.M.; Chea, L.; Nuon, S.; Bak, N.; Skull, S.A.; Biggs, B.A. Undiagnosed and potentially lethal parasite infections among immigrants and refugees in Australia. *J. Travel Med.* **2006**, *13*, 233–239. [CrossRef] [PubMed]

37. De Silva, S.; Saykao, P.; Kelly, H.; MacIntyre, C.R.; Ryan, N.; Leydon, J.; Biggs, B.A. Chronic *Strongyloides stercoralis* infection in Laotian immigrants and refugees 7–20 years after resettlement in Australia. *Epidemiol. Infect.* **2002**, *128*, 439–444. [CrossRef] [PubMed]

38. Einsiedel, L.; Spelman, D. *Strongyloides stercoralis*: Risks posed to immigrant patients in an Australian tertiary referral centre. *Intern. Med. J.* **2006**, *36*, 632–637. [CrossRef] [PubMed]

39. Speare, R.; Bradbury, R.S.; Croese, J. A case of *Ancylostoma ceylanicum* infection occurring in an Australian soldier returned from Solomon Islands. *Korean J. Parasitol.* **2016**, *54*, 533–536. [CrossRef] [PubMed]

40. Rahmanian, H.; MacFarlane, A.C.; Rowland, K.E.; Einsiedel, L.J.; Neuhaus, S.J. Seroprevalence of *Strongyloides stercoralis* in a South Australian Vietnam veteran cohort. *Aust. N. Z. J. Public Health* **2015**, *39*, 331–335. [CrossRef] [PubMed]

41. Pattison, D.A.; Speare, R. Strongyloidiasis in personnel of the Regional Assistance Mission to Solomon Islands (RAMSI). *Med. J. Aust.* **2008**, *189*, 203–206. [PubMed]

42. Crowe, A.L.; Smith, P.; Ward, L.; Currie, B.J.; Baird, R. Decreasing prevalence of *Trichuris trichiura* (whipworm) in the Northern Territory from 2002 to 2012. *Med. J. Aust.* **2014**, *200*, 286–289. [CrossRef] [PubMed]

43. Davies, J.; Majumdar, S.S.; Forbes, R.T.; Smith, P.; Currie, B.J.; Baird, R.W. Hookworm in the Northern Territory: Down but not out. *Med. J. Aust.* **2013**, *198*, 278–281. [CrossRef] [PubMed]

44. Chaves, N.J.; Gibney, K.B.; Leder, K.; O'Brien, D.P.; Marshall, C.; Biggs, B.-A. Screening practices for infectious diseases among Burmese refugees in Australia. *Emerg. Infect. Dis.* **2009**, *15*, 1769–1772. [CrossRef] [PubMed]

45. Biggs, B.A.; Caruana, S.; Mihrshahi, S.; Jolley, D.; Leydon, J.; Chea, L.; Nuon, S. Management of chronic strongyloidiasis in immigrants and refugees: Is serologic testing useful? *Am. J. Trop. Med. Hyg.* **2009**, *80*, 788–791. [PubMed]

46. Mounsey, K.; Kearns, T.; Rampton, M.; Llewellyn, S.; King, M.; Holt, D.; Currie, B.J.; Andrews, R.; Nutman, T.; McCarthy, J. Use of dried blood spots to define antibody response to the *Strongyloides stercoralis* recombinant antigen NIE. *Acta Trop.* **2014**, *138*, 78–82. [CrossRef] [PubMed]

47. Shield, J.; Aland, K.; Kearns, T.; Gongdjalk, G.; Holt, D.; Currie, B.; Prociv, P. Intestinal parasites of children and adults in a remote Aboriginal community of the Northern Territory, Australia, 1994. *West. Pac. Surveill. Response J.* **2015**, *6*, 44–51. [CrossRef]

48. Lim, L.; Biggs, B.A. Fatal disseminated strongyloidiasis in a previously-treated patient. *Med. J. Aust.* **2001**, *174*, 355–356. [PubMed]

49. Koehler, A.V.; Bradbury, R.S.; Stevens, M.A.; Haydon, S.R.; Jex, A.R.; Gasser, R.B. Genetic characterization of selected parasites from people with histories of gastrointestinal disorders using a mutation scanning-coupled approach. *Electrophoresis* **2013**, *34*, 1720–1728. [CrossRef] [PubMed]

50. Traub, R.J. *Ancylostoma ceylanicum*, a re-emerging but neglected parasitic zoonosis. *Int. J. Parasitol.* **2013**, *43*, 1009–1015. [CrossRef] [PubMed]

51. Traub, R.J.; Inpankaew, T.; Sutthikornchai, C.; Sukthana, Y.; Thompson, R.C.A. PCR-based coprodiagnostic tools reveal dogs as reservoirs of zoonotic ancylostomiasis caused by *Ancylostoma ceylanicum* in temple communities in Bangkok. *Vet. Parasitol.* **2008**, *155*, 67–73. [CrossRef] [PubMed]

52. Schär, F.; Inpankaew, T.; Traub, R.J.; Khieu, V.; Dalsgaard, A.; Chimnoi, W.; Chhoun, C.; Sok, D.; Marti, H.; Muth, S.; et al. The prevalence and diversity of intestinal parasitic infections in humans and domestic animals in a rural Cambodian village. *Parasitol. Int.* **2014**, *63*, 597–603. [CrossRef] [PubMed]

53. Bradbury, R.; Traub, R.J. Hookworm Infection in Oceania. In *Neglected Tropical Diseases—Oceania*; Loukas, A., Ed.; Springer International Publishing: Cham, Switzerland, 2016; pp. 33–68.

54. Ngui, R.; Mahdy, M.A.; Chua, K.H.; Traub, R.; Lim, Y.A. Genetic characterization of the partial mitochondrial cytochrome oxidase c subunit I (*cox 1*) gene of the zoonotic parasitic nematode, *Ancylostoma ceylanicum* from humans, dogs and cats. *Acta Trop.* **2013**, *128*, 154–157. [CrossRef] [PubMed]

55. Hookworm biology. Available online: https://www.cdc.gov/parasites/hookworm/biology.html (accessed on 18 August 2017).

56. Whipworm biology. Available online: https://www.cdc.gov/parasites/whipworm/biology.html (accessed on 18 August 2017).

57. Ascariasis biology. Available online: https://www.cdc.gov/parasites/ascariasis/biology.html (accessed on 18 August 2017).

58. Strongyloidiasis biology. Available online: https://www.cdc.gov/dpdx/strongyloidiasis/index.html (accessed on 18 August 2017).

59. Yamada, M.; Matsuda, S.; Nakazawa, M.; Arizono, N. Species-specific differences in heterogonic development of serially transferred free-living generations of *Strongyloides planiceps* and *Strongyloides stercoralis*. *J. Parasitol.* **1991**, *77*, 592–594. [CrossRef] [PubMed]

60. Viney, M.E.; Lok, J.B. The biology of *Strongyloides spp.*. *WormBook Online Rev. C Elegans Biol.* **2015**, 1–17. [CrossRef] [PubMed]

61. Toxocariasis biology. Available online: https://www.cdc.gov/parasites/toxocariasis/biology.html (accessed on 18 August 2017).

62. Quattrocchi, G.; Nicoletti, A.; Marin, B.; Bruno, E.; Druet-Cabanac, M.; Preux, P.M. Toxocariasis and epilepsy: Systematic review and meta-analysis. *PLoS Negl. Trop. Dis.* **2012**, *6*, e1775. [CrossRef] [PubMed]

63. Jex, A.R.; Lim, Y.A.; Bethony, J.M.; Hotez, P.J.; Young, N.D.; Gasser, R.B. Soil-transmitted helminths of humans in Southeast Asia - towards integrated control. *Adv. Parasitol.* **2011**, *74*, 231–265. [PubMed]

64. Brooker, S.J.; Bundy, D.A.P. 55—Soil-transmitted Helminths (Geohelminths). In *Manson's Tropical Infectious Diseases (Twenty-Third Edition)*; Farrar, J., Hotez, P.J., Junghanss, T., Kang, G., Lalloo, D., White, N.J., Eds.; W.B. Saunders: London, UK, 2014.

65. De Silva, N.R.; Brooker, S.; Hotez, P.J.; Montresor, A.; Engels, D.; Savioli, L. Soil-transmitted helminth infections: Updating the global picture. *Trends Parasitol.* **2003**, *19*, 547–551. [CrossRef] [PubMed]

66. Gordon, C.A.; McManus, D.P.; Acosta, L.P.; Olveda, R.; Williams, M.; Ross, A.G.; Gray, D.J.; Gobert, G.N. Multiplex real-time PCR monitoring of intestinal helminths in humans reveals widespread polyparasitism in Northern Samar, the Philippines. *Int. J. Parasitol.* **2015**, *45*, 477–483. [CrossRef] [PubMed]

67. Laymanivong, S.; Hangvanthong, B.; Keokhamphavanh, B.; Phommasansak, M.; Phinmaland, B.; Sanpool, O.; Maleewong, W.; Intapan, P.M. Current status of human hookworm infections, ascariasis, trichuriasis, schistosomiasis mekongi and other trematodiases in Lao People's Democratic Republic. *Am. J. Trop. Med. Hyg.* **2014**, *90*, 667–669. [CrossRef] [PubMed]

68. Rim, H.-J.; Chai, J.-Y.; Min, D.-Y.; Cho, S.; Eom, K.S.; Hong, S.; Sohn, W.; Yong, T.; Deodato, G.; Standgaard, H.; et al. Prevalence of intestinal parasite infections on a national scale among primary schoolchildren in Laos. *Parasitol. Res.* **2003**, *91*, 267–272. [CrossRef] [PubMed]

69. Conlan, J.V.; Khamlome, B.; Vongxay, K.; Elliot, A.; Pallant, L.; Sripa, B.; Blacksell, S.D.; Fenwick, S.; Thompson, R.C. Soil-transmitted helminthiasis in Laos: A community-wide cross-sectional study of humans and dogs in a mass drug administration environment. *Am. J. Trop. Med. Hyg.* **2012**, *86*, 624–634. [CrossRef] [PubMed]

70. Meurs, L.; Polderman, A.M.; Vinkeles Melchers, N.V.; Brienen, E.A.; Verweij, J.J.; Groosjohan, B.; Mendes, F.; Mechendura, M.; Hepp, D.H.; Langenberg, M.C.; et al. Diagnosing polyparasitism in a high-prevalence setting in Beira, Mozambique: Detection of intestinal parasites in fecal samples by microscopy and real-time PCR. *PLoS Negl. Trop. Dis.* **2017**, *11*, e0005310. [CrossRef] [PubMed]

71. Elyana, F.N.; Al-Mekhlafi, H.M.; Ithoi, I.; Abdulsalam, A.M.; Dawaki, S.; Nasr, N.A.; Atroosh, W.M.; Abd-Basher, M.H.; Al-Areeqi, M.A.; Sady, H.; et al. A tale of two communities: Intestinal polyparasitism among Orang Asli and Malay communities in rural Terengganu, Malaysia. *Parasit. Vectors* **2016**, *9*, 398. [CrossRef] [PubMed]

72. Fleming, F.M.; Brooker, S.; Geiger, S.M.; Caldas, I.R.; Correa-Oliveira, R.; Hotez, P.J.; Bethony, J.M. Synergistic associations between hookworm and other helminth species in a rural community in Brazil. *Trop. Med. Int. Health* **2006**, *11*, 56–64. [CrossRef] [PubMed]

73. Mehta, R.S.; Rodriguez, A.; Chico, M.; Guadalupe, I.; Broncano, N.; Sandoval, C.; Tupiza, F.; Mitre, E.; Cooper, P.J. Maternal geohelminth infections are associated with an increased susceptibility to geohelminth infection in children: A case-control study. *PLoS Negl. Trop. Dis.* **2012**, *6*, e1753. [CrossRef] [PubMed]

74. Menzies, S.K.; Rodriguez, A.; Chico, M.; Sandoval, C.; Broncano, N.; Guadalupe, I.; Cooper, P.J. Risk Factors for soil-transmitted helminth infections during the first 3 years of life in the tropics; findings from a birth cohort. *PLoS Negl. Trop. Dis.* **2014**, *8*, e2718. [CrossRef] [PubMed]

75. Olsen, A.; van Lieshout, L.; Marti, H.; Polderman, T.; Polman, K.; Steinmann, P.; Stothard, R.; Thybo, S.; Verweij, J.J.; Magnussen, P. Strongyloidiasis–the most neglected of the neglected tropical diseases? *Trans. R. Soc. Trop. Med. Hyg.* **2009**, *103*, 967–972. [CrossRef] [PubMed]

76. Ngui, R.; Halim, N.A.; Rajoo, Y.; Lim, Y.A.; Ambu, S.; Rajoo, K.; Chang, T.S.; Woon, L.C.; Mahmud, R. Epidemiological characteristics of strongyloidiasis in inhabitants of indigenous communities in Borneo island, Malaysia. *Korean J. Parasitol.* **2016**, *54*, 673–678. [CrossRef] [PubMed]

77. Requena-Mendez, A.; Chiodini, P.; Bisoffi, Z.; Buonfrate, D.; Gotuzzo, E.; Munoz, J. The laboratory diagnosis and follow up of strongyloidiasis: A systematic review. *PLoS Negl. Trop. Dis.* **2013**, *7*, e2002. [CrossRef] [PubMed]

78. Verweij, J.J.; Canales, M.; Polman, K.; Ziem, J.; Brienen, E.A.T.; Polderman, A.M.; van Lieshout, L. Molecular diagnosis of *Strongyloides stercoralis* in faecal samples using real-time PCR. *Trans. R. Soc. Trop. Med. Hyg.* **2009**, *103*, 342–346. [CrossRef] [PubMed]

79. Intapan, P.M.; Maleewong, W.; Wongsaroj, T.; Singthong, S.; Morakote, N. Comparison of the quantitative formalin ethyl acetate concentration technique and agar plate culture for diagnosis of human strongyloidiasis. *J. Clin. Microbiol.* **2005**, *43*, 1932–1933. [CrossRef] [PubMed]

80. Boonjaraspinyo, S.; Boonmars, T.; Kaewsamut, B.; Ekobol, N.; Laummaunwai, P.; Aukkanimart, R.; Wonkchalee, N.; Juasook, A.; Sriraj, P. A cross-sectional study on intestinal parasitic infections in rural communities, northeast Thailand. *Korean J. Parasitol.* **2013**, *51*, 727–734. [CrossRef] [PubMed]

81. Kling, K.; Kuenzli, E.; Blum, J.; Neumayr, A. Acute strongyloidiasis in a traveller returning from South East Asia. *Travel Med. Infect. Dis.* **2016**, *14*, 535–536. [CrossRef] [PubMed]

82. Nguyen, T.; Cheong, F.W.; Liew, J.W.; Lau, Y.L. Seroprevalence of fascioliasis, toxocariasis, strongyloidiasis and cysticercosis in blood samples diagnosed in Medic Medical Center Laboratory, Ho Chi Minh City, Vietnam in 2012. *Parasit. Vectors* **2016**, *9*, 486. [CrossRef] [PubMed]

83. Nontasut, P.; Muennoo, C.; Sa-nguankiat, S.; Fongsri, S.; Vichit, A. Prevalence of *Strongyloides* in Northern Thailand and treatment with ivermectin vs albendazole. *Southeast Asian J. Trop. Med. Public Health* **2005**, *36*, 442–444. [PubMed]

84. Schär, F.; Trostdorf, U.; Giardina, F.; Khieu, V.; Muth, S.; Marti, H.; Vounatsou, P.; Odermatt, P. *Strongyloides stercoralis*: Global distribution and risk factors. *PLoS Negl. Trop. Dis.* **2013**, *7*, e2288. [CrossRef] [PubMed]

85. Smout, F.A.; Skerratt, L.F.; Butler, J.R.A.; Johnson, C.N.; Congdon, B.C.; Thompson, R.C.A. The hookworm *Ancylostoma ceylanicum*: An emerging public health risk in Australian tropical rainforests and Indigenous communities. *One Health (Amsterdam, Netherlands)* **2017**, *3*, 66–69. [CrossRef] [PubMed]

86. Smout, F.A.; Thompson, R.C.A.; Skerratt, L.F. First report of *Ancylostoma ceylanicum* in wild canids. *Int. J. Parasitol. Parasites Wildl.* **2013**, *2*, 173–177. [CrossRef] [PubMed]

87. Lee, A. Internal parasites of pigs. Available online: https://www.dpi.nsw.gov.au/__data/assets/pdf_file/0019/433018/internal-parasites-of-pigs.pdf (accessed on 4 July 2017).

88. Prociv, P.; Luke, R.A. The changing epidemiology of human hookworm infection in Australia. *Med. J. Aust.* **1995**, *162*, 150–154. [PubMed]

89. Health, V. Ascariasis (roundworm infection). Available online: https://www2.health.vic.gov.au/public-health/infectious-diseases/disease-information-advice/ascariasis-roundworm-infection (accessed on 27 July 2017).

90. Johnston, F.H.; Morris, P.S.; Speare, R.; McCarthy, J.; Currie, B.; Ewald, D.; Page, W.; Dempsey, K. Strongyloidiasis: A review of the evidence for Australian practitioners. *Aust. J. Rural Health* **2005**, *13*, 247–254. [CrossRef] [PubMed]

91. Jones, H.I. Intestinal parasite infections in Western Australian Aborigines. *Med. J. Aust.* **1980**, *2*, 375–380. [PubMed]

92. Prociv, P.; Luke, R. Observations on strongyloidiasis in Queensland aboriginal communities. *Med. J. Aust.* **1993**, *158*, 160–163. [PubMed]

93. Speare, R.; Miller, A.; Page, W.A. Strongyloidiasis: A case for notification in Australia? *Med. J. Aust.* **2015**, *202*, 523–524. [CrossRef] [PubMed]

94. Page, W.; Speare, R. Chronic strongyloidiasis—Don't look and you won't find. *Aust. Fam. Physician* **2016**, *45*, 40–44. [PubMed]

95. Hsu, Y.; Lin, J. Intestinal Infestation with *Ancylostoma ceylanicum*. *N. Engl. J. Med.* **2012**, *366*. [CrossRef] [PubMed]

96. Inpankaew, T.; Schar, F.; Dalsgaard, A.; Khieu, V.; Chimnoi, W.; Chhoun, C.; Sok, D.; Marti, H.; Muth, S.; Odermatt, P.; et al. High prevalence of *Ancylostoma ceylanicum* hookworm infections in humans, Cambodia, 2012. *Emerg. Infect. Dis.* **2014**, *20*, 976–982. [CrossRef] [PubMed]

97. Liu, Y.; Zheng, G.; Alsarakibi, M. The zoonotic risk of *Ancylostoma ceylanicum* isolated from stray dogs and cats in Guangzhou, South China. *BioMed Res. Int.* **2014**, *2014*, 208759. [CrossRef] [PubMed]

98. Mahdy, M.A.; Lim, Y.A.; Ngui, R.; Siti Fatimah, M.R.; Choy, S.H.; Yap, N.J.; Al-Mekhlafi, H.M.; Ibrahim, J.; Surin, J. Prevalence and zoonotic potential of canine hookworms in Malaysia. *Parasit. Vectors* **2012**, *5*, 88. [CrossRef] [PubMed]

99. Mohd Zain, S.N.; Sahimin, N.; Pal, P.; Lewis, J.W. Macroparasite communities in stray cat populations from urban cities in Peninsular Malaysia. *Vet. Parasitol.* **2013**, *196*, 469–477. [CrossRef] [PubMed]

100. Ngui, R.; Lim, Y.A.; Chua, K.H. Rapid detection and identification of human hookworm infections through high resolution melting (HRM) analysis. *PLoS ONE* **2012**, *7*, e41996. [CrossRef] [PubMed]

101. Ngui, R.; Lim, Y.A.; Ismail, W.H.; Lim, K.N.; Mahmud, R. Zoonotic *Ancylostoma ceylanicum* infection detected by endoscopy. *Am. J. Trop. Med. Hyg.* **2014**, *91*, 86–88. [CrossRef] [PubMed]

102. Pa Pa Aung, W.; Htoon, T.T.; Tin, H.H.; Sanpool, O.; Jongthawin, J.; Sadaow, L.; Phosuk, I.; Ropai, R.; Intapan, P.M.; Maleewong, W. First molecular identifications of *Necator americanus* and *Ancylostoma ceylanicum* infecting rural communities in lower Myanmar. *Am. J. Trop. Med. Hyg.* **2017**, *96*, 214–216. [CrossRef] [PubMed]

103. Palmer, C.S.; Traub, R.J.; Robertson, I.D.; Hobbs, R.P.; Elliot, A.; While, L.; Rees, R.; Thompson, R.C. The veterinary and public health significance of hookworm in dogs and cats in Australia and the status of *A. ceylanicum*. *Vet. Parasitol.* **2007**, *145*, 304–313. [CrossRef] [PubMed]

104. Traub, R.J.; Pednekar, R.P.; Cuttell, L.; Porter, R.B.; Abd Megat Rani, P.A.; Gatne, M.L. The prevalence and distribution of gastrointestinal parasites of stray and refuge dogs in four locations in India. *Vet. Parasitol.* **2014**, *205*, 233–238. [CrossRef] [PubMed]

105. Traub, R.J.; Robertson, I.D.; Irwin, P.; Mencke, N.; Thompson, R.C. Application of a species-specific PCR-RFLP to identify *Ancylostoma* eggs directly from canine faeces. *Vet. Parasitol.* **2004**, *123*, 245–255. [CrossRef] [PubMed]

106. Tun, S.; Ithoi, I.; Mahmud, R.; Samsudin, N.I.; Kek Heng, C.; Ling, L.Y. Detection of helminth eggs and identification of hookworm species in stray cats, dogs and soil from Klang Valley, Malaysia. *PLoS ONE* **2015**, *10*, e0142231. [CrossRef] [PubMed]

107. Kaya, D.; Yoshikawa, M.; Nakatani, T.; Tomo-Oka, F.; Fujimoto, Y.; Ishida, K.; Fujinaga, Y.; Aihara, Y.; Nagamatsu, S.; Matsuo, E.; et al. *Ancylostoma ceylanicum* hookworm infection in Japanese traveler who presented chronic diarrhea after return from Lao People's Democratic Republic. *Parasitol. Int.* **2016**, *65*, 737–740. [CrossRef] [PubMed]

108. George, S.; Levecke, B.; Kattula, D.; Velusamy, V.; Roy, S.; Geldhof, P.; Sarkar, R.; Kang, G. Molecular identification of hookworm isolates in humans, dogs and soil in a tribal area in Tamil Nadu, India. *PLoS Negl. Trop. Dis.* **2016**, *10*, e0004891. [CrossRef] [PubMed]

109. Pumidonming, W.; Salman, D.; Gronsang, D.; Abdelbaset, A.E.; Sangkaeo, K.; Kawazu, S.I.; Igarashi, M. Prevalence of gastrointestinal helminth parasites of zoonotic significance in dogs and cats in lower Northern Thailand. *J. Vet. Med. Sci.* **2017**, *78*, 1779–1784. [CrossRef] [PubMed]

110. Brunet, J.; Lemoine, J.P.; Lefebvre, N.; Denis, J.; Pfaff, A.W.; Abou-Bacar, A.; Traub, R.J.; Pesson, B.; Candolfi, E. Bloody diarrhea associated with hookworm infection in traveler returning to France from Myanmar. *Emerg. Infect. Dis.* **2015**, *21*, 1878–1879. [CrossRef] [PubMed]

111. Ng-Nguyen, D.; Hii, S.F.; Nguyen, V.A.; Van Nguyen, T.; Van Nguyen, D.; Traub, R.J. Re-evaluation of the species of hookworms infecting dogs in Central Vietnam. *Parasit. Vectors* **2015**, *8*, 401. [CrossRef] [PubMed]

112. Hu, W.; Yu, X.G.; Wu, S.; Tan, L.P.; Song, M.R.; Abdulahi, A.Y.; Wang, Z.; Jiang, B.; Li, G.Q. Levels of *Ancylostoma* infections and phylogenetic analysis of *cox 1* gene of *A. ceylanicum* in stray cat faecal samples from Guangzhou, China. *J. Helminthol.* **2016**, *90*, 392–397. [CrossRef] [PubMed]

113. George, S.; Kaliappan, S.P.; Kattula, D.; Roy, S.; Geldhof, P.; Kang, G.; Vercruysse, J.; Levecke, B. Identification of *Ancylostoma ceylanicum* in children from a tribal community in Tamil Nadu, India using a semi-nested PCR-RFLP tool. *Trans. R. Soc. Trop. Med. Hyg.* **2015**, *109*, 283–285. [CrossRef] [PubMed]

114. Jiraanankul, V.; Aphijirawat, W.; Mungthin, M.; Khositnithikul, R.; Rangsin, R.; Traub, R.J.; Piyaraj, P.; Naaglor, T.; Taamasri, P.; Leelayoova, S. Incidence and risk factors of hookworm infection in a rural community of central Thailand. *Am. J. Trop. Med. Hyg.* **2011**, *84*, 594–598. [CrossRef] [PubMed]

115. Sato, M.; Sanguankiat, S.; Yoonuan, T.; Pongvongsa, T.; Keomoungkhoun, M.; Phimmayoi, I.; Boupa, B.; Moji, K.; Waikagul, J. Copro-molecular identification of infections with hookworm eggs in rural Lao PDR. *Trans. R. Soc. Trop. Med. Hyg.* **2010**, *104*, 617–622. [CrossRef] [PubMed]

116. Scholz, T.; Uhlirova, M.; Ditrich, O. Helminth parasites of cats from the Vientiane province, Laos, as indicators of the occurrence of causative agents of human parasitoses. *Parasite* **2003**, *10*, 343–350. [CrossRef] [PubMed]

117. Chung, C.S.; Lin, C.K.; Su, K.E.; Liu, C.Y.; Lin, C.C.; Liang, C.C.; Lee, T.H. Diagnosis of *Ancylostoma ceylanicum* infestation by single-balloon enteroscopy (with video). *Gastrointest. Endosc.* **2012**, *76*, 671–672. [CrossRef] [PubMed]

118. Einsiedel, L.J.; Pham, H.; Woodman, R.J.; Pepperill, C.; Taylor, K.A. The prevalence and clinical associations of HTLV-1 infection in a remote Indigenous community. *Med. J. Aust.* **2016**, *205*, 305–309. [CrossRef] [PubMed]

119. Einsiedel, L.; Woodman, R.J.; Flynn, M.; Wilson, K.; Cassar, O.; Gessain, A. Human T-Lymphotropic Virus type 1 infection in an Indigenous Australian population: Epidemiological insights from a hospital-based cohort study. *BMC Public Health* **2016**, *16*, 787. [CrossRef] [PubMed]

120. Al Maslamani, M.A.; Al Soub, H.A.; Al Khal, A.L.M.; Al Bozom, I.A.; Abu Khattab, M.J.; Chacko, K.C. *Strongyloides stercoralis* hyperinfection after corticosteroid therapy: A report of two cases. *Ann. Saudi Med.* **2009**, *29*, 397–401. [PubMed]

121. Koticha, A.; Kuyare, S.; Nair, J.; Athvale, A.; Mehta, P. *Strongyloides stercoralis* hyperinfection syndrome in patients on prolonged steroid treatment: Two case reports. *J. Indian Med. Assoc.* **2013**, *111*, 272–274. [PubMed]

122. Aru, R.G.; Chilcutt, B.M.; Butt, S.; deShazo, R.D. Novel findings in HIV, immune reconstitution disease and *Strongyloides stercoralis* Infection. *Am. J. Med. Sci.* **2017**, *353*, 593–596. [CrossRef] [PubMed]

123. Llenas-Garcia, J.; Fiorante, S.; Salto, E.; Maseda, D.; Rodriguez, V.; Matarranz, M.; Hernando, A.; Rubio, R.; Pulido, F. Should we look for *Strongyloides stercoralis* in foreign-born HIV-infected persons? *J. Immigr. Minor. Health* **2013**, *15*, 796–802. [CrossRef] [PubMed]

124. Mobley, C.M.; Dhala, A.; Ghobrial, R.M. *Strongyloides stercoralis* in solid organ transplantation: Early diagnosis gets the worm. *Curr. Opin. Organ Transplant.* **2017**, *22*, 336–344. [CrossRef] [PubMed]

125. Medicinewise, N. Albendazole (Zentel) listing extended to treat hookworm and strongyloidiasis. Available online: https://www.nps.org.au/radar/articles/albendazole-zentel-listing-extended-to-treat-hookworm-and-strongyloidiasis (accessed on 4 July 2017).

126. Refugee health services. Available online: https://www.health.qld.gov.au/public-health/groups/multicultural/refugee-services (accessed on 27 September 2017).

127. Refugee and asylum seeker health and wellbeing. Available online: https://www2.health.vic.gov.au/about/populations/refugee-asylum-seeker-health (accessed on 27 September 2017).

128. NSW refugee health service. Available online: https://www.swslhd.health.nsw.gov.au/refugee/ (accessed on 27 September 2017).

129. Humanitarian entrant health service. Available online: http://ww2.health.wa.gov.au/Articles/F_I/Humanitarian-Entrant-Health-Service (accessed on 27 September 2017).

130. Refugee Health Program. Available online: https://www.ntphn.org.au/refugee-health (accessed on 27 September 2017).

131. Statistics, A.B.O. Migration, Australia, 2015–2016. Available online: http://www.abs.gov.au/ausstats/abs@.nsf/mf/3412.0 (accessed on 4 July 2017).

132. Bradbury, R.S.; Hii, S.F.; Harrington, H.; Speare, R.; Traub, R. *Ancylostoma ceylanicum* hookworm in the Solomon Islands. *Emerg. Infect. Dis.* **2017**, *23*, 252–257. [CrossRef] [PubMed]

133. Hanieh, S.; Ryan, N.; Biggs, B. Assessing enteric helminths in refugees, asylum seekers and new migrants. *Microbiol. Aust.* **2016**, 15–19. [CrossRef]

134. Mayer-Coverdale, J.K.; Crowe, A.; Smith, P.; Baird, R.W. Trends in *Strongyloides stercoralis* faecal larvae detections in the Northern Territory, Australia: 2002 to 2012. *Trop. Med. Infect. Dis.* **2017**, *2*. [CrossRef]

135. Montes, M.; Sawhney, C.; Barros, N. *Strongyloides stercoralis*: There but not seen. *Curr. Opin. Infect. Dis.* **2010**, *23*, 500–504. [CrossRef] [PubMed]

136. Knopp, S.; Salim, N.; Schindler, T.; Voules, D.A.K.; Rothen, J.; Lweno, O.; Mohammed, A.S.; Singo, R.; Benninghoff, M.; Nsojo, A.A.; et al. Diagnostic accuracy of Kato-Katz, FLOTAC, Baermann, and PCR methods for the detection of light-intensity hookworm and *Strongyloides stercoralis* infections in Tanzania. *Am. J. Trop. Med. Hyg.* **2014**, *90*, 535–543. [CrossRef] [PubMed]

137. Knopp, S.; Speich, B.; Hattendorf, J.; Rinaldi, L.; Mohammed, K.A.; Khamis, I.S.; Mohammed, A.S.; Albonico, M.; Rollinson, D.; Marti, H.; et al. Diagnostic accuracy of Kato-Katz and FLOTAC for assessing anthelmintic drug efficacy. *PLoS Negl. Trop. Dis.* **2011**, *5*, e1036. [CrossRef] [PubMed]

138. Lin, D.-D.; Liu, J.-X.; Liu, Y.-M.; Hu, F.; Zhang, Y.-Y.; Xu, J.-M.; Li, J.-Y.; Ji, M.-J.; Bergquist, R.; Wu, G.-L.; et al. Routine Kato-Katz technique underestimates the prevalence of *Schistosoma japonicum*: A case study in an endemic area of the People's Republic of China. *Parasitol. Int.* **2008**, *57*, 281–286. [CrossRef] [PubMed]

139. McCarthy, J.S.; Lustigman, S.; Yang, G.-J.; Barakat, R.M.; García, H.H.; Sripa, B.; Willingham, A.L.; Prichard, R.K.; Basáñez, M.-G. A researcha genda for helminth diseases of humans: Diagnostics for control and elimination programmes. *PLoS Negl. Trop. Dis.* **2012**, *6*, e1601. [CrossRef] [PubMed]

140. Dacombe, R.J.; Crampin, A.C.; Floyd, S.; Randall, A.; Ndhlovu, R.; Bickle, Q.; Fine, P.E.M. Time delays between patient and laboratory selectively affect accuracy of helminth diagnosis. *Trans. R. Soc. Trop. Med. Hyg.* **2007**, *101*, 140–145. [CrossRef] [PubMed]

141. Cringoli, G. FLOTAC, a novel apparatus for a multivalent faecal egg count technique. *Parassitologica* **2006**, *48*, 381–384.

142. Glinz, D.; Silué, K.D.; Knopp, S.; Lohouringnon, L.K.; Yao, K.P.; Steinmann, P.; Rinaldi, L.; Cringoli, G.; N'Goran, E.K.; Utzinger, J. Comparing diagnostic accuraccy of Kato-Katz, koga agar plate, ether-concentration, and FLOTAC for *Schistosoma mansoni* and soli-transmitted helminths. *PLoS Negl. Trop. Dis.* **2010**, *4*, e754. [CrossRef] [PubMed]

143. Habtamu, K.; Degarege, A.; Ye-Ebiyo, Y.; Erko, B. Comparison of the Kato-Katz and FLOTAC techniques for the diagnosis of soil-transmitted helminth infections. *Parasitol. Int.* **2011**, *60*, 398–402. [CrossRef] [PubMed]

144. Knopp, S.; Rinaldi, R.; Khamis, I.S.; Stothard, J.R.; Rollinson, D.; Maurelli, M.P.; Steinmann, P.; Marti, H.; Cringoli, G.; Utzinger, J. A single FLOTAC is more sensitive than triplicate Kato-Katz for the diagnosis of low intensity soil-transmitted helminth infections. *Trans. R. Soc. Trop. Med. Hyg.* **2009**, *103*, 347–354. [CrossRef] [PubMed]

145. Speich, B.; Knopp, S.; Mohammed, A.K.; Khamis, I.S.; Rinaldi, L.; Cringoli, G.; Rollinson, D.; Utzinger, J. Comparative cost assessment of the Kato-Katz and FLOTAC techniques for soil-transmitted helminth diagnosis in epidemiological surveys. *Parasit. Vectors* **2010**, *3*. [CrossRef] [PubMed]

146. Buonfrate, D.; Formenti, F.; Perandin, F.; Bisoffi, Z. Novel approaches to the diagnosis of *Strongyloides stercoralis* infection. *Clin. Microbiol. Infect.* **2015**, *21*, 543–552. [CrossRef] [PubMed]

147. Buonfrate, D.; Perandin, F.; Formenti, F.; Bisoffi, Z. A retrospective study comparing agar plate culture, indirect immunofluorescence and real-time PCR for the diagnosis of *Strongyloides stercoralis* infection. *Parasitology* **2017**, 1–5. [CrossRef] [PubMed]

148. Van Doorn, H.R.; Koelewijn, R.; Hofwegen, H.; Gilis, H.; Wetsteyn, J.C.; Wismans, P.J.; Sarfati, C.; Vervoort, T.; van Gool, T. Use of enzyme-linked immunosorbent assay and dipstick assay for detection of *Strongyloides stercoralis* infection in humans. *J. Clin. Microbiol.* **2007**, *45*, 438–442. [CrossRef] [PubMed]

149. Anderson, N.W.; Klein, D.M.; Dornink, S.M.; Jespersen, D.J.; Kubofcik, J.; Nutman, T.B.; Merrigan, S.D.; Couturier, M.R.; Theel, E.S. Comparison of three immunoassays for detection of antibodies to *Strongyloides stercoralis*. *Clin. Vaccine Immunol. CVI* **2014**, *21*, 732–736. [CrossRef] [PubMed]

150. Gordon, C.A.; Gray, D.J.; Gobert, G.N.; McManus, D.P. DNA amplification approaches for the diagnosis of key parasitic helminth infections of humans. *Mol. Cell. Probes* **2011**, *25*, 143–152. [CrossRef] [PubMed]

151. Kumagai, T.; Furushima-Shimogawara, R.; Ohmae, H.; Wang, T.P.; Lu, S.; Chen, R.; Wen, L.; Ohta, N. Detection of early and single infections of *Schistosoma japonicum* in the intermediate host snail, *Oncomelania hupensis*, by PCR and loop-mediated isothermal amplification (LAMP) assay. *Am. J. Trop. Med. Hyg.* **2010**, *83*, 542–548. [CrossRef] [PubMed]

152. Mugambi, R.M.; Agola, E.L.; Mwangi, I.N.; Kinyua, J.; Shiraho, E.A.; Mkoji, G.M. Development and evaluation of a loop mediated isothermal amplification (LAMP) technique for the detection of hookworm (*Necator americanus*) infection in fecal samples. *Parasit. Vectors* **2015**, *8*, 574. [CrossRef] [PubMed]

153. Weerakoon, K.G.; Gordon, C.A.; Cai, P.; Gobert, G.N.; Duke, M.; Williams, G.M.; McManus, D.P. A novel duplex ddPCR assay for the diagnosis of schistosomiasis japonica: Proof of concept in an experimental mouse model. *Parasitology* **2017**, *144*, 1005–1015. [CrossRef] [PubMed]

154. Weerakoon, K.G.; Gordon, C.A.; Gobert, G.N.; Cai, P.; McManus, D.P. Optimisation of a droplet digital PCR assay for the diagnosis of *Schistosoma japonicum* infection: A duplex approach with DNA binding dye chemistry. *J. Microbiol. Methods* **2016**, *125*, 19–27. [CrossRef] [PubMed]

155. WHO. *KITS*; WHO: Geneva, Switzerland, 1998.

156. Pilotte, N.; Papaiakovou, M.; Grant, J.R.; Bierwert, L.A.; Llewellyn, S.; McCarthy, J.S.; Williams, S.A. Improved PCR-based detection of soil transmitted helminth infections using a next-generation sequencing approach to assay design. *PLoS Negl. Trop. Dis.* **2016**, *10*, e0004578. [CrossRef] [PubMed]

157. Belizario, V.Y.; Totanes, F.I.; de Leon, W.U.; Matias, K.M. School-based control of soil-transmitted helminthiasis in western Visayas, Philippines. *Southeast Asian J. Trop. Med. Public Health* **2014**, *45*, 556–567. [PubMed]

158. Insetta, E.R.; Soriano, A.J.; Totanes, F.I.; Macatangay, B.J.; Belizario, V.Y., Jr. Fear of birth defects is a major barrier to soil-transmitted helminth treatment (STH) for pregnant women in the Philippines. *PLoS ONE* **2014**, *9*, e85992. [CrossRef] [PubMed]

159. Ross, A.; Olveda, R.; Olveda, D.; Harn, D.; Gray, D.J.; McManus, D.P.; Tallo, V.; Chau, T.; Williams, G. Can mass drug administration lead to the sustainable control of schistosomiasis in the Philippines? *J. Infect. Dis.* **2015**, *211*, 283–289. [CrossRef] [PubMed]

160. Sanza, M.; Totanes, F.I.; Chua, P.L.; Belizario, V.Y., Jr. Monitoring the impact of a mebendazole mass drug administration initiative for soil-transmitted helminthiasis (STH) control in the Western Visayas Region of the Philippines from 2007 through 2011. *Acta Trop.* **2013**, *127*, 112–117. [CrossRef] [PubMed]

161. Geerts, S.; Gryseels, B. Drug resistance in human helminths: Current situation and lessons from livestock. *Clin. Microbiol. Rev.* **2000**, *13*, 207–222. [CrossRef] [PubMed]

162. WHO. *Monitoring Anthelmintic Efficacy for Soil Transmitted Helminths (STH)*; WHO: Geneva, Switzerland, 2008.

163. WHO. Soil-transmitted helminthiases: Number of children treated in 2014. *Wkly. Epidemiol. Rec.* **2015**, *90*, 701–712.

164. Gyorkos, T.W.; MacLean, J.D.; Viens, P.; Chheang, C.; Kokoskin-Nelson, E. Intestinal parasite infection in the Kampuchean refugee population 6 years after resettlement in Canada. *J. Infect. Dis.* **1992**, *166*, 413–417. [CrossRef] [PubMed]

165. Zaha, O.; Hirata, T.; Kinjo, F.; Saito, A.; Fukuhara, H. Efficacy of ivermectin for chronic strongyloidiasis: Two single doses given 2 weeks apart. *J. Infect. Chemother.* **2002**, *8*, 94–98. [CrossRef] [PubMed]

166. Hu, Y.; Miller, M.M.; Derman, A.I.; Ellis, B.L.; Monnerat, R.G.; Pogliano, J.; Aroian, R.V. *Bacillus subtilis* strain engineered for treatment of soil-transmitted helminth diseases. *Appl. Environ. Microbiol.* **2013**, *79*, 5527–5532. [CrossRef] [PubMed]

167. Osei-Atweneboana, M.Y.; Awadzi, K.; Attah, S.K.; Boakye, D.A.; Gyapong, J.O.; Prichard, R.K. Phenotypic evidence of emerging ivermectin resistance in *Onchocerca volvulus*. *PLoS Negl. Trop. Dis.* **2011**, *5*, e998. [CrossRef] [PubMed]

168. Diawara, A.; Schwenkenbecher, J.M.; Kaplan, R.M.; Prichard, R.K. Molecular and biological diagnostic tests for monitoring benzimidazole resistance in human soil-transmitted helminths. *Am. J. Trop. Med. Hyg.* **2013**, *88*, 1052–1061. [CrossRef] [PubMed]

169. Brockwell, Y.M.; Elliott, T.P.; Anderson, G.R.; Stanton, R.; Spithill, T.W.; Sangster, N.C. Confirmation of *Fasciola hepatica* resistant to triclabendazole in naturally infected Australian beef and dairy cattle. *Int. J. Parasitol. Drugs Drug Resist.* **2014**, *4*, 48–54. [CrossRef] [PubMed]

170. Wolstenholme, A.J.; Fairweather, I.; Prichard, R.; von Samson-Himmelstjerna, G.; Sangster, N.C. Drug resistance in veterinary helminths. *Trends Parasitol.* **2004**, *20*, 469–476. [CrossRef] [PubMed]

171. Vercruysse, J.; Albonico, M.; Behnke, J.M.; Kotze, A.C.; Prichard, R.K.; McCarthy, J.S.; Montresor, A.; Levecke, B. Is anthelmintic resistance a concern for the control of human soil-transmitted helminths? *Int. J. Parasitol. Drugs Drug Resist.* **2011**, *1*, 14–27. [CrossRef] [PubMed]

172. Bieri, F.A.M.; Gray, D.J.P.; Williams, G.M.P.; Raso, G.P.; Li, Y.-S.P.; Yuan, L.P.; He, Y.M.P.H.; Li, R.S.B.; Guo, F.-Y.B.A.; Li, S.-M.B.A.; et al. Health-education package to prevent worm infections in Chinese schoolchildren. *N. Engl. J. Med.* **2013**, *368*, 1603–1612. [CrossRef] [PubMed]

173. McManus, D.P.; Bieri, F.A.; Li, Y.S.; Williams, G.M.; Yuan, L.P.; Henglin, Y.; Du, Z.W.; Clements, A.C.; Steinmann, P.; Raso, G.; et al. Health education and the control of intestinal worm infections in China: A new vision. *Parasit. Vectors* **2014**, *7*, 344. [CrossRef] [PubMed]

174. Clarke, N.E.; Clements, A.C.; Bryan, S.; McGown, J.; Gray, D.; Nery, S.V. Investigating the differential impact of school and community-based integrated control programmes for soil-transmitted helminths in Timor-Leste: The (S)WASH-D for Worms pilot study protocol. *Pilot Feasibility Stud.* **2016**, *2*, 69. [CrossRef] [PubMed]

175. Nery, S.V.; McCarthy, J.S.; Traub, R.; Andrews, R.M.; Black, J.A.; Gray, D.J.; Weking, E.; Atkinson, J.A.; Campbell, S.; Francis, N.; et al. A cluster-randomised controlled trial integrating a community-based water, sanitation and hygiene programme, with mass distribution of albendazole to reduce intestinal parasites in Timor-Leste: The WASH for WORMS research protocol. *Br. Med. J.* **2015**, *5*. [CrossRef] [PubMed]

176. Yap, P.; Du, Z.W.; Wu, F.W.; Jiang, J.Y.; Chen, R.; Zhou, X.N.; Hattendorf, J.; Utzinger, J.; Steinmann, P. Rapid re-infection with soil-transmitted helminths after triple-dose albendazole treatment of school-aged children in Yunnan, People's Republic of China. *Am. J. Trop. Med. Hyg.* **2013**, *89*, 23–31. [CrossRef] [PubMed]

177. Mascarini-Serra, L. Prevention of soil-transmitted helminth infection. *J. Glob. Infect. Dis.* **2011**, *3*, 175–182. [CrossRef] [PubMed]

178. Hotez, P.J.; Bundy, D.A.P.; Beegle, K.; Brooker, S.; Drake, L.; de Silva, N.; Montresor, A.; Engels, D.; Jukes, M.; Chitsulo, L.; et al. Helminth infections: soil-transmitted helminth infections and schistosomiasis. In *Disease Control Priorities in Developing Countries*; Jamison, D.T., Breman, J.G., Measham, A.R., Alleyne, G., Claeson, M., Evans, D.B., Jha, P., Mills, A., Musgrove, P., Eds.; World Bank, The International Bank for Reconstruction and Development/The World Bank Group: Washington, DC, USA, 2006.

179. Conlan, J.V.; Sripa, B.; Attwood, S.; Newton, P.N. A review of parasitic zoonoses in a changing Southeast Asia. *Vet. Parasitol.* **2011**, *182*, 22–40. [CrossRef] [PubMed]

180. Overgaauw, P.A.M.; van Zutphen, L.; Hoek, D.; Yaya, F.O.; Roelfsema, J.; Pinelli, E.; van Knapen, F.; Kortbeek, L.M. Zoonotic parasites in fecal samples and fur from dogs and cats in The Netherlands. *Vet. Parasitol.* **2009**, *163*, 115–122. [CrossRef] [PubMed]

181. Overgaauw, P.A.M.; van Knapen, F. Veterinary and public health aspects of *Toxocara* spp. *Vet. Parasitol.* **2013**, *193*, 398–403. [CrossRef] [PubMed]

182. Simonato, G.; Frangipane di Regalbono, A.; Cassini, R.; Traversa, D.; Beraldo, P.; Tessarin, C.; Pietrobelli, M. Copromicroscopic and molecular investigations on intestinal parasites in kenneled dogs. *Parasitol. Res.* **2015**, *114*, 1963–1970. [CrossRef] [PubMed]

183. Paoletti, B.; Traversa, D.; Iorio, R.; De Berardinis, A.; Bartolini, R.; Salini, R.; Di Cesare, A. Zoonotic parasites in feces and fur of stray and private dogs from Italy. *Parasitol. Res.* **2015**. [CrossRef] [PubMed]

184. Roddie, G.; Stafford, P.; Holland, C.; Wolfe, A. Contamination of dog hair with eggs of *Toxocara canis*. *Vet. Parasitol.* **2008**, *152*, 85–93. [CrossRef] [PubMed]

185. Heyworth, J.S.; Cutt, H.; Glonek, G. Does dog or cat ownership lead to increased gastroenteritis in young children in South Australia? *Epidemiol. Infect.* **2006**, *134*, 926–934. [CrossRef] [PubMed]

186. Walker, N.I.; Croese, J.; Clouston, A.D.; Parry, M.; Loukas, A.; Prociv, P. Eosinophilic enteritis in northeastern Australia. Pathology, association with *Ancylostoma caninum*, and implications. *Am. J. Surg. Pathol.* **1995**, *19*, 328–337. [CrossRef] [PubMed]

187. Croese, J.; Loukas, A.; Opdebeeck, J.; Prociv, P. Occult enteric infection by *Ancylostoma caninum*: A previously unrecognized zoonosis. *Gastroenterology* **1994**, *106*, 3–12. [CrossRef]

188. Loukas, A.; Croese, J.; Opdebeeck, J.; Prociv, P. Detection of antibodies to secretions of *Ancylostoma caninum* in human eosinophilic enteritis. *Trans. R. Soc. Trop. Med. Hyg.* **1992**, *86*, 650–653. [CrossRef]

189. Loukas, A.; Opdebeeck, J.; Croese, J.; Prociv, P. Immunologic incrimination of *Ancylostoma caninum* as a human enteric pathogen. *Am. J. Trop. Med. Hyg.* **1994**, *50*, 69–77. [CrossRef] [PubMed]

190. Prociv, P.; Croese, J. Human enteric infection with *Ancylostoma caninum*: Hookworms reappraised in the light of a 'new' zoonosis. *Acta Trop.* **1996**, *62*, 23–44. [CrossRef]

191. Prociv, P.; Croese, J. Human eosinophilic enteritis caused by dog hookworm *Ancylostoma caninum*. *Lancet* **1990**, *335*, 1299–1302. [CrossRef]

192. Croese, J.; Fairley, S.; Loukas, A.; Hack, J.; Stronach, P. A distinctive aphthous ileitis linked to *Ancylostoma caninum*. *J. Gastroenterol. Hepatol.* **1996**, *11*, 524–531. [CrossRef] [PubMed]

193. McGuinness, S.L.; Leder, K. Global burden of toxocariasis: A common neglected infection of poverty. *Curr. Trop. Med. Rep.* **2014**, *1*, 52–61. [CrossRef]

194. Le, T.H.; Anh, N.T.; Nguyen, K.T.; Nguyen, N.T.; Thuy do, T.T.; Gasser, R.B. *Toxocara malaysiensis* infection in domestic cats in Vietnam—An emerging zoonotic issue? *Infect. Genet. Evol.* **2016**, *37*, 94–98. [CrossRef] [PubMed]

195. Li, M.W.; Lin, R.Q.; Song, H.Q.; Wu, X.Y.; Zhu, X.Q. The complete mitochondrial genomes for three *Toxocara* species of human and animal health significance. *BMC Genom.* **2008**, *9*, 224. [CrossRef] [PubMed]

196. Mohd Zain, S.N.; Rahman, R.; Lewis, J.W. Stray animal and human defecation as sources of soil-transmitted helminth eggs in playgrounds of Peninsular Malaysia. *J. Helminthol.* **2015**, *89*, 740–747. [CrossRef] [PubMed]

197. Arevalo, J.F.; Espinoza, J.V.; Arevalo, F.A. Ocular toxocariasis. *J. Pediatr. Ophthalmol. Strabismus* **2013**, *50*, 76–86. [CrossRef] [PubMed]

198. Blake, R.T.; Overend, D.J. The prevalence of *Dirofilaria immitis* and other parasites in urban pound dogs in north-eastern Victoria. *Aust. Vet. J.* **1982**, *58*, 111–114. [CrossRef] [PubMed]

199. Dunsmore, J.D.; Thompson, R.C.A.; Bates, I.A. Prevalence and survival of *Toxocara canis* eggs in the urban environment of Perth, Australia. *Vet. Parasitol.* **1984**, *16*, 303–311. [CrossRef]

200. Carden, S.M.; Meusemann, R.; Walker, J.; Stawell, R.J.; MacKinnon, J.R.; Smith, D.; Stawell, A.M.; Hall, A.J. *Toxocara canis*: Egg presence in Melbourne parks and disease incidence in Victoria. *Clin. Exp. Ophthalmol.* **2003**, *31*, 143–146. [CrossRef] [PubMed]

201. Nicholas, W.L.; Stewart, A.C.; Walker, J.C. Toxocariasis: A serological survey of blood donors in the Australian Capital Territory together with observations on the risks of infection. *Trans. R. Soc. Trop. Med. Hyg.* **1986**, *80*, 217–221. [CrossRef]

202. Nejsum, P.; Bertelsen, M.F.; Betson, M.; Stothard, J.R.; Murrell, K.D. Molecular evidence for sustained transmission of zoonotic *Ascaris suum* among zoo chimpanzees (*Pan Troglodytes*). *Vet. Parasitol.* **2010**, *171*, 273–276. [CrossRef] [PubMed]

203. Zhou, C.; Li, M.; Yuan, K.; Hu, N.; Peng, W. Phylogeography of *Ascaris lumbricoides* and *A. suum* from China. *Parasitol. Res.* **2011**, *109*, 329–338. [CrossRef] [PubMed]

204. Zhou, C.; Li, M.; Yuan, K.; Deng, S.; Peng, W. Pig *Ascaris*: An important source of human ascariasis in China. *Infect. Genet. Evol.* **2012**, *12*, 1172–1177. [CrossRef] [PubMed]

205. Traub, R.J.; Robertson, I.D.; Irwin, P.J.; Mencke, N.; Thompson, R.C.A.A. Canine gastrointestinal parasitic zoonoses in India. *Trends Parasitol.* **2005**, *21*, 42–48. [CrossRef] [PubMed]

206. Controlling worms in pigs. Available online: https://www.daf.qld.gov.au/animal-industries/pigs/pig-health-and-diseases/disease-prevention/controlling-worms-in-pigs (accessed on 11 October 2017).

207. Graves, S. Human infection with '*Ascaris suum*' in Tasmania? *Ann. ACTM* **2005**, *6*, 16.

208. Steinmann, P.; Yap, P.; Utzinger, J.; Du, Z.W.; Jiang, J.Y.; Chen, R.; Wu, F.W.; Chen, J.X.; Zhou, H.; Zhou, X.N. Control of soil-transmitted helminthiasis in Yunnan province, People's Republic of China: Experiences and lessons from a 5-year multi-intervention trial. *Acta Trop.* **2015**, *141*, 271–280. [CrossRef] [PubMed]

209. Tang, N.; Luo, N.J. A cross-sectional study of intestinal parasitic infections in a rural district of west China. *Can. J. Infect. Dis.* **2003**, *14*, 159–162. [CrossRef] [PubMed]

210. Yang, G.-J.; Liu, L.; Zhu, H.-R.; Griffiths, S.M.; Tanner, M.; Bergquist, R.; Utzinger, J.; Zhou, X.-N. China's sustained drive to eliminate neglected tropical diseases. *Lancet Infect. Dis.* **2014**, *14*, 881–892. [CrossRef]

211. Dunn, J.J.; Columbus, S.T.; Aldeen, W.E.; Davis, M.; Carroll, K.C. *Trichuris vulpis* recovered from a patient with chronic diarrhea and five dogs. *J. Clin. Microbiol.* **2002**, *40*, 2703–2704. [CrossRef] [PubMed]

212. Ravasi, D.F.; O'Riain, M.J.; Davids, F.; Illing, N. Phylogenetic evidence that two distinct *Trichuris* genotypes infect both humans and non-human primates. *PLoS ONE* **2012**, *7*, e44187. [CrossRef] [PubMed]

213. Hawash, M.B.F.; Andersen, L.O.; Gasser, R.B.; Stensvold, C.R.; Nejsum, P. Mitochondrial genome analyses suggest multiple *Trichuris* species in humans, baboons, and pigs from different geographical regions. *PLoS Negl. Trop. Dis.* **2015**, *9*, e0004059. [CrossRef] [PubMed]

214. Liu, G.H.; Zhou, W.; Nisbet, A.J.; Xu, M.J.; Zhou, D.H.; Zhao, G.H.; Wang, S.K.; Song, H.Q.; Lin, R.Q.; Zhu, X.Q. Characterization of *Trichuris trichiura* from humans and *T. suis* from pigs in China using internal transcribed spacers of nuclear ribosomal DNA. *J. Helminthol.* **2014**, *88*, 64–68. [CrossRef] [PubMed]

215. Liu, G.-H.; Gasser, R.B.; Su, A.; Nejsum, P.; Peng, L.; Lin, R.-Q.; Li, M.-W.; Xu, M.-J.; Zhu, X.-Q. Clear genetic distinctiveness between human- and pig-derived *Trichuris* based on analyses of mitochondrial datasets. *PLoS Negl. Trop. Dis.* **2012**, *6*, e1539. [CrossRef] [PubMed]

216. Bager, P.; Kapel, C.; Roepstorff, A.; Thamsborg, S.; Arnved, J.; Rønborg, S.; Kristensen, B.; Poulsen, L.K.; Wohlfahrt, J.; Melbye, M. Symptoms after ingestion of pig whipworm *Trichuris suis* eggs in a randomized placebo-controlled double-blind clinical trial. *PLoS ONE* **2011**, *6*, e22346. [CrossRef] [PubMed]

217. Helmby, H. Human helminth therapy to treat inflammatory disorders-where do we stand? *BMC Immunol.* **2015**, *16*, 12. [CrossRef] [PubMed]

218. Jackson, J.A.; Friberg, I.M.; Little, S.; Bradley, J.E. Review series on helminths, immune modulation and the hygiene hypothesis: Immunity against helminths and immunological phenomena in modern human populations: Coevolutionary legacies? *Immunology* **2009**, *126*, 18–27. [CrossRef] [PubMed]

219. Hewitson, J.P.; Grainger, J.R.; Maizels, R.M. Helminth immunoregulation: The role of parasite secreted proteins in modulating host immunity. *Mol. Biochem. Parasitol.* **2009**, *167*, 1–11. [CrossRef] [PubMed]

220. Feary, J.R.; Venn, A.J.; Mortimer, K.; Brown, A.P.; Hooi, D.; Falcone, F.H.; Pritchard, D.I.; Britton, J.R. Experimental hookworm infection: A randomized placebo-controlled trial in asthma. *Clin. Exp. Allergy* **2010**, *40*, 299–306. [CrossRef] [PubMed]

221. TOS. Available online: http://wormswell.com/science-research (accessed on 17 July 2017).

222. The helminthic therapy. Available online: https://tanawisa.com/ (accessed on 17 July 2017).

223. Turner, K.J.; Quinn, E.H.; Anderson, H.R. Regulation of asthma by intestinal parasites. Investigation of possible mechanisms. *Immunology* **1978**, *35*, 281–288. [PubMed]

224. Mpairwe, H.; Ndibazza, J.; Webb, E.L.; Nampijja, M.; Muhangi, L.; Apule, B.; Lule, S.; Akurut, H.; Kizito, D.; Kakande, M.; et al. Maternal hookworm modifies risk factors for childhood eczema: Results from a birth cohort in Uganda. *Pediatr. Allergy Immunol.* **2014**, *25*, 481–488. [CrossRef] [PubMed]

225. McSorley, H.J.; Gaze, S.; Daveson, J.; Jones, D.; Anderson, R.P.; Clouston, A.; Ruyssers, N.E.; Speare, R.; McCarthy, J.S.; Engwerda, C.R.; et al. Suppression of inflammatory immune responses in celiac disease by experimental hookworm infection. *PLoS ONE* **2011**, *6*, e24092. [CrossRef] [PubMed]

226. Daveson, A.J.; Jones, D.M.; Gaze, S.; McSorley, H.; Clouston, A.; Pascoe, A.; Cooke, S.; Speare, R.; Macdonald, G.A.; Anderson, R.; et al. Effect of hookworm infection on wheat challenge in celiac disease—A randomised double-blinded placebo controlled trial. *PLoS ONE* **2011**, *6*, e17366. [CrossRef] [PubMed]

227. Giacomin, P.; Zakrzewski, M.; Jenkins, T.P.; Su, X.; Al-Hallaf, R.; Croese, J.; de Vries, S.; Grant, A.; Mitreva, M.; Loukas, A.; et al. Changes in duodenal tissue-associated microbiota following hookworm infection and consecutive gluten challenges in humans with coeliac disease. *Sci. Rep.* **2016**, *6*, 36797. [CrossRef] [PubMed]

228. Cooper, P.; Walker, A.W.; Reyes, J.; Chico, M.; Salter, S.J.; Vaca, M.; Parkhill, J. Patent human infections with the whipworm, *Trichuris trichiura*, are not associated with alterations in the faecal microbiota. *PLoS ONE* **2013**, *8*, e76573. [CrossRef] [PubMed]

229. Williams, A.R.; Dige, A.; Rasmussen, T.K.; Hvas, C.L.; Dahlerup, J.F.; Iversen, L.; Stensvold, C.R.; Agnholt, J.; Nejsum, P. Immune responses and parasitological observations induced during probiotic treatment with medicinal *Trichuris suis* ova in a healthy volunteer. *Immunol. Lett.* **2017**, *188*, 32–37. [CrossRef] [PubMed]

230. Ruyssers, N.E.; De Winter, B.Y.; De Man, J.G.; Loukas, A.; Herman, A.G.; Pelckmans, P.A.; Moreels, T.G. Worms and the treatment of inflammatory bowel disease: Are molecules the answer? *Clin. Dev. Immunol.* **2008**, *2008*, 567314. [CrossRef] [PubMed]

231. Giacomin, P.; Croese, J.; Krause, L.; Loukas, A.; Cantacessi, C. Suppression of inflammation by helminths: A role for the gut microbiota? *Philos. Trans. R. Soc. Lond. B. Biol. Sci.* **2015**, *370*. [CrossRef] [PubMed]

232. Hays, R.; Esterman, A.; McDermott, R. Control of chronic *Strongyloides stercoralis* infection in an endemic community may be possible by pharmacological means alone: Results of a three-year cohort study. *PLoS Negl. Trop. Dis.* **2017**, *11*, e0005825. [CrossRef] [PubMed]

233. Flannery, G.; White, N. *Immunological Parameters in Northeast Arnhem Land Aborigines: Consequences of Changing Settlement and Lifestyles*; Cambridge University Press: New York, NY, USA, 1993; pp. 202–220.

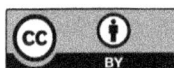

Tropical Medicine and
Infectious Disease

MDPI

Article

Trends in *Strongyloides stercoralis* Faecal Larvae Detections in the Northern Territory, Australia: 2002 to 2012

Johanna K. Mayer-Coverdale [1], Amy Crowe [2], Pamela Smith [3] and Robert W. Baird [3],*

[1] Department of Microbiology, Pathology Queensland, Royal Brisbane and Women's Hospital, Queensland 4001, Australia; johannak.mayer@gmail.com
[2] Infectious Diseases Physician, St Vincent's Hospital, 41 Victoria Pde, Fitzroy 3065, Australia; amy.crowe@svha.org.au
[3] Microbiology, Territory Pathology, Royal Darwin Hospital, Tiwi 0810, Australia; pam.smith@nt.gov.au
* Correspondence: rob.baird@nt.gov.au; Tel.: +61-8-8922-8888

Academic Editors: Patricia Graves and Peter Leggat
Received: 19 April 2017; Accepted: 13 June 2017; Published: 19 June 2017

Abstract: *Strongyloides stercoralis* is a soil-transmitted helminth (STH) endemic to tropical and subtropical areas. We reviewed the temporal detection trends in patients with *S. stercoralis* larvae present in faecal samples, in Northern Territory (NT) Government Health facilities, between 2002 and 2012. This was a retrospective observational study of consecutive patients with microbiologically confirmed detection of *S. stercoralis* in faeces. The presence of anaemia, eosinophilia, polyparasitism, and geographic and demographic data, were included in the assessment. *S. stercoralis* larvae were present in 389 of 22,892 faecal samples (1.7%) collected across the NT over 11 years, examined by microscopy after formol ethyl acetate concentration. 97.7% of detections were in Indigenous patients. Detections, by number, occurred in a biphasic age distribution. Detections per number of faecal samples collected, were highest in the 0–5 year age group. Anaemia was present in 44.8%, and eosinophilia in 49.9% of patients. Eosinophilia was present in 65.5% of the ≤5 age group, compared to 40.8% of >5 year age ($p < 0.0001$). Polyparasitism was present in 31.4% of patients. There was an overall downward trend in larvae detections from 2.64% to 0.99% detections/number of faecal samples year between 2002 and 2012, consistent with the trends observed for other local STHs. *S. stercoralis* remains an important NT-wide pathogen.

Keywords: Strongyloides; anaemia; eosinophilia; polyparasitism; indigenous; Northern Territory; Australia

---

1. Introduction

Strongyloides stercoralis is a soil-transmitted helminth (STH) endemic to tropical and subtropical regions around the world. There are very wide estimates, between 3 and 100 million people [1], of the number of persons infected with *S. stercoralis* globally, because the true incidence is difficult to determine as many infections occur in regions with economic and health hardware disadvantage, and poor access to laboratory diagnostic services.

S. stercoralis infection has been estimated to occur disproportionately in Australian Indigenous people living in the northern parts of Australia, not only compared to the rest of Australia, but also to ecologically similar regions around the world [2–6]. Indigenous Australians experience substantially poorer health, social, and economic outcomes compared to other Australians, including overcrowding and poor sanitary conditions [7], both of which are of importance in the transmission of *S. stercoralis*. The Northern Territory (NT) is a large but sparsely populated area covering 1.5 million square kilometers, with numerous remote Indigenous communities. Cases of intestinal obstruction complicating *S. stercoralis* infection in children have been documented in the NT since the 1970s [2], and a 1993 study documented *S. stercoralis* endemicity in Indigenous patients over a 12-month period [3]. An association between HTLV-1 and *S. stercoralis* has been documented in central Australia where HTLV-1 is endemic [4]. *S. stercoralis* detections have been described across the tropical and subtropical areas of Western Australia and Queensland, including to latitudes below the Tropic of Capricorn (latitude 23° S) [5,6].

S. *stercoralis* has a complex life cycle [8]. The most common way of becoming infected is by direct contact with soil, as the filariform larvae penetrate the host skin from soil that is contaminated with *S. stercoralis* larvae. High risk activities include walking with bare feet, direct contact with human waste or sewage, as well as occupations such as farming. The larvae migrate via the venous circulation to the lungs, where they ascend the bronchial tree and eventually are swallowed, thus entering the digestive tract. Once established in the small bowel they become adults. The female worms produce eggs by parthenogenesis, which subsequently hatch in the small bowel, as rhabditiform larvae, (non-infectious), then are deposited, and develop to filariform (infectious) larvae in the soil over several days. Larvae that are not passed in the faeces have the ability to develop in the bowel to filariform larvae, that can either penetrate the bowel wall directly, or the perianal mucosa repeating the infective cycle potentially indefinitely. This process of auto-infection is characteristic of *S. stercoralis* and can lead to hyperinfection even in individuals who have not been in endemic areas for decades. Clinically, strongyloidiasis may present as a range of syndromes, ranging from asymptomatic or mild abdominal discomfort, to Crohn's-like colitis, primarily pulmonary symptoms (Loeffler's syndrome), cutaneous larva currens, and disseminated infection with high associated mortality [9]. The latter is particularly associated with immunosuppressed patients, especially those taking corticosteroids. The ability to establish ongoing, potentially life-long infection coupled with the risk of dissemination that is associated with high mortality makes screening, and in some instances empiric treatment, for *S. stercoralis* infection in people who are about to undergo immunosuppression essential, not only in endemic areas, but also in selected populations such as migrants from endemic regions and refugees [10].

Our aim was to describe the temporal trends in *S. stercoralis* larvae detection in faecal samples collected in NT Government Health facilities over a period of 11 years, and review associated demographic and laboratory features, in this population.

2. Results

Between 2002 and 2012, 22,892 faecal samples were assessed for ova, cysts, and parasites (OCP) across NT Government Health facilities. The number of annual faecal microscopy samples examined remained relatively constant throughout this time period, approximately 2000 samples/year, though 2578 and 2919 faecal microscopy and concentrates were examined in 2011 and 2012, respectively. *S. stercoralis* larvae were detected in 389 (1.7%) of all faecal samples. Eleven patients had more than one episode, with one patient having three documented episodes.

Demographic and laboratory characteristics are summarised in Table 1.

Overall 381 (97.7%) patients were Indigenous, and 164 (42.2%) were five years old or younger. In the ≤5 year-old group, 163 (99.4%) patients were Indigenous, while in the >5 year-old group 218 (96.9%) were Indigenous. In total, 216 (55.5%) patients were male and 173 (44.5%) female. The male to female ratio in the ≤5 year-old group was 79 (48.2%) male, and 85 (51.8%) female compared to 137 (60.9%) and 88 (39.1%) respectively in the older group.

Figure 1 is a cumulative graph of 11 years data presenting cases, and cases by number of faecal specimens examined. The age distribution of actual cases was biphasic (Figure 1), with the highest number of detections occurring in patients less than five years of age, with a peak in the second year of life, and a second smaller peak in the 35–50-year-old group. However, reviewing larvae detections to number of faecal specimens examined revealed the peak detection age in the 4–5 year-old age group.

Cases were detected from across the NT, with the highest detection rates coming from West Arnhem, Tiwi Islands, and the Katherine regions (Figure 2).

Table 1. Demographic and laboratory parameters of patients with *S. stercoralis* larvae detection in the Northern Territory, 2002 to 2012.

Parameter		≤ 5 Years Old (%)	> 5 Years Old (%)	All Ages (%)	*p*-Value
Number [1]		164 (42.2)	224 (57.6)	389 (100)	
Sex					
	Male	79 (48.2)	137 (60.9)	216 (55.5)	0.012
	Female	85 (51.8)	88 (39.1)	173 (44.5)	
Indigenous status					
	Indigenous	163 (99.4)	218 (96.9)	381 (97.7)	<0.0001
	Non-indigenous	1 (0.6)	7 (3.1)	8 (2.3)	
Laboratory parameters [2]					
Median haemoglobin		114 (IQR 105–122)	111 (IQR 91–134)	113 (IQR 97.8–127)	0.48
Anaemia [3]		58 (38.6)	106 (49.1)	164 (44.8)	0.04
Median eosinophil count		1 (IQR 0.2–2.4)	0.3 (IQR 0.1–0.8)	0.5 (IQR 0.1–1.3)	<0.0001
Eosinophilia [4]		95 (65.5)	89 (40.8)	184 (49.9)	<0.0001
Polyparasitism [5]		61 (37.2)	61 (27.1)	122 (31.4)	0.03
Other intestinal helminths		13 (7.9)	29 (12.9)	42 (10.8)	0.12
Hymenolepis nana		18 (11)	4 (1.8)	22 (5.6)	<0.001
Other (eg. Protozoa)		40 (24.4)	36 (16)	76 (33.8)	0.04

[1] One Indigenous male, did not have age or haematological data. [2] 23 patients (4.3%) had no haematological data, of these 14 were ≤ 5 years old. An additional 6 patients had no data for eosinophilia (5.4%), 5 were ≤ 5 years old. [3] Anaemia: Haemoglobin ≤110 g/L. [4] Eosinophilia: eosinophils > 0.5×10^9 /L. [5] Intestinal helminths were hookworm and *T. trichiura*. *Ascaris* species were not detected.

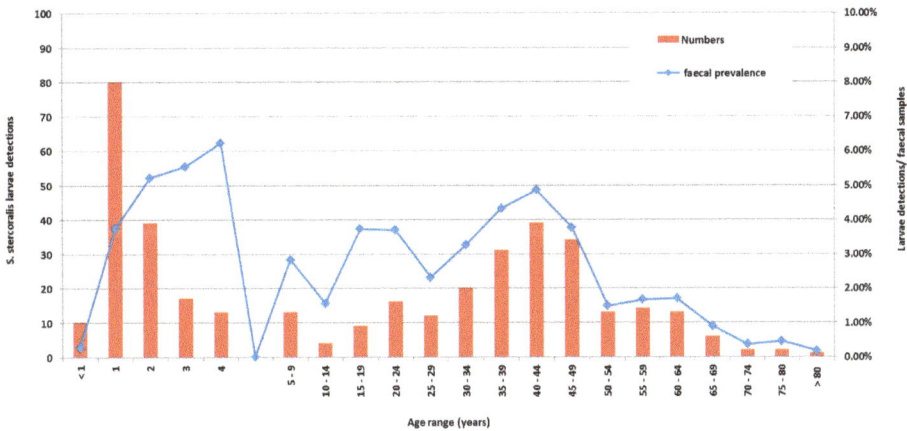

Figure 1. *S. stercoralis* larvae detections by age and diagnostic prevalence in the Northern Territory, 2002–2012.

The lowest detection rates were seen in the Darwin and the Gulf country, east of Katherine area. Anaemia was present in 164 (44.8%) of patients, with a median Hb of 113 g/L (interquartile range (IQR) 97.8–127) across both groups, and 114 g/L (IQR 105–122) and 111 g/L (IQR 91–134) in the younger and older groups respectively (*p* = 0.48). Anaemia was present in 38.6% of the younger group, compared to 49.1% in the greater than five-year-old cohort (*p* = 0.04). 184 (49.9%) patients had eosinophilia, with a median eosinophil count of 0.5×10^9/L across both groups. Eosinophilia was more common in the younger group: 65.5% compared to 40.8% ($p < 0.0001$), and the median eosinophil count in ≤ 5 year-old cohort was 1×10^9/L (Figure 3), while in >5 year-old group the median was 0.3×10^9/L ($p < 0.001$).

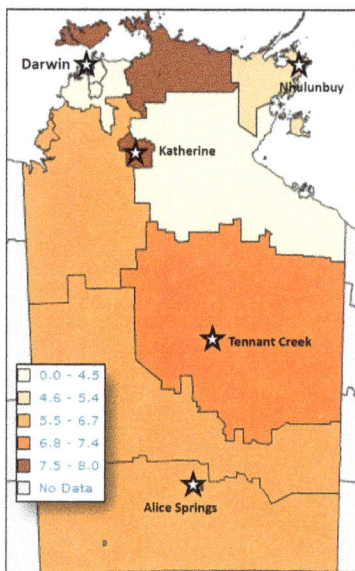

Figure 2. Geographic distribution of *S. stercoralis* larvae detection from patients in Northern Territory public healthcare facilities by geographic area of residence from 2002 to 2012. Prevalence figures are *S. stercoralis* larvae diagnostic detections in public health laboratories/10,000 Indigenous population/year.

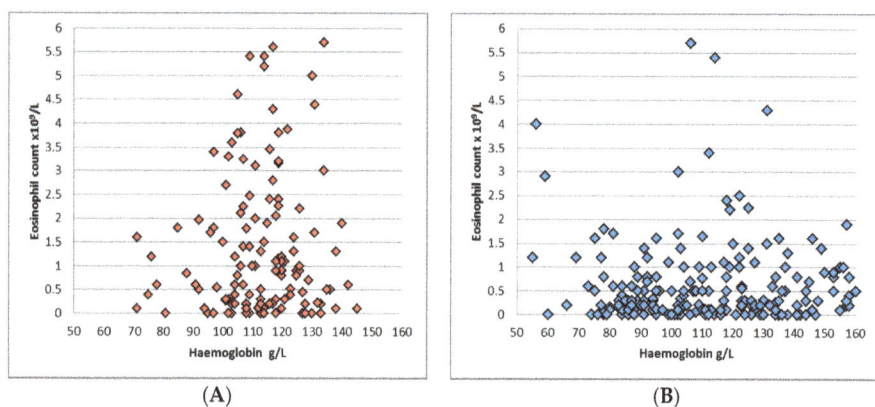

Figure 3. Distribution of contemporaneous haemoglobin and eosinophil counts in patients with *S. stercoralis* larvae detection. (**A**) Patients five-years-old and under (red diamonds represent the individual data points). (**B**) Patients aged older than five years of age (blue diamonds represent individual data points).

A normal haemoglobin and normal eosinophil count was present in 19% of the younger group, and 29.6% of the older cohort. The combination of anaemia and eosinophilia was present in 22% of the ≤5 year-old age group, compared to 18% in the older cohort.

Polyparasitism was observed in 122 (31.4%) of all patients with *S. stercoralis* larvae detections. In the younger cohort 61 (37.2%) patients had at least one other parasite identified in their faecal specimen, while in the older group 61 (27.1%) of patients had at least one other parasite identified. Overall, 42 (10.8%) patients had co-infection with at least one other STH, 22 (5.6%) also had *Hymenolepis nana* identified, while 76 (33.8%) had co-infection with intestinal protozoa.

Over the 11 years of this study, there was a downward trend in *S. stercoralis* detections from 2.64% (in 2012) to 0.99% (in 2012) larvae detections/stool specimens examined. (Figure 4), mirroring the results for hookworm and *T. trichiura* over the same time period from the same cohort. This downward trend in detections was due to a three-fold reduction in detections in children under the age of five, while detection of larvae in patients over the age of five, remained relatively constant. 10,208 samples from children less than five were examined during this time period, with a median 882 samples/year (IQR 883–1003); with no significant variation in faecal numbers during the study period to account for the three-fold reduction.

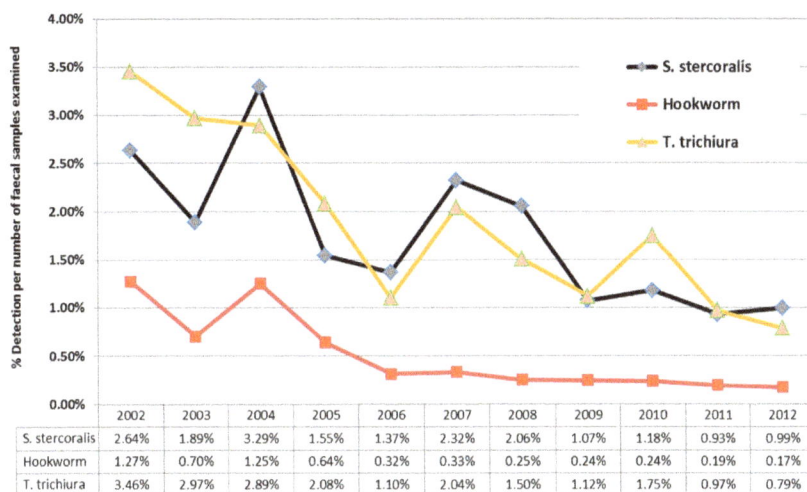

	2002	2003	2004	2005	2006	2007	2008	2009	2010	2011	2012
S. stercoralis	2.64%	1.89%	3.29%	1.55%	1.37%	2.32%	2.06%	1.07%	1.18%	0.93%	0.99%
Hookworm	1.27%	0.70%	1.25%	0.64%	0.32%	0.33%	0.25%	0.24%	0.24%	0.19%	0.17%
T. trichiura	3.46%	2.97%	2.89%	2.08%	1.10%	2.04%	1.50%	1.12%	1.75%	0.97%	0.79%

Figure 4. Comparative yearly detection of soil-transmitted helminths in the Northern Territory public laboratories, 2002 to 2012, by yearly diagnostic prevalence.

3. Discussion

The main findings of this study include: (i) the declining rate of *S. stercoralis* detection over the 11 years of this study, which mirrors the previously noted decline of two other helminths, namely, hookworm, [11] and whipworm [12]; (ii) the biphasic age distribution of the patients with larvae detection; and (iii) *S. stercoralis* infections' poor correlation with the presence of eosinophilia, particularly in detections in patients over the age of five, where eosinophilia was present in only 40.8% of patients.

Our findings are consistent with other studies of STH detection in the same time period [11,12] from the same cohort, revealing a declining detection rate in the NT. Two additional factors, possibly influencing the rates of detection of STHs in NT health care facilities have to be considered before definitely attributing the reduction to a community-wide decline in helminth infections. Firstly, hookworm has been targeted by an Indigenous community children's deworming program (CCDP) in the NT since 1995, which administers single-dose albendazole to children aged 6 months to 16 years, twice a year [11]. This is a lower albendazole dose than current recommended for *S. stercoralis* treatment therapy, but may have a partial effect. The Central Australian Rural Practitioners Association (CARPA) [13] currently recommends for *S. stercoralis* therapy: albendazole daily for three days (children ≤5 years of age), or ivermectin, for children >5 years and adults. The albendazole given as part of the CCDP may still have some effect, as noted by decreases in the detection of whipworm [12] in the same population. Dwarf tapeworm (*Hymenolepis nana*), which is common, and not susceptible to albendazole, has not shown a temporal decrease in detection in the NT [14], from the same cohort, during this time period, suggesting the CCDP may possibly be associated with some additional STH reductions outside the targeted hookworm-infected population. Secondly, hospital paediatric admissions for diarrhea have reduced Australia-wide, since the introduction of rotavirus vaccine in 2006 [15]. This may have led to a decrease in detection of asymptomatic *S. stercoralis* infection in patients admitted with acute diarrhoeal diseases. However, the decreasing trend may reflect some improvement in socio-economic and sanitary circumstances, but this is speculative until formal prevalence studies are temporally conducted in a cross-section of the many remote communities spread across the 1.5 million square kilometers of the Northern Territory.

The biphasic age distribution of patients in raw detection numbers with a secondary age peak between 35 and 50 years of age, with a male predominance across the NT, is quite different to the pattern observed with whipworm [12] in the NT from the same cohort, where conversely, women had a statistically significant higher proportion of infections. It was postulated that adult women have higher rates of infection because they care for and live in closer proximity to infected children who contaminate the nearby environment. The adult male and female population is outside the target group for CCDP, so these infections detections do represent continuing NT wide endemic disease.

This study used a standard widely-used concentration method to detect *S. stercoralis* faecal larvae as the diagnostic, allowing the demographic and laboratory parameters in patients with current *S. stercoralis* infection to be accurately correlated with actual infection, rather than implied from serological results, that can remain positive after the infection is cleared [16]. The gold standard for the diagnosis of *S. stercoralis* remains serial stool examination [17]. However, traditional stool examinations are insensitive, and require up to seven stool exams to reach a sensitivity of 100%. Specialized stool exams include Harada-Mori filter paper culture, quantitative acetate concentration technique, and nutrient agar plate cultures [17]. Detection by nucleic acid amplification of faecal strongyloides DNA, is in development, but has not as yet been demonstrated to be superior to traditional methods for *S. stercoralis* infection [18,19] and is not yet widely available.

Of note in our study was the significant difference in eosinophilia observed between the ≤5 year-old group and the >5 year-old group. This observation supports local NT and Australia-wide guidelines endorsing ivermectin prophylaxis for all Indigenous adults undergoing immunosuppression, rather than just those with eosinophilia. Eosinophilia could also be more common in the younger age group related to factors such as more recent infection, presence of other nematodes or to a lesser extent, the cestode, *H. nana*. Our study emphasises that the presence or absence of eosinophilia is not an adequate proxy test for *S stercoralis* infection in a community where the infection is prevalent, particularly in patients over the age of five years. This finding supports an earlier study where *S. stercoralis* serology results and the presence of eosinophilia, were found to correlate poorly [20] though the correlation in patients with diabetes was somewhat better. The higher rates of anaemia, we noted in the Indigenous older age group has been documented previously, as anaemia is highly prevalent in Indigenous communities. A study in an Aboriginal community of Western Australia identified anaemia among 55% of women and 18% of men [21], the causes being multifactorial, and often associated with other comorbidities, including social disadvantage [22].

Our retrospective study has several limitations and several potential biases that require consideration when interpreting this data. This was not a formal prevalence study, as systematic sampling from individual communities was not undertaken, so the actual prevalence rates are undoubtedly much higher than the laboratory microscopically-diagnosed rates found in our study population. The study population mainly reflected inpatients of NT Government health facilities, reflecting a selection bias towards patients with acute illness and comorbid conditions. Bias may have been introduced in regards to Indigenous status (as Indigenous patients are over-represented amongst admissions to NT Health Care facilities) and the bias towards inclusion of hospitalised patients may have resulted in an inflated estimate of comorbid anaemia and co-infection. Reduced recovery of parasites due to delays incurred by transport of specimens to the laboratory from remote locations, and use of routine laboratory methods rather than specialised enrichment techniques, will have led to an underestimate of the actual number of infections.

The main findings of this study of *S. stercoralis* larvae detections from NT Government health care facilities include: detections occur almost exclusively from Indigenous patients, across the entire NT; the detection of larvae in all age groups, the geographic distribution of larvae detection, and the lack of active infections being associated with eosinophilia. This last finding has important implications for patients receiving immunosuppressive therapy and their need for prophylactic *S. stercoralis* therapy. The temporal trend over the 11 years of this study, reveals declining rates of *S. stercoralis* detection, which mirrors that of the other helminths, whipworm, and hookworm, though all remain endemic in the NT, and remain markers of social disadvantage.

4. Materials and Methods

We conducted a retrospective observational review of microbiologically detected *S. stercoralis* larvae in faecal samples collected at NT Government Health facilities between 2002 and 2012 inclusive. Ethical approval for the study was obtained from both the Top End HREC-2013-1978 and Central Australian ethics committees, HREC-14-267. Cases were identified from the NT government pathology laboratory information system, Labtrak (Intersystems), which covers all NT Government Health facilities, including 5 hospitals, 2 correctional centres, and over 50 remote clinics. Previous STH studies have shown the NT public laboratories identified 94% of all documented STHs, as compared to 6% from other pathology providers, during this time period [11]. Given the intermittent shedding of *S. stercoralis* larvae, all faecal microscopy specimens (including second and third samples) were included in the analysis, but only one episode of larvae detection was recorded, even if multiple positive larvae detections were recorded in an individual episode of hospitalisation. Repeated episodes in a single patient were counted, if the temporal spacing was greater than six months. The episodes were linked to NT government electronic databases via medical record number to obtain data on age, sex, Indigenous status, geographic residence, haemoglobin level, and eosinophil count. Anaemia was defined as a haemoglobin <110 g/L and eosinophilia as a count $\geq 0.5 \times 10^9$/L. Parasite identification was done by faecal specimen examination by wet mount microscopy followed by a formol ethyl-acetate concentration method [17]. Initially manual, the lab has also changed to use a proprietary product, namely Mini Parasep SF Faecal Concentrator (Apacor, Wolkingham, England). Local standard reporting procedures were followed. Quantitative assessment of parasite numbers was not performed. Detection of larvae allowed specific correlation of current infection with the haematological parameters, but is relatively insensitive compared to research methods [17].

5. Statistical Analysis

Data was collected in a Microsoft Excel 2010 (Microsoft Corporation, Redmond, Washington, DC, USA) database and analysed using the 'Real-statistics' plug in (Zaiontz C. 2015, www.real-statistics.com). Results are presented as medians and interquartile ranges (IQRs) for non-normally distributed parameters. Age range groups, and faecal detection rates were cumulated for presentation in Figure 1. Indigenous population data from the NT were obtained from Australian Bureau of Statistics data [23]. Bivariate analyses were performed using the Chi Square or Fisher exact test (if expected frequencies were less than 5). For non-parametric data, (median haemoglobin and eosinophil counts, as well as polyparasitism in patients above and below the age of 5 years), the Mann–Whitney *U* test was used, with *p* values of <0.05 considered significant. The age cut-off of five years was chosen based on previous studies of STH in a similar population [11].

Acknowledgments: Microbiology staff of the five public hospital laboratories of the Northern Territory for helminth identification over the 11 years of this study.

Author Contributions: J.M.-C. compiled and extracted data, and prepared the submission, A.C. wrote the ethics submissions, compiled and extracted data, and prepared the submission. P.S. supervised all the laboratory components and parasite identification, and assisted with manuscript preparation. R.B. oversaw the project, assisted with data and manuscript preparation, revisions, and aspects of the discussion.

Conflicts of Interest: The authors declare no conflict of interest.

References

1. Schar, F.; Trostdorf, U.; Giardina, F.; Khieu, V.; Muth, S.; Marti, H.; Vounatsou, P.; Odermatt, P. *Strongyloides stercoralis*: Global distribution and risk factors. *PLoS Negl. Trop. Dis.* **2013**, *7*, e2288. [CrossRef] [PubMed]
2. Walker, A.C.; Blake, G.; Downing, D. A syndrome of partial intestinal obstruction due to *Strongyloides stercoralis*. *Med. J. Aust.* **1976**, *6*, 47–48.
3. Fisher, D.; McCarry, F.; Currie, B. Strongyloidiasis in the Northern Territory. Under-recognised and under-treated. *Med. J. Aust.* **1993**, *159*, 88–90. [PubMed]
4. Einsiedel, L.J.; Pham, H.; Woodman, R.J.; Pepperill, C.; Taylor, K.A. The prevalence and clinical associations of HTLV-1 infection in a remote Indigenous community. *Med. J. Aust.* **2016**, *205*, 305–309. [CrossRef] [PubMed]
5. Holt, D.C.; McCarthy, J.S.; Carapetis, J.R. Parasitic diseases of remote Indigenous communities in Australia. *Int. J. Parasitol.* **2010**, *40*, 1119–1126. [CrossRef] [PubMed]
6. Prociv, P.; Luke, R. Observations on strongyloidiasis in Queensland aboriginal communities. *Med. J. Aust.* **1993**, *158*, 160–163. [PubMed]
7. Vos, T.; Barker, B.; Begg, S.; Stanley, L.; Lopez, A.D. Burden of disease and injury in Aboriginal and Torres Strait Islander Peoples: The Indigenous health gap. *Int. J. Epidemiol.* **2009**, *38*, 470–477. [CrossRef] [PubMed]
8. WHO. Intestinal Worms Strongyloidiasis. Available online: http://www.who.int/intestinal_worms/epidemiology/strongyloidiasis/en/ (accessed on 5 January 2017).
9. Lim, L.; Biggs, B. Fatal disseminated strongyloidiasis in a previously treated patient. *Med. J. Aust.* **2001**, *174*, 355–356. [PubMed]
10. Caruana, S.R.; Kelly, H.A.; Ngeow, J.Y.; Ryan, N.J.; Bennett, C.M.; Chea, L.; Nuon, S.; Bak, N.; Skull, S.A.; Biggs, B.A. Undiagnosed and potentially lethal parasite infections among immigrants and refugees in Australia. *J. Travel Med.* **2006**, *13*, 233–239. [CrossRef] [PubMed]
11. Davies, J.; Majumdar, S.S.; Forbes, R.T.; Smith, P.; Currie, B.J.; Baird, R.W. Hookworm in the Northern Territory: Down but not out. *Med. J. Aust.* **2013**, *198*, 278–281. [CrossRef] [PubMed]
12. Crowe, A.L.; Smith, P.; Ward, L.; Currie, B.J.; Baird, R.W. Decreasing prevalence of *Trichuris trichiura* (whipworm) in the Northern Territory from 2002 to 2012. *Med. J. Aust.* **2014**, *200*, 286–289. [CrossRef] [PubMed]
13. Remote Primary Health Care Manuals. CARPA Standard Treatment Manual. Available online: http://www.remotephcmanuals.com.au/publication/stm/CARPA_STM_home_page.html (accessed on 1 February 2017).
14. Willcocks, B.; McAuliffe, G.N.; Baird, R.W. Dwarf tapeworm (*Hymenolepis. nana*): Characteristics in the Northern Territory 2002–2013. *J. Paediatr. Child. Health* **2015**, *51*, 982–987. [CrossRef] [PubMed]
15. Buttery, J.P.; Lambert, S.B.; Grimwood, K.; Nissen, M.D.; Field, E.J.; Macartney, K.K.; Akikusa, J.D.; Kelly, J.J.; Kirkwood, C.D. Reduction in rotavirus-associated acute gastroenteritis following introduction of rotavirus vaccine into Australia's national childhood vaccine schedule. *Pediatr. Infect. Dis. J.* **2011**, *30*, S25–S29. [CrossRef] [PubMed]
16. Page, W.A.; Dempsey, K.; McCarthy, J.S. Utility of serological follow-up of chronic strongyloidiasis after anthelminthic chemotherapy. *Trans. R Soc. Trop Med. Hyg.* **2006**, *100*, 1056–1062. [CrossRef] [PubMed]
17. Garcia, L.S.; Bruckner, D. *Diagnostic Medical Parasitology*, 3rd ed.; ASM Press: Washington, DC, USA, 1997; pp. 615–618.

18. Llewellyn, S.; Inpankaew, T.; Nery, S.V.; Gray, D.J.; Verweij, J.J.; Clements, A.C.; Gomes, S.J.; Traub, R.; McCarthy, J.S. Application of a multiplex quantitative PCR to assess prevalence and intensity of intestinal parasite infections in a controlled clinical trial. *PLoS Negl. Trop. Dis.* **2016**, *10*, e0004380. [CrossRef] [PubMed]

19. Verweij, J.J.; Canales, M.; Polman, K.; Ziem, J.; Brienen, E.A.; Polderman, A.M.; Lieshout, L.V. Molecular diagnosis of *Strongyloides stercoralis* in faecal samples using real-time PCR. *Trans. R. Soc. Trop. Med. Hyg.* **2009**, *103*, 342–346. [CrossRef] [PubMed]

20. Hays, R.; Thompson, F.; Esterman, A.; McDermott, R. *Strongyloides stercoralis*, eosinophilia, and type 2 diabetes mellitus: The predictive value of eosinophilia in the diagnosis of *S. stercoralis* infection in an endemic community. *Open Forum. Infect. Dis.* **2016**, *3*, ofw029. [CrossRef] [PubMed]

21. Hopkins, R.M.; Gracey, M.S.; Hobbs, R.P.; Spargo, R.M.; Yates, M.; Thompson, R.C. The prevalence of hookworm infection, iron deficiency and anaemia in an Aboriginal community in north-west Australia. *Med. J. Aust.* **1997**, *166*, 241–244. [PubMed]

22. Beknazarova, M.; Whiley, H.; Ross, K. Strongyloidiasis: A disease of socioeconomic disadvantage. *Int. J. Environ. Res. Public Health* **2016**, *13*. [CrossRef] [PubMed]

23. Australian Bureau of Statistics. *Experimental Estimates and Projections, Aboriginal and Torres Strait Islander Australians, 1991 to 2021*; (ABS Cat. No. 3238.0.); ABS: Canberra, Australia, 2009. Available online: http://www.abs.gov.au/ausstats/abs@.nsf/mf/3238.0.55.001 (accessed on 5 January 2017).

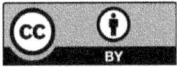

*Tropical Medicine and
Infectious Disease*

MDPI

Article

Soil-Transmitted Helminths in Children in a Remote Aboriginal Community in the Northern Territory: Hookworm is Rare but *Strongyloides stercoralis* and *Trichuris trichiura* Persist

Deborah C. Holt [1], Jennifer Shield [1,2] , Tegan M. Harris [1], Kate E. Mounsey [3], Kieran Aland [4], James S. McCarthy [5,6], Bart J. Currie [1] and Therese M. Kearns [1,*]

[1] Menzies School of Health Research, Charles Darwin University, Darwin NT 0811, Australia; deborah.holt@menzies.edu.au (D.C.H.); j.shield@latrobe.edu.au (J.S.); tegan.harris@menzies.edu.au (T.M.H.); bart.currie@menzies.edu.au (B.J.C.)
[2] Department of Pharmacy and Applied Science, La Trobe University, Bendigo VIC 3550, Australia
[3] School of Health and Sports Science, University of the Sunshine Coast, Maroochydore QLD 4558, Australia; kmounsey@usc.edu.au
[4] Queensland Museum, South Brisbane QLD 4101, Australia; bioscreenoz@gmail.com
[5] QIMR Berghofer Medical Research Institute, Herston QLD 4006, Australia; j.mcarthy@uq.edu.au
[6] School of Medicine, University of Queensland, Brisbane QLD 4072, Australia
* Correspondence: therese.kearns@menzies.edu.au; Tel.: +61-8-8946-6800

Received: 31 August 2017; Accepted: 30 September 2017; Published: 4 October 2017

Abstract: (1) Background: soil-transmitted helminths are a problem worldwide, largely affecting disadvantaged populations. The little data available indicates high rates of infection in some remote Aboriginal communities in Australia. Studies of helminths were carried out in the same remote community in the Northern Territory in 1994–1996 and 2010–2011; (2) Methods: fecal samples were collected from children aged <10 years and examined for helminths by direct smear microscopy. In the 2010–2011 study, some fecal samples were also analyzed by agar plate culture and PCR for *Strongyloides stercoralis* DNA. Serological analysis of fingerprick dried blood spots using a *S. stercoralis* NIE antigen was also conducted; (3) Results and Conclusions: a reduction in fecal samples positive for *S. stercoralis*, hookworm and *Trichuris trichiura* was seen between the studies in 1994–1996 and 2010–2011, likely reflecting public health measures undertaken in the region to reduce intestinal helminths. Comparison of methods to detect *S. stercoralis* showed that PCR of fecal samples and serological testing of dried blood spots was at least as sensitive as direct smear microscopy and agar plate culture. These methods have advantages for use in remote field studies.

Keywords: *Strongyloides stercoralis*; strongyloidiasis; *Trichuris trichiura*; *Rodentolepis nana*; Northern Territory; Aboriginal

---

1. Introduction

Soil-transmitted helminths are a worldwide problem generally affecting poor and vulnerable populations [1]. In Australia, there is a paucity of studies documenting the prevalence of soil-transmitted helminths due to the difficulties in diagnosing infection in communities, and timely transport to the nearest diagnostic laboratory. A cross-sectional survey in a remote Aboriginal community in the north of Western Australia in 1992 found hookworm infection in 77% of participants with the highest prevalence in children aged 5–14 years (93%) [2]. In a remote community in the Northern Territory (NT), a study in the mid-1990s of children and adults documented high rates of infection with hookworm, *Strongyloides stercoralis*, *Trichuris trichiura* and *Rodentolepis* (*Hymenolepis*) *nana* [3]. More recent surveys of *S. stercoralis* prevalence indicate that it is endemic in many northern Australian Aboriginal communities [4–6].

Currently, there is no gold standard test for diagnosing *S. stercoralis* [7,8]. Stool examination underestimates the prevalence of the parasite in population-based studies, while serological testing gives a higher prevalence [9]. When examining stools, the larval density is often low and output sporadic, resulting in variation in detection between samples in the same individuals [10]. Routine direct smear microscopy of single stool specimens has a low sensitivity in chronic cases and can fail to detect larvae in up to 70% of chronic infections [7,10]. The use of the agar culture plate technique has improved detection in chronic *S. stercoralis*, with a sensitivity of 96% when compared with direct fecal smear, formalin-ethyl acetate concentration and Harada-Mori filter paper culture [7]. A practical problem for the agar plate technique is that viable larvae are required for culture, which can be problematic for specimens that involve long delays (transport or otherwise) in reaching the laboratory. Serological examination for *S. stercoralis* antibodies improves detection in those with chronic infection. However, it may not readily detect those with acute infection as the prepatent period can be up to 28 days [8,11].

A study in a remote NT Aboriginal community in 1994–1996 revealed a high level of intestinal helminths by formol-ether concentration of fecal samples [3]. Concern of residents in this community about high rates of *S. stercoralis* infection resulted in a project in 2010–2011 to investigate the utility of mass drug administration to reduce the endemic prevalence of *S. stercoralis* and scabies [6,12]. The aim of this study was to compare the prevalence of intestinal parasites identified by direct smear microscopy between the 1994–1996 and 2010–2011 studies. In addition, due to the logistical challenges of handling and processing fecal samples during remote field studies, we also investigated the utility of alternative methods of *S. stercoralis* diagnosis during the 2010–2011 study. Serological testing of eluted dried blood spots and PCR were shown to be at least as sensitive as microscopy and culture, and have considerable advantages for use in remote community settings.

2. Materials and Methods

2.1. Sample Population

Samples were collected from consenting participants during two separate projects in a remote Aboriginal community with an estimated population of 2000, located 550 km east of Darwin, NT Australia. Ninety-four percent of the resident population are Australian Aboriginal with an average of 6.3 members per household, and 19.9% of the population are aged <10 years [13]. Each project received ethical approval from the Human Research Ethics Committee of the Northern Territory Department of Health and Menzies School of Health Research (EC00153; approvals 94/19 and 09/34).

2.2. Fecal Sample Collection and Processing

In the first study, surveys of intestinal parasites were conducted in the community from 1994–1996 [3]. Fecal samples were collected into disposable plastic containers by a parent or carer and collected by the researchers the following morning. Direct smears for the identification of intestinal parasites were undertaken in a field laboratory. Quantitative formol-ether counts conducted on fecal samples preserved in 4% formaldehyde were previously reported [3]. Treatment was administered by the local primary health care service and was not recorded as part of the study.

The 2010–2011 study consisted of two population censuses and mass drug administrations (MDAs) conducted 12 months apart in a staged roll-out. The full study design has been previously reported [6,12]. Fecal samples were collected from children by a parent or carer into disposable plastic containers and returned to the researchers. Direct smear microscopy on approximately 0.005 g of feces was performed on the majority of samples on site in a field laboratory within four hours of receipt. A small number of samples from 2011 were fixed in SAF (sodium acetate, acetic acid, formalin) and transported by aircraft to a commercial pathology laboratory for microscopic analysis the day after receipt. Only the results of the first fecal sample collected from each participant aged <10 years are reported here.

Fisher exact probability tests were performed at the VassarStats website [14].

2.3. Agar Plate Culture

For samples with sufficient fecal matter, agar plate culture was conducted, based on the method of Garcia [15], except that nutrient-deficient Mueller-Hinton agar plates were used, with the aim of reducing fungal growth. Specifically, a patch of ~2 cm diameter of feces was applied to the center of a nutrient-deficient Mueller-Hinton agar plate, sealed, and incubated at room temperature (~25 °C) overnight. The plates were then transported by aircraft to the research laboratory the following day in a foam container with a sweated ice brick to maintain a temperature of 17–25 °C. The plates were maintained in the research laboratory at 25 °C and examined macroscopically for larval tracks marked by bacterial colonies daily for up to five days after plating. Once tracks were observed, or after five days had elapsed, the plate was flooded with 10% formalin for five minutes, the liquid aspirated and centrifuged at 500× *g*, and the sediment examined microscopically for *S. stercoralis* and hookworm infective larvae.

2.4. Fecal DNA Extraction and PCR

Any remaining fecal material was transported to the research laboratory, where it was stored in ethanol at −20 °C. DNA extraction using up to 30 mg of stored fecal samples was performed using a PowerSoil® DNA isolation kit (MoBio Laboratories Inc, Carlsbad, CA, USA), according to the manufacturer's instructions. The PowerSoil kit is designed for use with complex samples and has been shown to be superior to four other DNA extraction methods in terms of sensitivity and ease of use, for extraction and detection of *Strongyloides ratti* DNA in spiked human stool samples [16]. DNA samples were tested using a published real-time PCR based method for the detection of *S. stercoralis* 18S rDNA [17]. Due to a high percentage of positive samples in 2010 that were detected using this method (34/39), the real-time PCR products were analyzed by agarose gel electrophoresis. Many samples did not have the correct 101 bp product, but had a smaller DNA fragment, possibly primer dimer, that presumably reacted with the probe to produce fluorescence in the real-time PCR. As a result, we designed an alternative forward primer (Stro18S-altF 5′ GGGCCGGACACTATAAGGAT 3′), which produced a 471 bp product with the published Stro18S-1630R primer (5′ TGCCTCTGGATATTGCTCAGTTC 3′) [17]. The original Stro18S-1530F and Stro18S-1630R primer set was shown to be highly specific for *S. stercoralis* [17]; however, the specificity when using the alternative forward primer designed here was not systematically tested. End-point PCR using this alternative primer combination was conducted using 2 µL of DNA extraction, 20 pmol each primer, 100 µM dNTPs, 1.5 mM Mg^{2+} and 1 U *Taq* polymerase in a total volume of 20 µL. Cycling conditions were 35 cycles of 95 °C for 30 s, 58 °C for 30 s, and 72 °C 30 s. A positive control plasmid was constructed by cloning a PCR product obtained from an agar plate culture-positive sample into pBlueScript II SK. The efficiency of the PCR was optimized using the plasmid control and a culture-positive fecal sample.

2.5. Blood Spot Collection and Serological Testing

Dried blood spots were collected by fingerprick onto filter paper cards, air dried and stored in zip-lock bags with silica desiccant at 4–8 °C. Serum was eluted from the dried blood spots and analyzed by ELISA using a recombinant *S. stercoralis* NIE antigen [18] as previously reported [19]. Briefly, dried blood spots were eluted in 150 µL phosphate buffered saline and 0.05% Tween 20 (PBS-T) overnight at room temperature. A 1:500 dilution of this eluate was used in the NIE ELISA. Plates were coated with 100 µL of 125 ng/mL NIE antigen, and blocked with 5% skim milk powder in PBS-T. Dried blood spot elutions were added and incubated at 37 °C for two hours. Alkaline phosphatase conjugated goat anti-human IgG was used as the secondary antibody at a dilution of 1:2500. Plates were developed with phosphatase substrate and optical density read at 405 nm. The assay was initially established and validated using a panel of sera from participants that were either positive or negative for *S. stercoralis* by fecal culture. Each ELISA assay included positive and negative control dried blood spots, which were used to validate the assay and normalize optical density (OD) results [19]. Normalized ODs were calculated by the ratio of test sample OD to positive control dried blood spot OD. The result of the first sample collected from each participant is reported here.

3. Results

3.1. Comparison of Intestinal Parasites Identified in Children <10 Years in 1994–1996 and 2010–2011

Fecal samples were collected from children aged <10 years and examined by direct smear. Samples were collected from 84 participants in 1994–1996 (mean age 5.6 years) and 85 children in 2010–2011 (mean age 3.7 years). The percentage of samples positive for hookworm and *T. trichiura* in 2010–2011 was significantly less than that reported in 1994–1996 ($p = 0.002$ and 0.012 respectively). The percentage of samples positive for *S. stercoralis* also reduced, however *R. nana* remained unchanged (Table 1). The mean number of intestinal parasites identified per fecal sample was 1.5 in 1994–1996 and 2 in 2010–2011 (data not shown).

Table 1. Intestinal parasites identified in fecal samples by direct smear microscopy.

n	1994–1996 84	2010–2011 85	Fisher Exact Probability Test p (Two-tail)
Average age (years)	5.6	3.7	
Strongyloides stercoralis	11 (13.1%)	4 (4.7%)	0.063
Hookworm	11 (13.1%)	1 (1.2%)	0.002 *
Rodentolepis nana	20 (23.8%)	19 (22.4%)	0.857
Trichuris trichiura	57 (67.9%)	41 (48.2%)	0.012 *

* $p < 0.05$.

3.2. Comparison of Diagnostic Methods for S. stercoralis

In addition to the direct smears, in the 2010–2011 study agar plate culture for helminth larvae, and PCR for *S. stercoralis* DNA was conducted on a subset of fecal samples, and serology was performed on sera eluted from dried blood spots (Table 2). *S. stercoralis* larvae were detected in five of 77 (6.5%) samples examined by agar plate culture and formalin sedimentation (Figure 1). Four of these samples were positive for *S. stercoralis* by direct smear, while one was negative. No hookworm larvae were detected. End point PCR for *S. stercoralis* 18S rDNA was positive for six (7.2%) of 83 samples tested, which included the five agar plate-positive samples. The percentage of samples considered positive by serology was higher than for the other methods with 25 (16.2%) of the dried blood spot samples considered positive.

Table 2. Comparison of *Strongyloides stercoralis* diagnostic methods in children aged <10 years in 2010–2011.

Method	+ve/n (%)
Direct smear	4/85 (4.7%)
Culture and formalin sedimentation	5/77 (6.5%)
S. stercoralis 18S rDNA PCR	6/83 (7.2%)
Serology on dried blood spots	25/154 (16.2%)

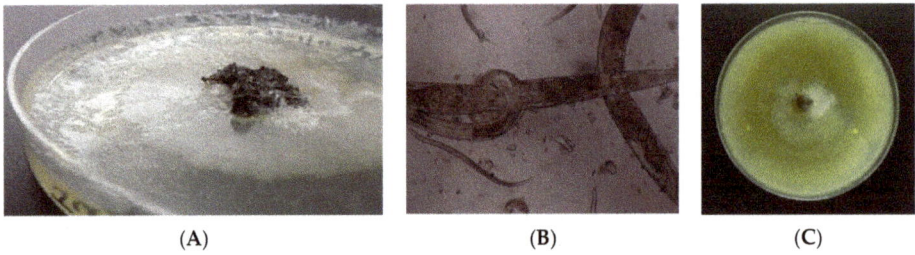

Figure 1. Identification of *S. stercoralis* larvae by agar plate culture and formalin sedimentation: (**A**) Bacterial growth on Mueller-Hinton agar in tracks made by helminth larvae; (**B**) *S. stercoralis* adults and filariform larvae in formalin sediment of agar culture; (**C**) Fungal overgrowth may have obscured larval tracks on some plates.

There were 28 blood spot samples for which a fecal sample had also been analyzed by agar plate culture at the same time point. Of these, 20 participants were negative for both methods, and five were positive by serology but negative by culture. It is unknown if these children had recent infections or if results were false positives, as children are rarely tested for *Strongyloides* in this setting. For three participants who were positive by agar plate culture and had blood spots collected, one was also positive by serology, but the other two were negative by serology. This indicates that this serological method may not detect some acute infections.

4. Discussion

This is one of the first NT studies to examine and compare helminth infections in a remote Aboriginal community using three different diagnostic methods. Aboriginal Australians are traditionally hunter-gatherer societies, and there has been a rapid and often problematic transition to permanent settlement since European colonization. Aboriginal Australians have a higher burden of disease compared with non-Aboriginal Australians, with the largest difference seen in remote communities [20]. In remote community settings in northern Australia, government programs concentrating on the provision of infrastructure alone have been shown to have limited impact on community-level crowding and hygiene [21] or common childhood infectious diseases [22,23].

The introduction of a deworming program using albendazole in 1995 [24] is likely to have contributed to the reduction in samples positive for *S. stercoralis* (not statistically significant), hookworm and *T. trichiura* between the two study periods. The observed low rate of hookworm in 2010–2011 is supported by a downward trend in hookworm infections seen in a hospital-based study conducted during the same time period, which reported 14 cases per 100,000 in 2002 and 2.2 cases per 100,000 in 2012 [25]. The percentage of fecal samples positive for *S. stercoralis* dropped from 13.1% in 1994–1996 to 4.7% in 2010–2011, which reflects an overall reduction in the NT [26]. The single-dose albendazole used in the NT deworming program may have had a partial effect despite being lower than the recommended dose for treating *S. stercoralis* infection [26]. Serology on blood spots was positive for 16.2% of children tested in 2010–2011, higher than for fecal detection methods. The community-wide mass drug administration at the time of this study was shown to reduce the rate of seropositivity in treated participants 12 months later [6]. The reduction in participants positive for *T. trichiura* between the 1994–1996 study and the 2010–2011 study is consistent with overall data for the NT [27]; however, the percentage of participants positive for *T. trichiura* remained high in 2010–2011 at 48.2%. This may be due to the fact that single-dose albendazole reduces egg counts but has a low cure rate for *T. trichiura* infection [28–30]. The prevalence of *R. nana* infection remained unchanged between the study periods, consistent with a recent analysis of infections in the NT, which showed that infections were predominantly in Aboriginal children aged under 5 years [31]. Single-dose albendazole

Trop. Med. Infect. Dis. **2017**, *2*, 51

does not appear to produce a significant cure rate for *R. nana* [28] and the recommended treatment, praziquantel [32], is rarely stocked in health services in rural and remote communities.

As *S. stercoralis* larval output is often low and intermittent in chronic cases [10], a limitation of this study is the examination of a single fecal specimen for diagnosis. Agar plate culture and formalin sedimentation yielded only a single additional *S. stercoralis* positive sample compared with the direct smear method in 2010–2011, and this method is reported to have greater sensitivity than both direct smear and formol-ether concentration [33]. Fungal growth on the agar culture plates was common, and may have hindered the identification of larval tracks. It is also possible, that in spite of the care taken to maintain the temperature of agar plates within the tolerance range of *S. stercoralis* larvae, some larval death may have occurred during transport. The sensitivity of the direct smear microscopy may have also been high due to large numbers of parasites present and/or an experienced microscopist.

As collection, processing and analysis of fecal samples presents a number of logistical challenges, we undertook three different methods for the diagnosis of *S. stercoralis* that might be more suited to studies in remote field sites. PCR on DNA extractions of ethanol-preserved fecal samples was at least as sensitive as agar plate culture and formalin sedimentation. PCR has the advantage of reducing the handling of fecal specimens in the field, and allowed samples to be batched for testing. This method could be modified to have greater utility in remote field settings. Alternative methods of fecal preservation that allow storage at room temperature [34] could be used, avoiding the need for cold storage. Methods utilizing loop-mediated isothermal amplification (LAMP) require only a single temperature incubation and have the possibility of incorporating visualization of positive results by color or turbidity change [35,36] that could be conducted in a field laboratory. Detection of multiple intestinal parasite species can also be achieved with PCR, using multi-parallel [37] or multiplexed reactions [38,39]. The sensitivity of DNA amplification methods may further be improved by targeting high copy number sequences identified by whole genome sequence analysis [40].

Serology was positive for 16.2% of samples in 2010–2011, higher than for the other diagnostic methods used, and consistent with previous reports [9,41]. In endemic areas, serology has a high positive predictive value due to the high prevalence of infection [8] but may not identify all acute infections, and may be of most use in monitoring the effect of treatment in an individual or population over time [6,19].

5. Conclusions

PCR of fecal samples and serological testing of dried blood spots were shown to be at least as sensitive as microscopy and culture for the diagnosis of *S. stercoralis* in this setting. These methods have considerable advantages for use in remote field studies and may be useful for the ongoing assessment of efforts to reduce the prevalence of *S. stercoralis* in remote communities.

Despite a reduction in the percentage of children aged <10 years positive for *S. stercoralis*, hookworm and *T. trichiura* in 2010–2011 compared to 1994–1996 in this remote Aboriginal community in Australia, the rates of *S. stercoralis* and *T. trichiura* remained high at 4.7% and 48.2% respectively. The percentage of children positive for *R. nana* was unchanged. The reduction is consistent with public health measures in the region to reduce intestinal helminths but requires further investigation to assess the impact that these infections are having on child health and development.

Acknowledgments: The 1994–1996 study was funded by a National Health and Medical Research Council grant through the Public Health Research and Development Committee. K.A. was supported by a Commonwealth Postgraduate Scholarship at the University of Queensland. The 2010–2011 study was funded by a National Health and Medical Research Council Project Grant (605804). We thank all of the study participants in both studies and Professor Ross Andrews and other investigators involved in these projects for their support.

Author Contributions: D.C.H., J.S., T.M.H., K.E.M., K.A., J.S.M., B.J.C. and T.M.K. conceived and designed the experiments; D.C.H., J.S., T.M.H., K.E.M., K.A., T.M.K. performed the experiments; D.C.H., J.S., T.M.H., K.E.M., K.A. and T.M.K analyzed the data; D.C.H., J.S., T.M.H., K.E.M., J.S.M., B.J.C. and T.M.K wrote the paper.

Conflicts of Interest: The authors declare no conflict of interest.

References

1. World Health Organization. Available online: http://www.who.int/mediacentre/factsheets/fs366/en/ (accessed on 17 July 2017).
2. Hopkins, R.M.; Gracey, M.S.; Hobbs, R.P.; Spargo, R.M.; Yates, M.; Thompson, R.C. The prevalence of hookworm infection, iron deficiency and anaemia in an aboriginal community in north-west Australia. *Med. J. Aust.* **1997**, *166*, 241–244. [PubMed]
3. Shield, J.; Aland, K.; Kearns, T.; Gongdjalk, G.; Holt, D.; Currie, B.; Prociv, P. Intestinal parasites of children and adults in a remote Aboriginal community of the Northern Territory, Australia, 1994–1996. *Western Pac. Surveill. Response J.* **2015**, *6*, 44–51. [CrossRef] [PubMed]
4. Fryar, D.; Hagan, S. Pilot screening program for intestinal parasites and anaemia in adults in a Top End Aboriginal community. *NT Comm Dis Bull.* **1997**, *4*, 20–21.
5. Johnston, F.H.; Morris, P.S.; Speare, R.; McCarthy, J.; Currie, B.; Ewald, D.; Page, W.; Dempsey, K. Strongyloidiasis: A review of the evidence for Australian practitioners. *Aust. J. Rural Health* **2005**, *13*, 247–254. [CrossRef] [PubMed]
6. Kearns, T.M.; Currie, B.J.; Cheng, A.C.; McCarthy, J.; Carapetis, J.R.; Holt, D.C.; Page, W.; Shield, J.; Gundjirryirr, R.; Mulholland, E.; et al. *Strongyloides* seroprevalence before and after an ivermectin mass drug administration in a remote Australian Aboriginal community. *PLoS Negl. Trop. Dis.* **2017**, *11*, e0005607. [CrossRef] [PubMed]
7. Siddiqui, A.A.; Berk, S.L. Diagnosis of *Strongyloides stercoralis* infection. *Clin. Infect. Dis.* **2001**, *33*, 1040–1047. [CrossRef] [PubMed]
8. Speare, R.; Durrheim, D.N. *Strongyloides* serology – useful for diagnosis and management of strongyloidiasis in rural Indigenous populations, but important gaps in knowledge remain. *Rural Remote Health* **2004**, *4*, 264. [PubMed]
9. Grove, D.I. Human strongyloidiasis. *Adv. Parasitol.* **1996**, *38*, 251–309. [PubMed]
10. Dreyer, G.; Fernandes-Silva, E.; Alves, S.; Rocha, A.; Albuquerque, R.; Addiss, D. Patterns of detection of *Strongyloides stercoralis* in stool specimens: Implications for diagnosis and clinical trials. *J. Clin. Microbiol.* **1996**, *34*, 2569–2571. [PubMed]
11. Tanaka, H. Experimental and epidemiological studies on strongyloidiasis of Amami Oshima island. *Jpn. J. Exp. Med.* **1958**, *28*, 159–182. [PubMed]
12. Kearns, T.M.; Speare, R.; Cheng, A.C.; McCarthy, J.; Carapetis, J.R.; Holt, D.C.; Currie, B.J.; Page, W.; Shield, J.; Gundjirryirr, R.; et al. Impact of an ivermectin mass drug administration on scabies prevalence in a remote Australian Aboriginal community. *PLoS Negl. Trop. Dis.* **2015**, *9*, e0004151. [CrossRef] [PubMed]
13. Australian Bureau of Statistics. Available online: http://www.censusdata.abs.gov.au/census_services/getproduct/census/2016/quickstat/SSC70106 (accessed on 31 August 2017).
14. VassarStats: Website for Statistical Computation. Available online: http://vassarstats.net/ (accessed on 30 September 2017).
15. Garcia, L. *Diagnostic Medical Parasitology*, 5th ed.; American Society for Microbiology Press: Washington DC, USA, 2007; pp. 837–840.
16. Sultana, Y.; Jeoffreys, N.; Watts, M.R.; Gilbert, G.L.; Lee, R. Real-time polymerase chain reaction for detection of *Strongyloides stercoralis* in stool. *Am. J. Trop. Med. Hyg.* **2013**, *88*, 1048–1051. [CrossRef] [PubMed]
17. Verweij, J.J.; Canales, M.; Polman, K.; Ziem, J.; Brienen, E.A.; Polderman, A.M.; van Lieshout, L. Molecular diagnosis of *Strongyloides stercoralis* in faecal samples using real-time PCR. *Trans. R. Soc. Trop. Med. Hyg.* **2009**, *103*, 342–346. [CrossRef] [PubMed]
18. Ravi, V.; Ramachandran, S.; Thompson, R.W.; Andersen, J.F.; Neva, F.A. Characterization of a recombinant immunodiagnostic antigen (NIE) from *Strongyloides stercoralis* L3-stage larvae. *Mol. Biochem. Parasitol.* **2002**, *125*, 73–81. [CrossRef]
19. Mounsey, K.; Kearns, T.; Rampton, M.; Llewellyn, S.; King, M.; Holt, D.; Currie, B.J.; Andrews, R.; Nutman, T.; McCarthy, J. Use of dried blood spots to define antibody response to the *Strongyloides stercoralis* recombinant antigen NIE. *Acta Trop.* **2014**, *138*, 78–82. [CrossRef] [PubMed]
20. Vos, T.; Barker, B.; Begg, S.; Stanley, L.; Lopez, A.D. Burden of disease and injury in Aboriginal and Torres Strait Islander Peoples: the Indigenous health gap. *Int. J. Epidemiol.* **2009**, *38*, 470–477. [CrossRef] [PubMed]

21. Bailie, R.S.; McDonald, E.L.; Stevens, M.; Guthridge, S.; Brewster, D.R. Evaluation of an Australian indigenous housing programme: Community level impact on crowding, infrastructure function and hygiene. *J. Epidemiol. Community Health* **2011**, *65*, 432–437. [CrossRef] [PubMed]

22. Bailie, R.S.; Stevens, M.; McDonald, E.L. The impact of housing improvement and socio-environmental factors on common childhood illnesses: A cohort study in Indigenous Australian communities. *J. Epidemiol. Community Health* **2012**, *66*, 821–831. [CrossRef] [PubMed]

23. McDonald, E.; Bailie, R. Hygiene improvement: Essential to improving child health in remote Aboriginal communities. *J. Paediatr. Child. Health* **2010**, *46*, 491–496. [CrossRef] [PubMed]

24. Central Australian Rural Practitioners Association. *CARPA Standard Treatment Manual*, 2nd ed.; Central Australian Rural Practitioners Association: Alice Springs, NT, Australia, 1994.

25. Davies, J.; Majumdar, S.S.; Forbes, R.T.; Smith, P.; Currie, B.J.; Baird, R.W. Hookworm in the Northern Territory: down but not out. *Med. J. Aust.* **2013**, *198*, 278–281. [CrossRef] [PubMed]

26. Mayer-Coverdale, J.K.; Crowe, A.; Smith, P.; Baird, R.W. Trends in *Strongyloides stercoralis* faecal larvae detections in the Northern Territory, Australia: 2002–2012. *Trop. Med. Infect. Dis.* **2017**, *2*, 18. [CrossRef]

27. Crowe, A.L.; Smith, P.; Ward, L.; Currie, B.J.; Baird, R. Decreasing prevalence of *Trichuris trichiura* (whipworm) in the Northern Territory from 2002 to 2012. *Med. J. Aust.* **2014**, *200*, 286–289. [CrossRef] [PubMed]

28. Horton, J. Albendazole: A review of anthelmintic efficacy and safety in humans. *Parasitology* **2000**, *121*, S113–S132. [CrossRef] [PubMed]

29. Keiser, J.; Utzinger, J. Efficacy of current drugs against soil-transmitted helminth infections: systematic review and meta-analysis. *J.A.M.A.* **2008**, *299*, 1937–1948. [CrossRef] [PubMed]

30. Steinmann, P.; Utzinger, J.; Du, Z.W.; Jiang, J.Y.; Chen, J.X.; Hattendorf, J.; Zhou, H.; Zhou, X.N. Efficacy of single-dose and triple-dose albendazole and mebendazole against soil-transmitted helminths and *Taenia* spp.: A randomized controlled trial. *PLoS One* **2011**, *6*, e25003. [CrossRef] [PubMed]

31. Willcocks, B.; McAuliffe, G.N.; Baird, R.W. Dwarf tapeworm (*Hymenolepis nana*): Characteristics in the Northern Territory 2002–2013. *J. Paediatr. Child. Health* **2015**, *51*, 982–987. [CrossRef] [PubMed]

32. Central Australian Rural Practitioners Association. *CARPA Standard Treatment Manual*, 5th ed.; Central Australian Rural Practitioners Association: Alice Springs, NT, Australia, 2014.

33. Sato, Y.; Kobayashi, J.; Toma, H.; Shiroma, Y. Efficacy of stool examination for detection of *Strongyloides* infection. *Am. J. Trop. Med. Hyg.* **1995**, *53*, 248–250. [CrossRef] [PubMed]

34. Beknazarova, M.; Millsteed, S.; Robertson, G.; Whiley, H.; Ross, K. Validation of DESS as a DNA preservation method for the detection of *Strongyloides* spp. in canine feces. *Int. J. Environ. Res. Public Health* **2017**, *14*. [CrossRef]

35. Watts, M.R.; James, G.; Sultana, Y.; Ginn, A.N.; Outhred, A.C.; Kong, F.; Verweij, J.J.; Iredell, J.R.; Chen, S.C.; Lee, R. A loop-mediated isothermal amplification (LAMP) assay for *Strongyloides stercoralis* in stool that uses a visual detection method with SYTO-82 fluorescent dye. *Am. J. Trop. Med. Hyg.* **2014**, *90*, 306–311. [CrossRef] [PubMed]

36. Fernandez-Soto, P.; Sanchez-Hernandez, A.; Gandasegui, J.; Bajo Santos, C.; Lopez-Aban, J.; Saugar, J.M.; Rodriguez, E.; Vicente, B.; Muro, A. Strong-LAMP: A LAMP Assay for *Strongyloides* spp. detection in stool and urine samples. Towards the diagnosis of human strongyloidiasis starting from a rodent model. *PLoS Negl. Trop. Dis.* **2016**, *10*, e0004836. [CrossRef]

37. Mejia, R.; Vicuna, Y.; Broncano, N.; Sandoval, C.; Vaca, M.; Chico, M.; Cooper, P.J.; Nutman, T.B. A novel, multi-parallel, real-time polymerase chain reaction approach for eight gastrointestinal parasites provides improved diagnostic capabilities to resource-limited at-risk populations. *Am. J. Trop. Med. Hyg.* **2013**, *88*, 1041–1047. [CrossRef] [PubMed]

38. Basuni, M.; Muhi, J.; Othman, N.; Verweij, J.J.; Ahmad, M.; Miswan, N.; Rahumatullah, A.; Aziz, F.A.; Zainudin, N.S.; Noordin, R. A pentaplex real-time polymerase chain reaction assay for detection of four species of soil-transmitted helminths. *Am. J. Trop. Med. Hyg.* **2011**, *84*, 338–343. [CrossRef] [PubMed]

39. Llewellyn, S.; Inpankaew, T.; Nery, S.V.; Gray, D.J.; Verweij, J.J.; Clements, A.C.; Gomes, S.J.; Traub, R.; McCarthy, J.S. Application of a multiplex quantitative PCR to assess prevalence and intensity of intestinal parasite infections in a controlled clinical trial. *PLoS Negl. Trop. Dis.* **2016**, *10*, e0004380. [CrossRef] [PubMed]

40. Pilotte, N.; Papaiakovou, M.; Grant, J.R.; Bierwert, L.A.; Llewellyn, S.; McCarthy, J.S.; Williams, S.A. Improved PCR-based detection of soil transmitted helminth infections using a next-generation sequencing approach to assay design. *PLoS Negl. Trop. Dis.* **2016**, *10*, e0004578. [CrossRef] [PubMed]

41. Buonfrate, D.; Perandin, F.; Formenti, F.; Bisoffi, Z. A retrospective study comparing agar plate culture, indirect immunofluorescence and real-time PCR for the diagnosis of *Strongyloides stercoralis* infection. *Parasitology* **2017**, *144*, 812–816. [CrossRef] [PubMed]

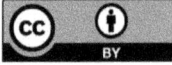

Tropical Medicine and Infectious Disease

MDPI

Article

Poverty, Dietary Intake, Intestinal Parasites, and Nutritional Status among School-Age Children in the Rural Philippines

Allen G. Ross [1,*]**, Keren Papier** [2]**, Ruby Luceres-Catubig** [3]**, Thao N. Chau** [4]**,
Marianette T. Inobaya** [1,3]**and Shu-Kay Ng** [1]

[1] Menzies Health Institute Queensland, Griffith University, Gold Coast, QLD 4222, Australia;
net_inobaya@yahoo.com (M.T.I.); s.ng@griffith.edu.au (S.-K.N.)
[2] National Centre for Epidemiology & Population Health, Australian National University,
Canberra, ACT 2601, Australia; keren.papier@anu.edu.au
[3] Department of Health, Research Institute for Tropical Medicine, Muntinlupa 1781,
Metro Manila, Philippines; ruby.luceres@yahoo.com
[4] Discipline of Public Health, School of Health Sciences, Flinders University, Adelaide, SA 5001, Australia;
tnpchau@gmail.com
* Correspondence: a.ross@griffith.edu.au; Tel.: +61-733-821-098

Received: 14 August 2017; Accepted: 17 September 2017; Published: 21 September 2017

Abstract: Intestinal helminths are endemic throughout the Philippines; however, there is limited evidence with respect to their prevalence, intensity, and impact on children's nutritional status. A cross-sectional survey was carried out on 693 children from five rural villages in Northern Samar, the Philippines. Data on dietary intake, nutritional status, and intestinal parasites were collected. Infection with *Schistosoma japonicum*, *Ascaris lumbricoides*, *Trichuris trichiura*, and hookworm was evident in 20.1, 54.4, 71.4, and 25.3% of the children. The majority (84.7%) was infected with one or more helminth species, with about one-quarter of the sample (24.7%) infected with three or more. About half (49.2%, $n = 341$) of the children were stunted and 27.8% ($n = 193$) were wasted. A lower prevalence of normal height-for-age (48.3%) appeared in those with polyparasitism, while the prevalence of stunted children increased with infection (46.7% monoparasitism and 51.7% polyparasitism). There was a decreasing trend between infection intensity and the mean values of HAZ and BAZ identified for *T. trichiura* or hookworm infections. Stunted children were more likely to be male (AOR = 1.58; 95% CI: 1.05–2.39; $p = 0.028$), older in age (10–14 years) (AOR = 1.93; 95% CI: 1.29–2.88; $p = 0.001$), and living in poorer households with palm leaves/nipa roof (AOR = 1.85; 95% CI: 1.14–3.01; $p = 0.013$). Intestinal parasitic treatment needs to be combined with nutrient supplements and health education in order to interrupt the parasite life cycle and achieve sustainable control.

Keywords: childhood; malnutrition; intestinal parasites; nutritional status; poverty

1. Introduction

More than a third of the world's population is infected with soil-transmitted helminths (STH), mainly in the developing nations of Asia, Africa, and Latin America [1]. STHs are intestinal parasitic nematode worms causing human disease. They are the most common of the 17 major neglected tropical diseases (NTDs) and the most widespread and disabling chronic infections globally [2]. *Ascaris lumbricoides* is the most prevalent STH with an estimated one billion infections; and *Trichuris trichiura* and hookworms (*Necator americanus* and *Ancylostoma duodenale*) each infect approximately 600–800 million [1]. STHs are a significant public health concern in the Philippines, particularly among school-aged children who, if infected, suffer from profound physical deficits, including anaemia and malnutrition, stunted growth, reduced fitness, and cognitive delays [2–8]. Sixteen out of 17 regions in the Philippines are endemic for STHs with a prevalence of $\geq$50% [9]. A nationwide survey performed over 10 years found the prevalence in children aged 2–14 years was 50–90%; and up to 30% of the 22 million children in the Philippines were infected with more than one of the three STH species [10,11].

The cornerstone of intestinal parasitic control is recurrent mass drug administration (MDA) with benzimidazole anthelmintics (e.g., 400 mg albendazole) that are cheap, safe, and effective. The current WHO strategy is to continually treat pre-school and school-age children, women of childbearing age, and adults at high risk, once or twice per year, depending on prevalence [8,9]. This is partially effective in achieving morbidity control; however, it does not prevent re-infection. A number of studies have shown that once treatment is stopped, prevalence returns to pre-treatment levels within 12–18 months [2,7–11]. Therefore, interventions that prevent re-infection and boost immunity (e.g., the use of micro/macronutrient supplements) are required to augment chemotherapy as part of an integrated approach. The global target is to eliminate morbidity due to soil-transmitted helminthiases in children by 2020 [8]. This will only be achieved by regularly treating at least 75% of the children in endemic areas (an estimated 873 million), who are free from malnutrition [8,9].

Nutritional deficiencies and infectious diseases can negatively impact the nutritional status of children and adolescents [12,13]. Intestinal helminth worm infections can damage a child's internal mucosa, leading to impaired digestion and poor absorption of nutrients [14]. Deficiencies in macro- and micronutrient intakes during childhood can impair both physical and cognitive growth as well as increase the risk of mortality [15]. Moreover, inadequate intake of selected micronutrients can cause immune deficiency and increase susceptibility to infection [16]. The micronutrients vitamin A, vitamin B_{12}, vitamin C, β-carotene, riboflavin, zinc, selenium, and iron all have immune-modulating functions, enabling them to influence the course of an infection [16]. Laboratory studies have shown that vitamin A deficiency can reduce schistosome (human blood fluke)-specific antibody responses, suggesting a possible link between vitamin A deficiency and susceptibility to schistosomiasis [12]. Deficiency of some nutrients may reduce the host's immune function, impairing the body's resistance to infectious diseases and increasing susceptibility to intestinal parasites [17]. Once present, parasitic infections can promote the further loss of nutrients, leading to reduced growth and poor nutritional status as part of a vicious cycle [18]. Children aged 5–14 years suffer from the highest burden of infectious disease [19], partly due to their increased behavioural risk, frequent outdoor exposure, and poor personal hygiene [20].

Intestinal helminths are endemic throughout the Philippines and efforts are underway to decrease their burden. However, there is limited evidence with regards to their prevalence, intensity and their impact on children's nutritional status. The purpose of this study was to examine the relationship between poverty, dietary intake, intestinal parasites, and childhood nutritional status in the rural Philippines.

2. Material and Methods

2.1. Study Population

A cross-sectional survey was conducted in 2013 on 693 children from five rural villages in Palapag [21], Northern Samar, the Philippines. Villagers there are typically poor rice farmers, with over 50% of the population living below the poverty line. Water, sanitation, and hygiene conditions are most often rudimentary. Most households typically have 6–10 children per family and the prevalence rates of parasitic diseases, acute respiratory infections, diarrhoeal diseases, and other communicable diseases, are high [22].

2.2. Study Procedures

Individuals were asked, over the course of a week, to provide two stool specimens from which six Kato–Katz thick smears were prepared on microscope slides. These slides were examined under a light microscope by experienced laboratory technicians who counted the number of STH and *Schistosoma japonicum* (SJ) eggs per slide. For quality control, 10% of slides were randomly selected and re-examined by a senior microscopist at the Research Institute for Tropical Medicine, Manila. Individual and head of household questionnaires were completed to collect the following information: occupation, level of education, home and land ownership, number of animals owned and raising practices, animal waste disposal practices, pasturing of animals, sanitation, and housing characteristics (roofing, wall, and floor materials). For wealth status, participants were classified as wealthy if their house had a cement floor, a galvanized roof, cement walls, and a tile/marble floor. Participants were classified as poor if they had a house with a nipa (palm) roof and a soil floor, and without cement walls. All other participants were classified as having a moderate wealth status.

2.3. Nutritional Assessment

Anthropometric measurements of height and weight were collected using standard procedures [23]. Weight was measured using a portable digital scale to the nearest 0.1 kg. Height was assessed to the nearest 0.1 cm using a tape measure. The Z values for weight-for-height (WAZ) (children aged <10 years only), body mass index (BMI)—for-age (BAZ), and height-for-age (HAZ) were calculated according to World Health Organization (WHO) guidelines using the new WHO growth standards [24,25]. Weight-for-height is considered an inappropriate indicator for monitoring child growth beyond the age of 10 due to its inability to distinguish between relative height and body mass. Therefore, BMI-for-age was used to assess thinness/wasting for children aged $\geq$10 and for adolescents. Based on the Z values, the children were categorized as 'thin/wasted' (BAZ < -2 and/or WAZ < -2) and 'stunted' (HAZ < -2). Children with Z values > -2 for BAZ, WAZ, and HAZ were categorized as 'normal'.

2.4. Dietary Intake Data

Dietary intake information was elicited using a 24-h recall method. Three qualified nutritionists together with 10 field nurses collected the data. Household food utensils were used to assist study participants quantify food portions and liquids consumed. In order to estimate food weights, macro- and micronutrient intakes were calculated for each child using food composition tables developed by the Food and Nutrition Research Institute [26]. These tables contained data on 17 food components of 1541 foods commonly consumed in the Philippines. Dietary intake data was evaluated against the national Filipino recommended energy and nutrient intake (RENI) values by age and sex [27].

2.5. Statistical Analysis

Data were double-entered into FoxPro (version 6.0), crosschecked, and subsequently analysed using STATA SE version 13.0 software (StataCorp LP, College Station, TX, USA). All variables including sex, age group, and endemic setting were explored individually by Chi-square statistics. Infection intensity was explored with the Student *t*-test and Kruskal–Wallis test. The standard error (SE) of each estimate was converted to a variance; all variances were summed to provide an overall variance, SE, and 95% confidence interval (CI). The Chi-square test and the Student *t*-test were used to explore associations of a participant's demographic and socio-economic characteristics and the likelihood of having *S. japonicum*, any STH, and any helminth infection. Significant demographic and socio-economic factors were entered into the mixed-effect logistic regression analysis to obtain the final model for predicting stunting. Random barangay (village) and household effects were included in the model to account for the correlation among observations within each barangay and household, respectively. Adaptive Gaussian quadrature with 10 points was adopted to approximate the log likelihood for all levels of both random effects in the mixed model. Factors that were not significantly relevant (cut-off for significance = 0.05) were removed in a stepwise backward regression elimination procedure.

2.6. Study Oversight

Ethical consent for the study was obtained from the ethics review boards of the Department of Health in the Philippines (IRB # 2012-13-0) and Griffith University, Australia. Written informed consent was obtained from the parents/legal guardians. All questionnaires were translated into the local dialect and back-translated into English. Individuals found positive for a STH or *S. japonicum* were treated according to the Department of Health clinical guidelines.

3. Results

3.1. Demographic, Household, and Nutritional Characteristics and Prevalence of Infection

A cross-sectional survey was carried out on 693 children, of whom 53% were male. A total of 41.7% of the study population was aged between 6–9 years with the remainder between 10–14 years. The majority of children (56%) lived in a house with a roof made from either palm leaves or nipa, an indirect indicator of lower socioeconomic status. Infection with *S. japonicum*, *Ascaris lumbricoides*, *Trichuris trichiura*, and hookworm was evident in 20.1, 54.4, 71.4, and 25.3% of the 667 children sampled for intestinal parasites. The majority of the children (84.7%) was infected with one or more helminth species, with about one-quarter of the study sample (24.7%) infected with three or more different worm species.

The demographic, household, and nutritional characteristics of the study sample are presented in Table 1. About half (49.2%, $n = 341$) of the study sample were stunted and 27.8% ($n = 193$) were thin. Both mean HAZ and BAZ scores were below world standard (-2.0 SD and -1.3 SD from world mean, respectively). SJ infection occurred more often for males (64.2%, $p = 0.003$) and higher age group (70.2%, $p = 0.002$). Children with *S. japonicum* infection also had lower BAZ scores (-1.603, $p = 0.039$). Children with any STH infection were more likely to be of higher age group (60.5%, $p = 0.019$) or living in houses with palm leaves/nipa roofs (57.5%, $p = 0.040$). There was no significant difference for the nutrition indicators between children with and without any STH infection. Age group and roof material were the only factors that differentiated the three children groups of non-infected, monoparasitism, and polyparasitism (proportion of polyparasitism was higher for the higher age group, $p = 0.018$, and for those with house roof materials of palm leaves or nipa, $p = 0.021$).

3.2. Demographic, Household, and Nutritional Characteristics and Intensity of Infection

Table 2 presents the demographic, household, and nutritional characteristics of the study sample, by intensity of infection. Significant results were found between negative, light, and moderate/heavy SJ infection. Males ($p = 0.01$) and older children ($p = 0.009$) were more likely to have *S. japonicum* infection. For *A. lumbricoides* infections, children in the household without toilets ($p = 0.009$) or without galvanized iron/cement roof ($p < 0.001$) were more likely to have moderate or heavy infections. These factors have the same impact for *T. trichiura* infections. Children in households without toilets ($p < 0.001$) or galvanized iron/cement roof ($p = 0.038$) were more likely to have moderate or heavy infections. Moreover, children with moderate or heavy *T. trichiura* infections had a significantly higher mean levels of vitamin C intake, compared to those with light infections ($p = 0.038$). Finally, children with light hookworm infections were more likely to be male (62.1% versus 49.4%, $p = 0.004$), to be stunted (61.5% versus 44.8%, $p < 0.001$), and had a higher proportion of households without toilets (25.7% versus 17.9%, $p = 0.028$), and lower mean HAZ Z-scores (-2.14 versus -1.92, $p = 0.014$) and BAZ Z-scores (-1.61 versus -1.37, $p = 0.013$).

Table 1. Demographic, household, and nutritional characteristics of the study sample ($n = 693$) according to *Schistosoma japonicum* (SJ) and/or soil-transmitted helminth (STH) infections.

Characteristic	All Children (n = 693)	Positive for SJ Infection (n = 134)	p value [a]	Positive for any STH Infection (n = 552)	p value [a]	Non-Infected (n = 102)	Monoparasitism (n = 184)	Polyparasitism (n = 381)	p Value [b]
Gender									
Male	365 (52.7%)	86 (64.2%)	0.003 *	294 (53.3%)	0.470	49 (48.0%)	90 (48.9%)	212 (55.6%)	0.195
Female	328 (47.3%)	48 (35.8%)		258 (46.7%)		53 (52%)	94 (51.1%)	169 (44.4%)	
Age group									
6–9	289 (41.7%)	40 (29.9%)	0.002 *	218 (39.5%)	0.019 *	55 (53.9%)	76 (41.3%)	146 (38.3%)	0.018 *
10–14	404 (58.3%)	94 (70.2%)		334 (60.5%)		47 (46.1%)	108 (58.7%)	235 (61.7%)	
Toilet									
Yes	547 (80.0%)	108 (81.2%)	0.726	434 (79.6%)	0.492	84 (83.2%)	149 (81.9%)	295 (78.5%)	0.451
No	137 (20.0%)	25 (18.8%)		111 (20.4%)		17 (16.8%)	33 (18.1%)	81 (21.5%)	
Own home									
Yes	620 (90.4%)	121 (91.0%)	0.965	497 (90.9%)	0.671	92 (91.1%)	170 (92.4%)	340 (90.4%)	0.746
No	66 (9.6%)	12 (9.0%)		50 (9.1%)		9 (8.9%)	14 (7.6%)	36 (9.6%)	
Roof material									
Palm leaves/nipa	380 (56.1%)	72 (54.1%)	0.692	312 (57.5%)	0.040 *	44 (44.9%)	97 (53.0%)	223 (59.8%)	0.021 *
Galvanized iron/cement	298 (43.9%)	61 (45.9%)		231 (42.5%)		54 (55.1%)	86 (47.0%)	150 (40.2%)	
Height for age									
Normal	352 (50.8%)	60 (44.8%)	0.108	274 (49.6%)	0.130	58 (56.9%)	98 (53.3%)	184 (48.3%)	0.235
Stunted	341 (49.2%)	74 (55.2%)		278 (50.4%)		44 (43.1%)	86 (46.7%)	197 (51.7%)	
BMI for age									
Normal	500 (72.2%)	89 (66.4%)	0.103	399 (72.4%)	0.667	71 (69.6%)	133 (72.3%)	276 (72.6%)	0.831
Thin	193 (27.8%)	45 (33.6%)		152 (27.6%)		31 (30.4%)	51 (27.7%)	104 (27.4%)	
Mean HAZ score	−1.985 (0.973)	−2.091 (0.976)	0.131	−1.999 (0.986)	0.196	−1.85 (0.92)	−1.98 (1.04)	−2.01 (0.96)	0.360
Mean BAZ score	−1.285 (3.961)	−1.603 (1.099)	0.039 *	−1.448 (1.082)	0.412	−1.39 (1)	−1.34 (1.14)	−1.49 (1.05)	0.291
Mean energy (kj)	7512 (3078)	7371 (2737)	0.577	7463 (3166)	0.531	7528 (2538)	7489 (2663)	7486 (3382)	0.992
Mean protein (g)	55.3 (52.3)	52.8 (20.8)	0.304	55.48 (57.80)	0.765	54.51 (20.13)	51.35 (18.45)	57.46 (68.38)	0.435
Mean total fat (g)	36.7 (31.6)	35.6 (22.8)	0.654	36.50 (34.04)	0.911	35.95 (17.61)	37.33 (21.74)	36.18 (38.17)	0.908
Mean carbohydrate (g)	310.7 (119.7)	307.4 (124.1)	0.764	308.0 (117.2)	0.313	314.6 (121.3)	311.9 (122.7)	308.1 (116.3)	0.864
Mean water (g)	1997 (699)	2016 (661)	0.614	2016 (661.246)	0.614	1989 (674)	1956 (736)	2006 (681)	0.725
Mean thiamin (g)	0.663 (1.33)	0.578 (0.292)	0.121	0.671 (1.480)	0.611	0.63 (0.33)	0.61 (0.33)	0.70 (1.77)	0.713
Mean riboflavin (mg)	0.583 (0.617)	0.532 (0.303)	0.108	0.586 (0.679)	0.769	0.59 (0.29)	0.54 (0.30)	0.60 (0.79)	0.571
Mean niacin (mg)	17.1 (10.9)	16.5 (8.5)	0.473	0.487 (11.448)	0.803	17.06 (8.77)	15.87 (7.21)	17.53 (12.84)	0.242
Mean vitamin C (mg)	36.0 (52.1)	30.4 (44.7)	0.110	36.62 (52.12)	0.645	33.94 (56.45)	39.62 (55.43)	35.13 (49.91)	0.569

Data are count (%) for categorical variables and mean (standard deviation) for continuous variables. [a] Test differences between participants with positive infection vs negative infection (using either *t*-test or Chi-square test). [b] Test differences among participants without infection, monoparasitism, and polyparasitism (2–4 infections of SJ or any STH) (using either *t*-test or Chi-square test). * Significance at the 0.05 level.

Table 2. Demographic, household, and nutritional characteristics of the study sample according to intensity of infection.

Characteristic	Schistosoma japonicum [a]			A. lumbricoides [b]			T. trichiura [c]			Hookworms [d]	
	Negative (n = 533)	Light (n = 124)	Mod-Heavy (n = 10)	Negative (n = 304)	Light (n = 241)	Mod-Heavy (n = 122)	Negative (n = 191)	Light (n = 392)	Mod-Heavy (n = 84)	Negative (n = 498)	Light (n = 169)
Gender [a,d]											
Male	265 (49.7%)	79 (63.7%)	7 (70.0%)	161 (53.0%)	131 (54.4%)	59 (48.4%)	99 (51.8%)	202 (51.5%)	50 (59.5%)	246 (49.4%)	105 (62.1%)
Female	268 (50.3%)	45 (36.3%)	3 (30.0%)	143 (47.0%)	110 (45.6%)	63 (51.6%)	92 (48.2%)	190 (48.5%)	34 (40.5%)	252 (50.6%)	64 (37.9%)
Age group [a]											
6–9	237 (44.5%)	37 (29.8%)	3 (30.0%)	128 (42.1%)	98 (40.7%)	51 (41.8%)	91 (47.6%)	151 (38.5%)	35 (41.7%)	211 (42.4%)	66 (39.1%)
10–14	296 (55.5%)	87 (70.2%)	7 (70.0%)	176 (57.9%)	143 (59.3%)	71 (58.2%)	100 (52.4%)	241 (61.5%)	49 (58.3%)	287 (57.6%)	103 (60.9%)
Toilet [b,c,d]											
Yes	420 (79.9%)	99 (80.5%)	9 (90.0%)	253 (84.1%)	190 (79.8%)	85 (70.8%)	153 (81.0%)	325 (83.6%)	50 (61.7%)	404 (82.1%)	124 (74.3%)
No	106 (20.1%)	24 (19.5%)	1 (10.0%)	48 (15.9%)	48 (20.2%)	35 (29.2%)	36 (19.0%)	64 (16.4%)	31 (38.3%)	88 (17.9%)	43 (25.7%)
Own home											
Yes	481 (91.1%)	113 (91.9%)	8 (80.0%)	278 (92.1%)	217 (90.8%)	107 (89.2%)	175 (92.1%)	353 (90.8%)	74 (90.2%)	452 (91.5%)	150 (89.8%)
No	47 (8.9%)	10 (8.1%)	2 (20.0%)	24 (7.9%)	22 (9.2%)	13 (10.8%)	15 (7.9%)	36 (9.2%)	8 (9.8%)	42 (8.5%)	17 (10.2%)
Roof material [b,c]											
Palm leaves/nipa	292 (56.1%)	67 (54.5%)	5 (50.0%)	142 (47.5%)	137 (57.8%)	85 (72.0%)	95 (51.1%)	214 (55.2%)	55 (68.8%)	264 (54.2%)	65 (38.5%)
Galvanized iron/cement	229 (43.9%)	56 (45.5%)	5 (50.0%)	157 (52.5%)	100 (42.2%)	33 (28.0%)	91 (48.9%)	174 (44.8%)	25 (31.2%)	223 (45.8%)	67 (40.1%)
Height for age [d]											
Normal	280 (52.5%)	56 (45.2%)	4 (40.0%)	160 (52.6%)	125 (51.9%)	55 (45.1%)	106 (55.5%)	196 (50.0%)	38 (45.2%)	275 (55.2%)	65 (38.5%)
Stunted	253 (47.5%)	68 (54.8%)	6 (60.0%)	144 (47.4%)	116 (48.1%)	67 (54.9%)	85 (44.5%)	196 (50.0%)	46 (54.8%)	223 (44.8%)	104 (61.5%)
BMI for age [d]											
Normal	391 (73.5%)	83 (66.9%)	6 (60.0%)	212 (69.7%)	176 (73.3%)	92 (75.4%)	136 (71.2%)	284 (72.6%)	60 (71.4%)	363 (72.9%)	117 (69.6%)
Thin	141 (26.5%)	41 (33.1%)	4 (40.0%)	92 (30.3%)	64 (26.7%)	30 (24.6%)	55 (28.8%)	107 (27.4%)	24 (28.6%)	135 (27.1%)	51 (30.4%)
Mean HAZ score [d]	−1.95 (1.0)	−2.09 (1.0)	−2.05 (1.0)	−1.98 (1.0)	−1.94 (0.9)	−2.05 (1.0)	−1.86 (1.0)	−2.00 (1.0)	−2.15 (1.0)	−1.92 (1.0)	−2.14 (0.9)
Mean BAZ score [d]	−1.39 (1.1)	−1.61 (1.1)	−1.56 (1.4)	−1.45 (1.1)	−1.47 (1.1)	−1.32 (0.9)	−1.35 (1.1)	−1.45 (1.1)	−1.54 (0.8)	−1.37 (1.1)	−1.61 (1.1)
Mean energy (kj)	7349 (2792)	7643 (2015)	7990 (3178)	7536 (2544)	7628 (3890)	7122 (2372)	7632 (2811)	7472 (3308)	7279 (2477)	7483 (3105)	7523 (2993)
Mean protein (g)	55.97 (38.6)	52.32 (20.8)	58.29 (20.7)	52.86 (19.0)	60.29 (84.6)	51.67 (20.1)	54.14 (20.7)	55.90 (67.2)	55.34 (21.3)	54.93 (34.8)	56.48 (48.3)
Mean totalfat (g)	36.68 (33.7)	35.80 (23.0)	32.93 (21.4)	36.57 (19.5)	38.59 (46.7)	31.99 (16.3)	38.76 (22.7)	36.65 (37.4)	30.36 (16.6)	36.73 (32.4)	35.67 (29.8)
Mean carbohydrate (g)	310.9 (117)	306.1 (126)	324.3 (99.3)	315.0 (120)	308.4 (120)	301.6 (113)	314.6 (128)	307.9 (114)	310.8 (119)	309.3 (119)	312.6 (119)
Mean water (g)	1982 (704)	2005 (672)	2158 (519)	1992 (681)	1984 (711)	1994 (705)	2005 (693)	1973 (690)	2028 (728)	1976 (694)	2028 (700)
Mean thiamin (g)	0.69 (1.51)	0.58 (0.30)	0.54 (0.22)	0.60 (0.29)	0.80 (2.22)	0.57 (0.26)	0.65 (0.38)	0.69 (1.74)	0.57 (0.24)	0.67 (1.39)	0.65 (1.24)
Mean riboflavin (mg)	0.60 (0.69)	0.53 (0.31)	0.51 (0.25)	0.54 (0.27)	0.64 (0.98)	0.57 (0.29)	0.59 (0.32)	0.57 (0.78)	0.61 (0.29)	0.58 (0.64)	0.60 (0.58)
Mean niacin (mg)	17.13 (11.5)	16.18 (8.1)	20.34 (12.3)	16.33 (7.8)	17.88 (15.0)	16.93 (7.8)	16.81 (8.4)	16.79 (12.4)	18.40 (8.7)	16.76 (11.1)	17.70 (10.8)
Mean vitamin C [c] (mg)	37.65 (54.2)	29.76 (44.0)	38.24 (35.0)	37.55 (55.4)	35.66 (49.1)	33.83 (51.8)	36.12 (53.2)	33.37 (47.3)	49.51 (69.7)	36.01 (51.2)	36.71 (56.2)

Data are count (%) for categorical variables and mean (standard deviation) for continuous variables. [a] Significant difference between negative, light, and moderate/heavy SJ infection in gender (p = 0.01) and age group (p = 0.009). [b] Significant difference between negative, light, and moderate/heavy A. lumbricoides infection in the proportions of owning toilet (p = 0.009) and galvanized iron/cement roof material (p < 0.001). [c] Significant difference between negative, light, and moderate/heavy T. trichiura infection in the proportions of owning toilet (p < 0.001) and galvanized iron/cement roof material (p = 0.028), and the mean level of vitamin C (p = 0.038). [d] Significant difference between negative and light hookworms infection in gender (p = 0.004), the proportions of owning toilet (p = 0.028) and stunted children (p < 0.001), and the mean levels of the HAZ Z-score (p = 0.014) and the BAZ Z-score (p = 0.013).

As depicted in Figure 1, a decreasing trend between infection intensity and the mean values of HAZ and BAZ was identified for *T. trichiura* or hookworm infections (that is, the heavier the intensity, the lower the HAZ and BAZ mean values). For SJ or *A. lumbricoides* infections, the trend was not so obvious.

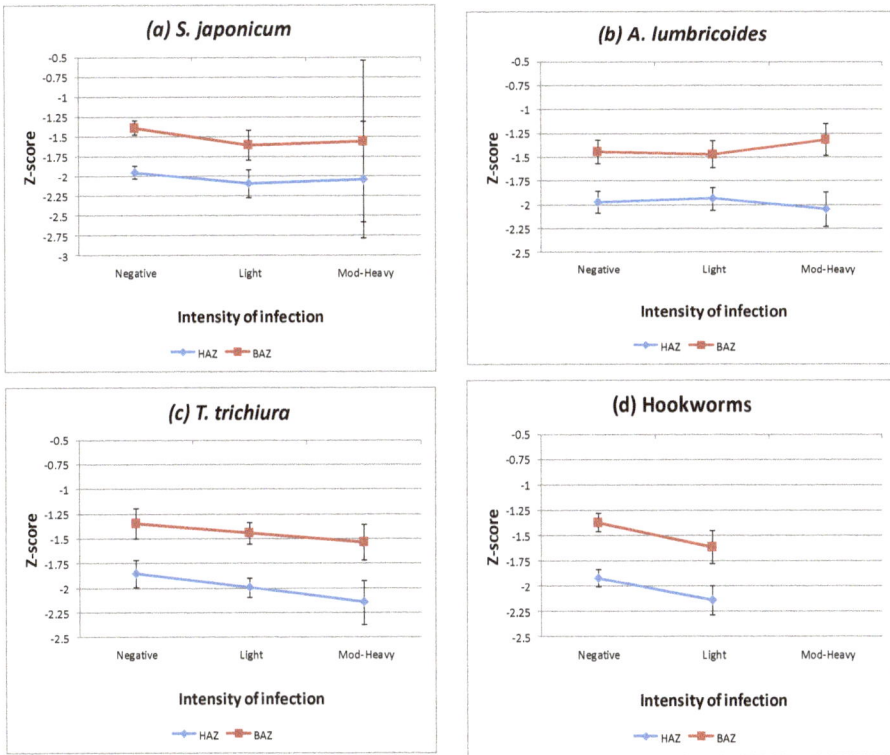

Figure 1. Plots of Z-scores for the anthropometric indicators versus (**a**) *Schistosoma japonicum*; (**b**) *T. trichiura*; (**c**) *A. lumbricoides*; (**d**) hookworms infection. Note HAZ: height for age Z-score; BAZ: BMI for age Z-score. Mod-Heavy: infections of moderate to heavy intensity.

3.3. Demographic, Socioeconomic Factors and Stunting

Table 3 displays the mixed-effect logistic regression model for stunting. Compared to children with normal height for age, stunted children were more likely to be male (AOR = 1.58; 95% CI: 1.05–2.39; $p = 0.028$), older in the age group of 10–14 (AOR = 1.93; 95% CI: 1.29–2.88; $p = 0.001$), and living in poorer households with palm leaves/nipa roofs (AOR = 1.85; 95% CI: 1.14–3.01; $p = 0.013$). All nutrition factors were not significantly associated with stunting. Variation among the predicted barangay-specific random effects for stunting was not statistically significant. However, there is significant household-specific random effects (estimated variance: 1.82, $p < 0.001$) in the probability of stunting, indicating that unknown household effects other than the identified household risk factor (roof materials) exist.

Table 3. Mixed-effect logistic regression analysis of the relationship between stunting with demographic and socio-economic variables.

Variable	Height for Age		Stunting Versus Normal	
	Normal (*n* = 352)	Stunted (*n* = 341)	Adjusted OR (95% CI)	*p*-Value
Gender				
Male	172 (48.9%)	193 (56.6%)	1.58 (1.05–2.39)	0.028
Female	180 (51.1%)	148 (43.4%)	Reference	
Age group				
6–9	167 (47.4%)	122 (35.8%)	Reference	
10–14	185 (52.6%)	219 (64.2%)	1.93 (1.29–2.88)	0.001
Roof material				
Palm leaves/nipa	173 (50.0%)	207 (62.4%)	1.85 (1.14–3.01)	0.013
Galvanized iron/cement	173 (50.0%)	125 (37.6%)	Reference	
Barangay variance			0.10 (0.01–1.25)	
Household variance			1.82 (0.91–3.64)	

4. Discussion

The current WHO strategy for intestinal helminths in children is to continually treat pre-school and school-age children at high risk once or twice per year depending on prevalence [8]. This is effective in achieving morbidity control; however, it does not prevent re-infection. Our study area has participated in national control efforts for over two decades yet the prevalence of helminth infection remains stubbornly high due largely to poverty and malnutrition. In our study, we found that approximately 85% of the rural children were infected with one or more helminth infections. *T. trichiura* infections (71.4%) were found to be more prevalent than *A. lumbricoides* (54.4%) infections. Moreover, about half (49%) of the study sample were stunted and almost a third (28%) were wasted. Stunted children were more likely to be male, older in age (10–14 years), and living in poorer households with palm leaves/nipa roofs.

In the mixed-effect logistic regression model for stunting all of the nutrition factors (i.e., grams) were found not to be significantly associated with stunting. However, we previously found a significant association between the coinfection of all four helminthiases and low intakes of energy, thiamine, and riboflavin among children, when the recommended energy and nutrient intake (RENI) for total calories was examined [21]. Thiamine and riboflavin deficiencies are common in Northern Samar, where dairy and meat intakes are low and mostly rice-based meals are consumed [21]. Iron deficiency has been associated with impairments in both adaptive and innate immunity and with lowering the body's resistance to infectious diseases [21]. Poor nutrient intake may increase susceptibility to parasitic diseases and together they negatively affect the nutritional status of children and adolescents [21].

We believe that a deworming program must be coupled with a nutrition program at the primary school level. Children are presently eating 1–2 meals per day at home and this is insufficient to meet their macro or micronutrient requirements. An additional meal at school appears to be of paramount importance for those severely malnourished. In order to address this problem the Philippine government has initiated the school-based feeding program called *'Gulayan sa Paaralan'*, which has been successfully piloted in approximately one percent of schools. However, to date it has not been formally evaluated in a clinical trial.

An appropriate eight-week micronutrient weaning period of 'ready-to-use therapeutic foods' (RUTF), with demonstrated immune-modulating functions—including iron, zinc, calcium, vitamin A, B and C, n-3 and n-6 fatty acids—also needs to be considered following the macronutrient school intervention. In a recent pilot study conducted at the Philippine General Hospital, the researchers created their modified version of RUTF from commercially-available ingredients including milk, sugar, coconut oil, and peanut butter [28]. A total of 100 children (aged 18 months to 10 years) was randomized to either a RUTF group, who received the supplement, and a control group, who did not [28]. The treatment group received RUTF on weekdays for five weeks. Changes in weight, height, and arm circumference were recorded for five weeks and two weeks after supplementation. Results of the study showed that RUTF was an effective, safe, and acceptable alternative supplement for children with mild to severe malnutrition [28].

Annual or biannual albendazole treatment (i.e., 400 mg) needs to be combined with macro/micronutrient supplements, WASH, and health education in order to interrupt the life cycles of STH diseases, prevent reinfection, and achieve sustainable control. A well-nourished population, with an intact immune system, has a better chance of warding off future parasitic infection. Simply providing drugs to malnourished populations, which is a common practice in the global control of STHs, is not the answer. Both poverty and malnutrition must be addressed if future MDA programs for NTDs are to have a lasting impact.

Acknowledgments: We thank the Australian National Health and Medical Research Council for providing financial support for this research in the Philippines.

Author Contributions: A.G.R. and K.P. conceived and designed the experiments; A.G.R., K.P. and R.L.-C. performed the field studies; S.-K.N, T.N.C. and M.T.I. analyzed and interpreted the data; all authors contributed to writing the paper.

Conflicts of Interest: The authors declare no conflict of interest.

References

1. Bethony, J.; Brooker, S.; Albonico, M.; Geiger, S.M.; Loukas, A.; Diemert, D.; Hotez, P.J. Soil-transmitted helminth infections: Ascariasis, trichuriasis, and hookworm. *Lancet* **2006**, *367*, 1521–1532. [CrossRef]
2. Hotez, P.J. Mass drug administration and integrated control for the world's high-prevalence neglected tropical diseases. *Clin. Pharmacol. Ther.* **2009**, *85*, 659–664. [CrossRef] [PubMed]
3. Brooker, S.; Hotez, P.J.; Bundy, D.A. Hookworm-related anaemia among pregnant women: A systematic review. *PLoS Negl. Trop. Dis.* **2008**, *2*, e291. [CrossRef] [PubMed]
4. Miguel, E.A.; Kremer, M. Worms: Identifying impacts on education and health in the presence of treatment externalities. *Econometrica* **2004**, *72*, 159–217. [CrossRef]
5. Sakti, H.; Nokes, C.; Hertanto, W.S.; Hendratno, S.; Hall, A.; Bundy, D.A. Evidence for an association between hookworm infection and cognitive function in Indonesia school children. *Trop. Med. Int. Health* **1999**, *4*, 322–334. [CrossRef] [PubMed]
6. Nokes, C.; Grantham-McGregor, S.M.; Sawyer, A.W.; Cooper, E.S.; Robinson, B.A.; Bundy, D.A. Moderate to heavy infections of *Trichuris trichiura* affect cognitive function in Jamaican school children. *Parasitology* **1992**, *104*, 539–547. [CrossRef] [PubMed]
7. Hotez, P. Hookworm and poverty. *Ann. N. Y. Acad. Sci.* **2008**, *1136*, 38–44. [CrossRef] [PubMed]
8. World Health Organization (WHO). *Deworming for Health and Development*; Report of the Third Global Meeting of the Partners for Parasite Control; World Health Organization: Geneva, Switzerland, 2005.
9. World Health Organization (WHO). *Priority Communicable Diseases: Health in Asian and the Pacific*; Chapter 7; World Health Organization: Geneva, Switzerland, 2008.
10. Belizario, V.Y., Jr.; de Leon, W.U.; Lumampao, Y.F.; Anastacio, M.B.; Tai, C.M. Sentinel surveillance of soil-transmitted helminthiases in selected local government units in the Philippines. *Asia Pac. J. Public Health* **2009**, *21*, 26. [CrossRef] [PubMed]
11. Easton, A. Intestinal worms impair child health in the Philippines. *BMJ* **1999**, *318*, 214. [CrossRef] [PubMed]
12. Reilly, L.; Nausch, N.; Midzi, N.; Mduluza, T.; Mutapi, F. Association between micronutrients (vitamin A, D, iron) and schistosome-specific cytokine responses in Zimbabweans exposed to *Schistosoma haematobium*. *J. Parasitol. Res.* **2012**, *2012*, 128628. [CrossRef] [PubMed]
13. Zhou, H.; Ohtsuka, R.; He, Y.; Yuan, L.; Yamauchi, T.; Sleigh, A.C. Impact of parasitic infections and dietary intake on child growth in the schistosomiasis-endemic Dongting Lake Region, China. *Am. J. Trop. Med. Hyg.* **2005**, *72*, 534–539. [PubMed]
14. Hesham, M.S.; Edariah, A.B.; Norhayati, M. Intestinal parasitic infections and micronutrient deficiency: A review. *Med. J. Malaysia* **2004**, *59*, 284–293. [PubMed]

15. Katona, P.; Katona-Apte, J. The interaction between nutrition and infection. *Clin. Infect. Dis.* **2008**, *46*, 1582–1588. [CrossRef] [PubMed]

16. Cunningham-Rundles, S.; McNeeley, D.F.; Moon, A. Mechanisms of nutrient modulation of the immune response. *J. Allergy Clin. Immunol.* **2005**, *115*, 1119–1128. [CrossRef] [PubMed]

17. Nga, T.T.; Winichagoon, P.; Dijkhuizen, M.A.; Khan, N.C.; Wasantwisut, E.; Wieringa, F.T. Decreased parasite load and improved cognitive outcomes caused by deworming and consumption of multi-micronutrient fortified biscuits in rural Vietnamese schoolchildren. *Am. J. Trop. Med. Hyg.* **2011**, *85*, 333–340. [CrossRef] [PubMed]

18. Amare, B.; Ali, J.; Moges, B.; Yismaw, G.; Belyhun, Y.; Gebretsadik, S.; Woldeyohannes, D.; Tafess, K.; Abate, E.; Endris, M.; et al. Nutritional status, intestinal parasite infection and allergy among school children in northwest Ethiopia. *BMC Pediatr.* **2013**, *13*, 7. [CrossRef] [PubMed]

19. Sanza, M.; Totanes, F.I.; Chua, P.L.; Belizario, V.Y., Jr. Monitoring the impact of a mebendazole mass drug administration initiative for soil transmitted helminthiasis (STH) control in the Western Visayas region of the Philippines from 2007 through 2011. *Acta Trop.* **2013**, *127*, 112–117. [CrossRef] [PubMed]

20. Belizario, V.Y., Jr.; Totanes, F.I.; de Leon, W.U.; Lumampao, Y.F.; Ciro, R.N. Soil transmitted helminth and other intestinal parasitic infections among school children in indigenous people communities in Davao del Norte, Philippines. *Acta Trop.* **2011**, *120* (Suppl. S1), S12–S18. [CrossRef] [PubMed]

21. Papier, K.; Williams, G.M.; Frauk, A.; Olveda, R.M.; McManus, D.P.; Harn, D.A.; Li, Y.S.; Gray, D.J.; Chau, T.N.P.; Ross, A.G. Chronic malnutrition and parasitic helminth interations. *Clin. Infect. Dis.* **2014**, *59*, 234–243. [CrossRef] [PubMed]

22. Ross, A.G.; Olveda, R.M.; Chy, D.; Olveda, D.U.; Li, Y.; Harn, D.A.; Gray, D.J.; McManus, D.P.; Tallo, V.; Chau, T.N.; et al. Can mass drug administration lead to the sustainable control of schistosomiasis? *J. Infect. Dis.* **2015**, *211*, 283–289. [CrossRef] [PubMed]

23. Gibson, R.S. *Principles of Nutritional Assessment*, 2nd ed.; Oxford University Press: New York, NY, USA, 2005.

24. World Health Organization (WHO). *WHO AnthroPlus for Personal Computers Manual: Software for Assessing Growth of the World's Children and Adolescent*; World Health Organization: Geneva, Switzerland, 2009.

25. World Health Organization (WHO). *WHO AnthroPlus Software: Software for Assessing Growth and Development of the World's Children*; World Health Organization: Geneva, Switzerland, 2007.

26. Philippine Statistics Authority. National Statistical Coordination Board, Department of Science and Technology: Taguig, Philippines, 1997; p. 163.

27. Food and Nutrition Research Institute. *Recommended Energy and Nutrient Intakes*; Department of Science and Technology: Taguig, Metro Manila, Philippines, 2002; p. 423.

28. Laylo-Navarr, C.; Limos, E. A randomized controlled trial on the efficacy and safety of a modified ready to use therapeutic food among malnourished children. *Acta Med. Philipp.* **2011**, *45*, 29–33.

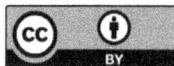

Tropical Medicine and Infectious Disease

MDPI

Article

Epidemiology and Characteristics of *Rickettsia australis* (Queensland Tick Typhus) Infection in Hospitalized Patients in North Brisbane, Australia

Adam Stewart [1,*], Mark Armstrong [1], Stephen Graves [2] and Krispin Hajkowicz [1,3]

[1]   Department of Infectious Diseases, Royal Brisbane and Women's Hospital, Butterfield St & Bowen Bridge Rd, Herston, Queensland 4029, Australia; mark.armstrong@health.qld.gov.au (M.A.); krispin.hajkowicz@health.qld.gov.au (K.H.)

[2]   Australian Rickettsial Reference Laboratory, Barwon Health, Geelong Hospital, Bellerine Street, PO BOX 281, Geelong, Victoria 3220, Australia; graves.rickettsia@gmail.com

[3]   School of Medicine, University of Queensland, St Lucia, Queensland 4072, Australia

*   Correspondence: adm_stewart@hotmail.com; Tel.: +61-421759716

Academic Editors: Patricia Graves, Thewarach Laha, Peter A. Leggat and Khin Saw Aye

Received: 22 March 2017; Accepted: 10 April 2017; Published: 15 April 2017

Abstract: Queensland tick typhus (QTT; *Rickettsia australis*) is a spotted fever group (SFG) rickettsial infection endemic to Australia. It is an underreported and often unrecognized illness with poorly-defined epidemiology. This article describes epidemiological features and the geographical distribution of QTT in hospitalized patients. Cases of QTT were identified retrospectively from 2000–2015 at five sites in Northern Brisbane through a pathology database. Included cases had a four-fold rise in SFG-specific titre, a single SFG-specific titre $\geq$256 or an SFG-specific titre $\geq$128 with a clinically consistent illness. Of the fifty cases identified by serology, 36 were included. Age ranged from 3–72 years (with a mean of 39.5 years) with a male-to-female ratio of 1:1.1. Fifteen of 36 (42%) study participants had hobbies and/or occupations linked with the acquisition of the disease. Seventeen of 36 (47%) identified a tick bite in the days preceding presentation to hospital, and reported exposure to a known animal host was minimal (25%). QTT infection occurred throughout the year, with half of the cases reported between April and July. Recent ecological and sociocultural changes have redefined the epidemiology of this zoonotic illness, with areas of higher infection risk identified. Heightened public health awareness is required to monitor QTT disease activity.

Keywords: tick-borne diseases; *Rickettsia* infections; epidemiology; Queensland; Australia

1. Introduction

Queensland tick typhus (QTT) is an important cause of febrile illness; particularly among those exposed to the eastern coastal bushlands in Australia [1]. Currently, a diagnosis of any rickettsial infection does not require compulsory reporting in Australia, making disease surveillance incredibly difficult and inaccurate [2,3]. Although its true epidemiological impact is unknown, recently identified socio-ecological drivers of rickettsial disease could re-define QTT as a public health threat [1]. In addition, recent serological surveys point to a disease burden along the eastern coast that is greater than previously realized [1,4]. The geographical distribution and boundaries of QTT infection continue to be pushed further along the coastline, as well as inland [5]. As our understanding of host-vector interactions and ecological factors that drive disease emergence improves, informed public health interventions will become pivotal.

2. Materials and Methods

Study patients were both adults and children identified retrospectively during the period of January 2000 to January 2015 at any of the five sites in Metropolitan North Hospital and Health Service (MNHSS) in Queensland, Australia via the local pathology database. Medical records were reviewed for each identified case. Epidemiological and clinical data were recorded onto a standardized electronic case report form. Clinical features were considered present only if their presence was documented in the medical record. Confirmed or probable cases of QTT included those with a greater or equal to a four-fold rise in spotted fever group (SFG)-specific serology; a single SFG-specific titre ≥256; or an SFG-specific titre ≥128 with a clinically consistent illness [5]. A clinically consistent illness was defined as a presentation typical for QTT, without a more likely diagnosis being apparent, as well as a good clinical response to doxycycline or another appropriate antibiotic. Cases were further excluded if serology results represented an old infection, an acute illness thought to be acquired overseas, or a known cause of antibody cross-reactivity to *Rickettsia*-specific antigens (e.g. autoimmune conditions). The indirect microimmunofluorescence assay (IFA) utilizing an SFG-specific *Rickettsia rickettsii* antigen was used in serological testing.

The study was conducted in accordance with the Declaration of Helsinki, and the protocol was approved by the Royal Brisbane & Women's Hospital Ethics Committee (HREC/14/QRBW/432).

3. Results

Of the 50 cases identified by serological criteria alone through the pathology database, 36 were included after the exclusion criteria were applied. Two patient's medical records were destroyed and thus inaccessible.

3.1. Demographics

Of the studied patients, age ranged from 3–72 years (with a mean of 39.5 years) and sex distribution was approximately equal between males and females with a male-to-female ratio of 1:1.1. Fifteen of 36 (42%) study participants had hobbies and/or occupations that were linked with the acquisition of the disease, including gardening, bushwalking/orienteering, camping, and working as a botanist, wildlife ranger, groundsman, or farm worker/grazier. Eleven of 36 (31%) patients acquired their infection in association with travel away from their primary residence. Four of 36 (11%) were noted to live on a property with dense surrounding bushland. Moreover, 17 out of 36 (47%) reported a tick bite in the days preceding presentation to hospital, and 3 out of 36 (8%) reported multiple tick bites in the past, usually associated with their occupation or place of residence. Reported exposure to vertebrate animals on history was only 9 out of 36 (25%), which included exposure to cattle, dogs and horses (Table 1). Of note, eight patients reported no known risk factors for acute rickettsial infection.

3.2. Distribution of Disease

Eighteen of 36 (50%) cases occurred between April and July; 10/36 (28%) occurred from September to December; and 8/36 (22%) occurred between January and March (Figure 1). To determine the distribution of disease, the postcode of the patient's primary residence was recorded, unless there was a clear history of preceding travel to another place where the tick bite had occurred; in this case, the postcode from the site where the infection was acquired was entered into the database. A high density of infection occurred in the Samford Valley, Woodford and Mount Nebo areas (Figure 2). Eleven of 36 (31%) infections were acquired in this area alone. Six of 36 (8%) were located in the Narangba and Morayfield areas, 5–10 kilometers from the coastal area of Samford. Other infections were sporadically distributed along the eastern coast of Queensland and northern New South Wales. Interestingly, of those requiring intensive care unit (ICU) admission (4/36), 75% lived or acquired their infection within a five-kilometer radius of each other, and presented during the March/April period.

Table 1. Demographic and historical features of 36 patients with Queensland tick typhus (QTT).

Characteristic	Value
Age	3–72 years (Mean 39.5, Median 36.1)
Sex	Male-to-female ratio 1:1.1
- Male	17/36 (47%)
- Female	19/36 (53%)
Occupation	
- Groundsman/ranger	3/36 (8%)
- Farming	3/36 (8%)
Hobby/activity	
- Camping	3/36 (8%)
- Gardening	3/36 (8%)
- Bushwalking	2/36 (6%)
- Other	1/36 (3%)
Residence on acreage/property	4/36 (11%)
Recent travel (e.g., holiday)	11/36 (31%)
Tick bite	17/36 (47%)
- Single	14/36 (39%)
- Multiple	3/36 (8%)
Frequency of known risk factors	
- 0	8/36 (22%)
- 1	13/36 (36%)
- 2	13/36 (36%)
- 3	3/36 (8%)

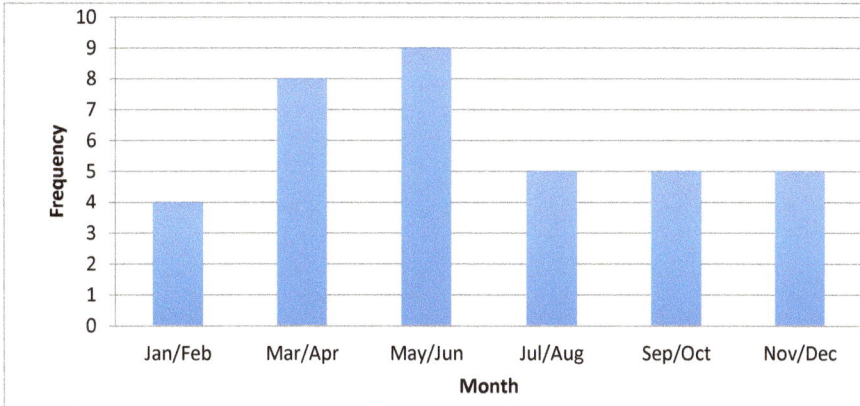

Figure 1. Seasonal variation in QTT infection in 36 hospitalized patients with Queensland tick typhus (QTT).

(A)

(B)

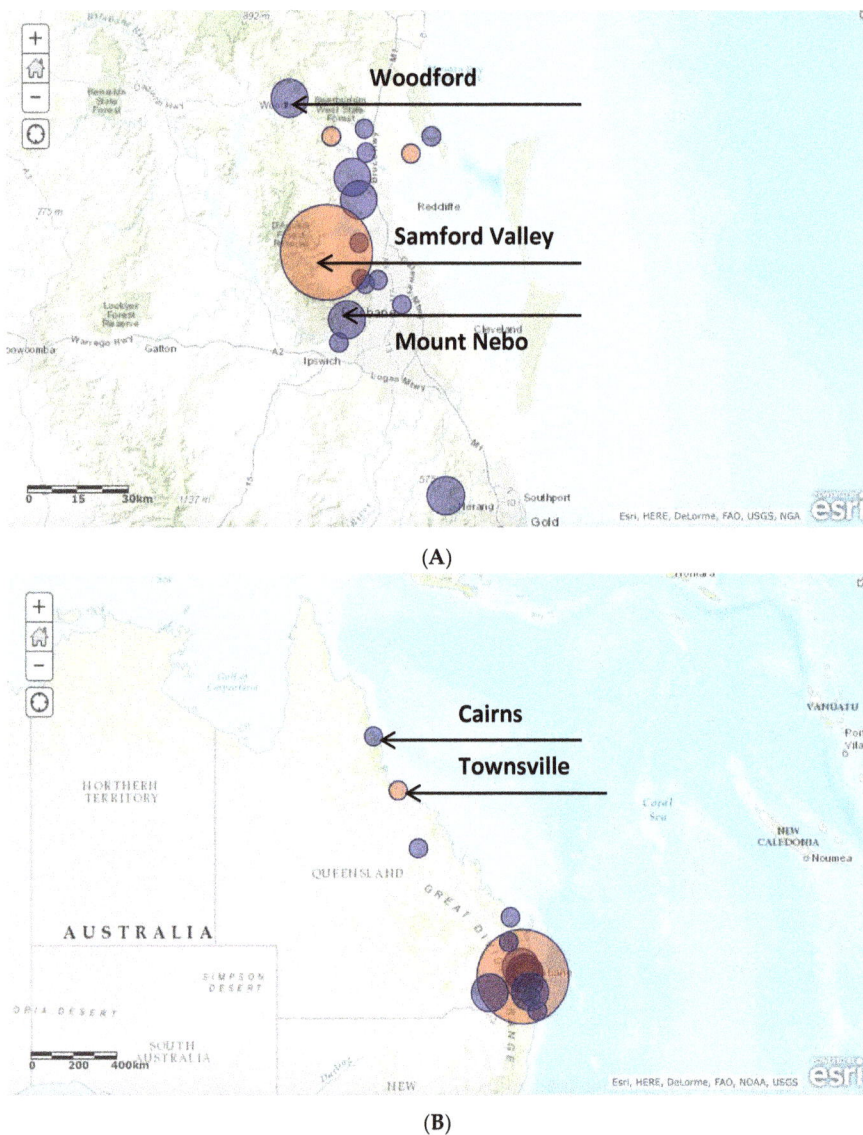

Figure 2. Location of the 36 patients who presented to the five study sites with acute *Rickettsia australis* infection within southeast (**A**) and greater Queensland (**B**) Note: Size of circle indicates relative frequency of infection; orange circles indicate where cases of severe infection occurred.

4. Discussion

Defining the distribution of each SFG rickettsial disease in Australia has been a difficult task [1]. This is largely due to inadequate reporting of infection, as well as low recognition and testing in the community and hospital settings [3,6]. In addition, there may be a larger pool of subclinical infection [1]. We relied on sporadic independent serological surveys to guide our current understanding; these are few and far between [3]. Even these can be unreliable due to assay cross-reactivity with other pathogenic and non-pathogenic rickettsia, as well as with bacteria (e.g., *Proteus species*) [7]. This report is among the few current studies documenting the features of *R. australis* infection; however, it carries significant limitations due to its retrospective nature.

Although *R. australis* infection can occur throughout the year, in this study half of the cases of QTT occurred between April and July, during the seasons of autumn and winter in Australia. This finding appeared to contradict previous reports of increasing incidence of QTT during the summer and spring months [8]. Adult female *Ixodes* spp. ticks (vector for *R. australis*) are most abundant in Queensland from October to December [9]. The reasons for this are unclear, although factors influencing vector distribution and behavior such as rainfall and climate change may play a role.

When mapping out the geographical distribution of QTT among the 36 identified cases, the postcode of the site where the infection or tick bite was thought to have occurred was recorded. If this was not immediately apparent on chart review, the patient's place of residence was used as a surrogate. The major limitation to this approach was that the tick bite was often not acquired from home, and often results from occupational or recreational exposures were not always elicited on history. Nonetheless, infection occurred along eastern coastal Queensland and northern New South Wales with none reported more than 20 kilometers inland—a finding that is consistent with previous reports [2]. A focal hyperendemic area of QTT infection was identified spanning the Samford Valley, Woodford and Mount Nebo regions, accounting for 31% of cases. A further 8% of cases were located within a 5–10 kilometer distance from this area. This identifies an area where ecological conditions for *Ixodes holocyclus* and mammalian hosts are optimal, causing increased infection among susceptible humans [1]. Increasing urbanization of this area over the last few decades has been a major contributor to this phenomenon [1]. It is likely that this will be seen in multiple locations along coastal Australia as population densities change and encroach into new areas.

The mean age of infection was 39.5 years (median 36.1 years), although there was a wide range observed (3–72 years). Extremes of age did not appear to increase the risk of infection. The male-to-female ratio was 1:1.1, which are in contrast to previous reports that revealed a male predominance (2:1) [8]. This could represent a change in occupation and recreational activities among women over the past half century, which is known to highly influence the risk of infection. Given the large number of mammalian host species for *Ixodes* spp. ticks and its predilection for wet forested areas in certain times of the year, certain human activities are high risk for acquiring infection [8,10]. Nearly half of the study participants acquired their infection through occupational or recreational activities, which was consistent with previous studies [8]. No new high-risk human behaviors were identified.

Tick bite is still a useful guide for identifying those with possible QTT, with nearly half reporting this in their history. Exposure to vertebrate animal hosts may be of less utility in diagnosis; although, this aspect of the patient's history was frequently missed or poorly documented. Multiple tick bites were reported by a minority of patients, especially those living in tick-dense areas, and may be particularly important for identifying those at risk of severe disease and sepsis [1]. Many patients discharged from hospital were given advice to avoid ticks, although none had documented lifestyle changes on follow-up; moreover, no reinfections occurred. It is difficult to conclude any benefit from this advice.

5. Conclusions

Rickettsia australis and QTT is an evolving disease with a growing public health importance [1]. A lack of current epidemiological data on its incidence and distribution limits our understanding of the disease and options for beneficial public health interventions. This study has demonstrated the current epidemiology of this infection and has identified a new area of intense QTT endemicity in eastern coastal Queensland. SFG rickettsial infections should be notifiable diseases in Australia. Furthermore, prospective studies refining our understanding of the risk of infection and hospitalization of QTT need to be carried out. In addition, serological surveys of both animal hosts and humans would identify potential hot-spot areas of QTT to limit future disease.

Trop. Med. Infect. Dis. **2017**, *2*, 10

Author Contributions: A.S. provided data, drafted and revised the manuscript. M.A. revised the manuscript and provided intellectual content. S.G. and K.H. provided clinical expertise and intellectual content. All authors have sighted and approved the final manuscript.

Conflicts of Interest: The authors declare no conflict of interest.

References

1. Derne, B.; Weinstein, P.; Musso, D.; Lau, C. Distribution of rickettsioses in Oceania: past patterns and implications for the future. *Acta Trop.* **2015**, *143*, 121–133. [CrossRef] [PubMed]
2. Australian Rickettsial Reference Laboratory. Disease Description and/or Epidemiology. 2015. Available online: http://www.rickettsialab.org.au/-!about (accessed on 22 July 2015).
3. NNDSS. Australia's Notifiable Disease Status: Annual Report of the National Notifiable Diseases Surveillance System. Department of Health and Ageing, 2013. Available online: http://www.commcarelink.health.gov.au/internet/main/publishing.nsf/Content/cda-pubs-annlrpt-nndssar.htm (accessed on 22 July 2015).
4. Faa, A.G.; Graves, S.R.; Stenos, J. A serological survey of rickettsial infections in the Gazelle Peninsula, East New Britain and a review of the literature. *PNG Med. J.* **2006**, *49*, 1–2.
5. Graves, S.; Stenos, J. Rickettsioses in Australia. In *Rickettsiology and Rickettsial Diseases*; Hechemy, K.E., Brouqui, P., Samuel, J.E., Raoult, D.A., Eds.; Wiley-Blackwell: Hoboken, NJ, USA, 2009; Volume 1166, pp. 151–155. [CrossRef] [PubMed]
6. Graves, S. Management of rickettsial diseases and Q Fever. *Med. Today* **2013**, *14*, 65–69.
7. Sexton, D.J.; Banks, J.; Graves, S.; Hughes, K.; Dwyer, B. Prevalence of antibodies to spotted fever group rickettsiae in dogs from south-eastern Australia. *Am. J. Trop. Reed. Hyg.* **1991**, *45*, 243–248.
8. Sexton, D.J.; Dwyer, B.; Kemp, R.; Graves, S. Spotted fever group rickettsial infections in Australia. *Rev. Infect. Dis.* **1991**, *13*, 876–886. [CrossRef] [PubMed]
9. Barker, S.C.; Walker, A.R. Ticks of Australia. The species that infect domestic animals and humans. *Zootaxa* **2014**, *3816*, 1–144. [CrossRef] [PubMed]
10. Derrick, E.H. The challenge of north Queensland fevers. *Australas. Ann. Med.* **1957**, *6*, 173–188. [PubMed]

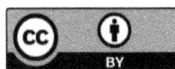

Tropical Medicine and Infectious Disease

MDPI

Article

Infection of Rodents by *Orientia tsutsugamushi*, the Agent of Scrub Typhus, in Relation to Land Use in Thailand

Kittipong Chaisiri [1], **Jean-François Cosson** [2] **and Serge Morand** [3,*]

[1] Department of Helminthology, Faculty of Tropical Medicine, Mahidol University, Bangkok 10400, Thailand; kittipong.cha@mahidol.ac.th
[2] NRA, Biologie Moléculaire et Immunologie Parasitaires et Fongiques, BIPAR, Ecole Nationale Vétérinaire d'Alfort, 94704 Maisons-Alfort Cedex, France; cosson@supagro.inra.fr
[3] CNRS ISEM-CIRAD ASTRE, Faculty of Veterinary Technology, Kasetsart University, Bangkok 10220, Thailand
* Correspondence: serge.morand@umontpellier.fr or serge.morand@cirad.fr; Tel.: +44-870-405-616

Received: 23 August 2017; Accepted: 4 October 2017; Published: 6 October 2017

Abstract: The relationship between land use structures and occurrence of the scrub typhus agent, *Orientia tsutsugamushi,* in small wild mammals was investigated in three provinces of Thailand: Buriram, Loei, and Nan. *O. tsutsugamushi* detection was performed using 16S ribosomal DNA (rDNA) amplicon sequencing approach using Miseq Illumina platform. In total, 387 animals (rodents and shrews) were examined for the infection. The 16S rDNA sequences of the bacterium were found in nine animals, namely *Bandicota savilei, Berylmys bowersi, Leopoldamys edwardsi, Rattus exulans, R. tanezumi,* and *Rattus* sp. phylogenetic clade 3, yielding 2.3% infection rate, with two new rodent species found infected by the bacterium in Thailand: *B. bowersi* and *L. edwardsi.* Using a generalized linear mixed model (GLMM) and Random Forest analyses for investigating the association between human-land use and occurrence of the bacterium, forest habitat appeared as a strong explicative variable of rodent infection, meaning that *O. tsutsugamushi*-infected animals were more likely found in forest-covered habitats. In terms of public health implementation, our results suggest that heterogenous forested areas including forest-converted agricultural land, reforestation areas, or fallows, are potential habitats for *O. tsutsugamushi* transmission. Further understanding of population dynamics of the vectors and their hosts in these habitats could be beneficial for the prevention of this neglected zoonotic disease.

Keywords: *Orientia tsutsugamushi*; scrub typhus; 16S rDNA amplicon sequencing; rodents; land use land cover; Thailand

---

1. Introduction

The obligate intracellular bacterium *Orientia tsutsugamushi* (Rickettsiales: Rickettsiaceae) is the causative agent of scrub typhus in humans, mainly reported in the Asia-Pacific region, and sporadically in some other regions of the world [1,2]. Approximately one million cases of scrub typhus occur annually in Asia, with a 7% to 10% fatality rate if the patients are not treated sufficiently and early in the course of illness [3,4]. Chiggers, the six-legged parasitic larval stage of mites belonging to the family Trombiculidae, are the disease vectors carrying and transmitting the bacterial agent through their bites. *O. tsutsugamushi* is strictly confined to this mite family [5], and potentially develops a symbiotic relationship with its mite host [6–8]. Chigger species from the genus *Leptotrombidium* are the main vectors of scrub typhus in Asia [9,10]. *O. tsutsugamushi* was also reported in other trombiculid species [11] but there is still a lack of supporting evidence to prove their vectorial role in disease transmission, or whether they attack humans. In terms of vertebrate hosts apart from humans, small terrestrial mammals such as rodents (rats, mice and ground squirrels), insectivores and tree-shrews have been reported as hosts of *Leptotrombidium* and are infected by the bacterium. They play important roles in the ecology of chigger mites and thus for the epidemiology of the disease [12,13]. In addition, some other vertebrates such as bats, birds or reptiles, can be also hosts for chigger mites [14,15]. It was hypothesized that their feeding activity on a wide range of hosts may explain the huge diversification of strains of *O. tsutsugamushi* [9,13].

A large diversity of chigger mites can infect Asian small mammals, particularly rodents [16,17] and similarly, a large number of rodent and other small mammal species have been found to be infected by *O. tsutsugamushi* [18]. In Thailand, more than 10 species of rodents (*Bandicota indica, B. savilei, Berylmys berdmorei, Menestes berdmorei, Mus caroli, Niviventer fulvescens, Rattus andamanensis, R. argentiventer, R. exulans, R. losea, R. norvegicus* and *R. tanezumi*) and one species of tree-shrew (*Tupaia glis*) have been reported to be infected by the bacterium [12,19–25]. According to these studies, *O. tsutsugamushi* was detected using serological methods (i.e., fluorescence antibody assay), or by detecting the genetic material of the bacterium via specific gene target polymerase chain reaction (PCR) assays (i.e., the 56-kD type-specific antigen gene).

With the advent of modern molecular tools in bacteriology, high throughput sequencing provides affordable costs, effective detection, and rapid generation of microbial profiling using two main approaches: 16S rDNA amplicon sequencing (sequencing the genome of particular gene targets) and microbiome metagenomics (sequencing the whole particular genome in a sample) [26]. Here in the present study, 16S rDNA amplicon sequencing was conducted to screen the 16S rDNA gene of *O. tsutsugamushi* alongside other bacterial profiles in wild rodents from Thailand.

Environmental factors, including land cover and land use, are known to influence the reproduction and survival of both trombiculid mites [27,28] and rodents [29], and ultimately the spatial heterogeneity of infection risk. The increasing incidence of scrub typhus in South China was associated with habitats characterized by forested areas and climate factors such as relative humidity [30]. In Taiwan, a significant correlation was observed between scrub typhus incidence and habitats characterized by a mosaic of cropland and vegetation [28], which represent transitional land cover use. Scrub typhus occurs in transitional habitats such as forest edges, fallows along streams or abandoned agricultural lands [9]. These habitats favor both chigger mites, because of soil moisture, and their rodent hosts, by providing food and shelters [31].

The present study proposes to investigate the relationships between the structure of landscape and *O. tsutsugamushi* incidence in rodents captured from human-dominated habitats in Thailand. The structure of landscapes may promote *O. tsutsugamushi* transmission in rodents, and consequently the risk of transmission to humans [32,33]. Heterogenic landscape affects the distribution and abundance of rodent species regarding their specialization to habitat [29]. We explored the relationship between the structure of the landscape at a fine environmental scale and individual rodents investigated for infection by *O. tsutsugamushi*. For this, we used the land covers developed for investigating other rodent-borne diseases for each locality investigated in this study [29]. Specifically, we hypothesized that heterogeneous habitats with high forest cover may favor the transmission ecology of *O. tsutsugamushi* among rodents and mites, and its potential transmission to humans.

2. Materials and Methods

2.1. Ethical Statement

Rodent species included in the study are neither on the Convention on International Trade in Endangered Species of Wild Fauna and Flora (CITES) list, nor the Red List (IUCN). Animals were treated in accordance with the guidelines of the American Society of Mammalogists, and within the European Union legislation guidelines (Directive 86/609/EEC). Each trapping campaign was validated by the national and local health authorities. Approval notices for trapping and investigation of rodents were provided by the Ethical Committee of Mahidol University, Bangkok, Thailand, number 0517.1116/661 (see [29] for more details), based on the CERoPath protocols for field and laboratory rodent studies [34].

2.2. Study Sites and Rodent Trappings

Three different sites in Thailand were investigated for the presence of *O. tsutsugamushi*. Rodents were trapped in the provinces of Buriram (14.89 N, 103.01 E), Loei (17.39 N, 101.77 E) and Nan (19.15 N, 100.83 E) in 2008 and 2009 (Figure 1). These sampling sites were part of the CERoPath project (www.ceropath.org). Reported human cases of scrub typhus were obtained from national statistics [35]. Reported cases of scrub typhus per 100,000 from 2003–2007 were 72.5 in Nan, 23.3 in Loei and less than 12.2 in Buriram. Nan and Loei belonged to the 10 leading provinces in the incidence rate of scrub typhus [35] (Bureau of Epidemiology, 2007).

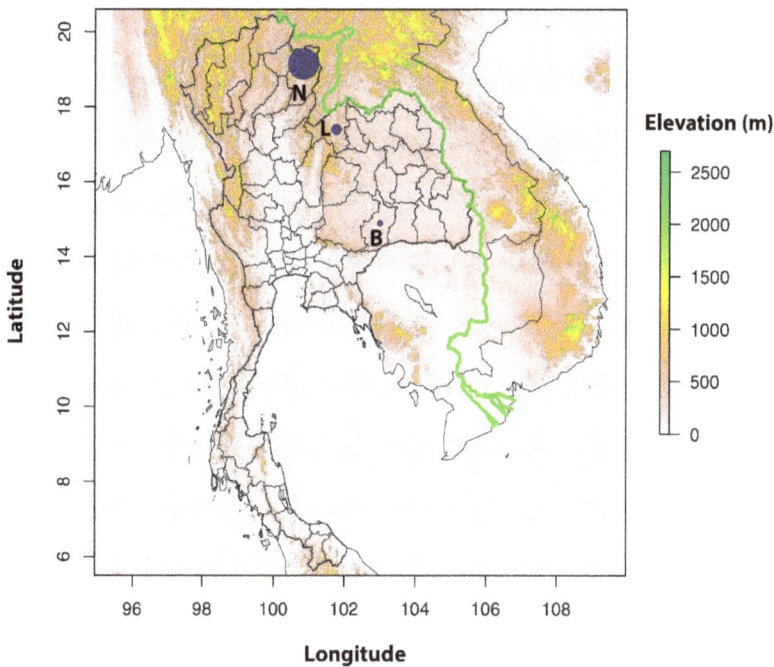

Figure 1. Map of Thailand with locations of the three sample sites in the provinces of Buriram (B), Loei (L) and Nan (N), with reported cases of scrub typhus per 100,000 from 2003–2007: 72.5 in Nan, 23.3 in Loei and <12.2 in Buriram. The relative size of the blue circles indicates average scrub typhus case numbers at each site. Nan and Loei belonged to the 10 leading provinces in the incidence rate of scrub typhus [35].

The methodology was described in Morand et al. [29]. Trapping sessions were conducted in each locality in both wet and dry seasons during 2008–2009. At each locality, the same trap-lines were trapped over a four-night period during each trapping session, with 30 lines of 10 traps (10 m between each trap) placed in three different habitats, namely: (1) forests and mature plantations (rubber trees, teak trees, palm trees, coffee trees), (2) non-flooded lands or fields (shrubby waste land, fallow, young plantations, orchards), (3) rain-fed or irrigated lowland paddy rice fields corresponding to a cultivated floodplain (irrigation allows several crop harvests per year). This corresponded to a total of 1200 night-traps per trapping session. Locally-made live cage-traps were used, and the lines were placed in the same positions during each trapping session using GPS coordinates. Villages and isolated houses, which corresponded to a fourth habitat category, human settlement, were also sampled opportunistically using cage-traps distributed to residents.

Rodent and shrew species were identified in the field using morphological criteria, but were confirmed using molecular methods if needed using a mitochondrial gene for barcoding of some rodent species [36]. Complete data on the animals used as reference specimens for the barcoding assignment are available on the 'Barcoding Tool/RodentSEA' section of the CERoPath project web site (www.ceropath.org).

2.3. Environmental Indices and Land Use

The methodology was described in Morand et al. [30] and Bordes et al. [33]. For each locality, recent (years 2007–2008) high spatial resolution (2.5 m in panchromatic mode and 10 m in multispectral mode) SPOT 5 satellite images were acquired (CNES 2009©, distributed by Astrium Services/Spot Image S.A., Toulouse, France). SPOT-digital elevation model (DEM) with a spatial resolution of 20 m together with SRTM (shuttle radar topography mission) was also acquired. For each locality, the SPOT scene was classified into different land-cover types using an object-based approach. The land-cover maps and the DEM were integrated into a geographic information system (GIS) in order to compute landscape metrics for each trapping site. In order to describe the landscape surrounding the trapping location of each individual rodent, landscape metrics were calculated within a 100 m radius. These metrics included: cover of agriculture on steep land, cover of agriculture on flat land, cover of irrigated agricultural land, cover of forest, cover of human settlement, cover of irrigated land, a proxy of habitat diversity (patch density), a proxy of habitat fragmentation (edge density), and all distances between each rodent trapped and each land-cover types.

2.4. Rodent Screening for O. tsutsugamushi

Rodent spleens were placed in RNAlater® storage solution (Sigma-Aldrich, Saint Louis, MO, USA) then stored at −20 °C until further analysis. Genomic DNA was then extracted from the spleen using the DNeasy®96 Tissue Kit (Qiagen, Germany). Spleen DNA samples were screened for the presence of bacteria using universal primers (16S-V4F [GTGCCAGCMGCCGCGGTAA] and 16S-V4R [GGACTACHVGGGTWTCTAATCC]) targeting the hypervariable region V4 of the 16S rRNA gene (251 bp) via Illumina MiSeq (Illumina) sequencing. The V4 region has been proven to have excellent taxonomic resolution at the genus level [37]. A multiplexing strategy enabled the identification of bacterial genera in each individual sample. We followed the method described in Kozich et al. [38] to perform PCR amplification, indexing, pooling, de-multiplexing and finally taxonomic identification using the SILVA SSU Ref NR 119 database as a reference [39] (http://www.arb-silva.de/projects/ssu-ref-nr/). We then used the trimming strategy of Galan et al. [39,40] in order to clean the raw data set and to estimate reliable rodent positivity for bacteria.

2.5. Statistical Analyses

To analyze the infection of rodents, we first modeled the probability of presence/absence of *O. tsutsugamushi* as a function of several environmental indices with logistic regression, GLMM with logit function and random effects (locality), using package 'lme4' [40,41] implemented in R freeware [41,42]. The binomial variable, infected or non-infected individual rodent, was used in the logistic regression. The initial model included the environmental indices related to the habitat structure, and calculated for a buffer of 100 m for each individual rodent trapped: cover of agriculture on steep land, cover of agriculture on flat land, cover of irrigated agricultural land, cover of forest, cover of human settlement, cover of irrigated land, a proxy of habitat diversity (patch density), and a proxy of habitat fragmentation (edge density). No interactions were added among the independent variables. We evaluated support for competing models, investigating the relationship between the prevalence of *O. tsutsugamushi* and all explanatory variables of interest. We used AIC adjusted for sample size (AICc) to assess the relative information content of the models. We quantified the uncertainty that the 'best' model would emerge as superior if different data were used with Akaike weights (w_r), the probability that a particular model is the best one from the available data. Selection of the best competing models was made using the package 'glmulti' (version 1.0.7 2) [42,43] implemented in R, which allows the exploration of all models using automated model selection and model-averaging procedure using a genetic algorithm.

We also modeled the probability of presence/absence of *O. tsutsugamushi* as a function of several environmental indices with statistical learning Random Forest [43,44] using the 'randomForest' package [44,45]. The measures of importance of each variable are given by values of mean decrease accuracy, i.e., the decrease of model accuracy when the variable is dropped and by values of mean decrease Gini impurity, an index measuring the importance of each variable. All statistical analyses were performed in R freeware [40,41].

3. Results

3.1. Micro-Mammal Identification and O. tsutsugamushi Screening

In total, 387 rodents and shrews were captured and identified at species level (Table 1). The 16S rDNA sequences of *O. tsutsugamushi* were found in only nine rodent individuals (representing 2.3% rate of infection of all the micro-mammals investigated), i.e., *B. savilei* (2), *B. bowersi* (1), *L. edwardsi* (1), *R. exulans* (1), *R. tanezumi* (2), and *Rattus* sp. clade 3 (2) (Table 1). Two rodent species were newly recorded in Thailand for infection by the bacterium: *B. bowersi* and *L. edwardsi*. *O. tsutsugamushi* was detected in all the three localities: Buriram (5), Loei (3), and Nan (1) (Table 1).

Table 1. List and number of host species infected by *O. tsutsugamushi* in three localities of Thailand.

Locality	Micro-Mammal Species	Number Tested	*O. tsutsugamushi* Positive
Buriram	*Bandicota indica*	2	0
	Bandicota savilei	10	2
	Menetes berdmorei	1	0
	Mus caroli	8	0
	Mus cervicolor	11	0
	Mus cookii	1	0
	Rattus argentiventer	1	0
	Rattus exulans	32	0
	Rattus sakaretensis	2	0
	Rattus tanezumi	3	1
	Rattus sp. clade 3	26	2
Loei	*Bandicota indica*	15	0
	Bandicota savilei	12	0
	Berylmys berdmorei	9	0
	Berylmys bowersi	14	1
	Cannomys badius	1	0
	Chiropodomys gliroides	2	0
	Crocidura attenuate	1	0
	Hapalomys delacouri	1	0
	Leopoldamys edwardsi	5	1
	Leopoldamys sabanus	5	0
	Maxomys surifer	15	0
	Mus caroli	5	0
	Mus cervicolor	5	0
	Mus cookii	6	0
	Mus fragilicauda	1	0
	Niviventer fulvescens	16	0
	Rattus exulans	26	1
	Rattus sakaretensis	30	0
	Rattus nitidus	1	0
	Rattus tanezumi	16	0
	R. tanezumi clade 3	2	0

Table 1. *Cont.*

Locality	Micro-Mammal Species	Number Tested	*O. tsutsugamushi* Positive
	Bandicota indica	30	0
	Berylmys berdmorei	8	0
	Berylmys bowersi	1	0
Nan	*Mus caroli*	1	0
	Mus cookiie	4	0
	Rattus exulans	24	0
	Rattus tanezumi	25	1

3.2. Individual Surrounding Habitat Characteristics and O. tsutsugamushi Infection

Infected rodents were trapped in forested and reforestation areas, fallows, cassava plantations, and rice fields.

Comparisons of models testing the effect of several surrounding habitat characteristics on individual rodent infection (GLMM with logit function) are given in Table 2 (best top 3 models) for the three sites in Thailand. Results of GLMM model-averaged importance of surrounding habitat characteristics explaining the infection of rodents by *O. tsutsugamushi* showed that only the explanatory variable forest cover is found in 100 per cent of the top best models (Figure 2).

Table 2. Comparison of models testing the effect of several surrounding habitat characteristics on individual rodent infection by *O. tsutsugamushi* [generalized linear mixed model (GLMM) with logit function] for the three localities (locality as random factor). Models are ranked from lowest to highest supported, according to corrected Akaike information criteria (AIC). Only localities with at least one individual infected rodent were kept for each analyzed dataset. The initial model included the following explanatory variables: cover of agriculture on steep land, cover of agriculture on flat land, cover of agriculture on irrigated land, cover of forest, cover of human settlement, habitat diversity (patch density), habitat fragmentation (edge density), slope, distance to agriculture on flat land, distance to agriculture on steep land, distance to forest, distance to human settlement (K is the number of estimated parameters, AICc is the selection criterion, and w_r are the Akaike weights)

Models (Best Top Three)	K	AICc	w_r
slope + cover of forest + distance to agriculture on flat land	4	84.70	0.033
slope + cover of forest	3	85.02	0.028
Slope+ cover of agriculture on steep land + cover of agriculture on flat land + cover of forest + distance to agriculture on flat land + distance to human settlement	6	85.22	0.025

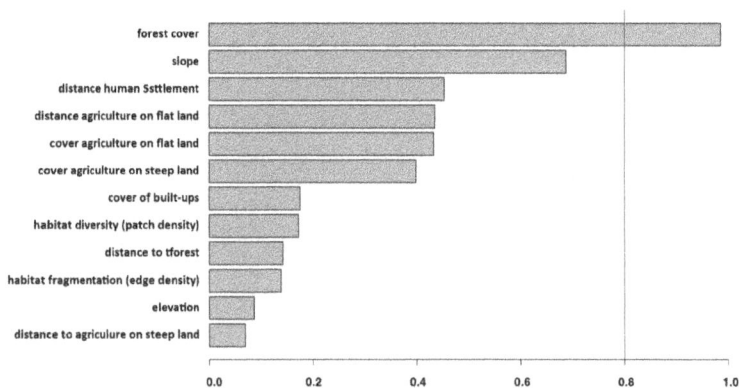

Figure 2. Results of GLMM model-averaged importance of surrounding habitat characteristics explaining the infection of rodents by *O. tsutsugamushi*. Note that only the explanatory variable forest cover is found in 100 per cent of the top best models.

Hence, the best top model selected using AICc values demonstrated that surrounding habitat characterized by large forest cover on slow slope, distant from agriculture on flat land, explained the occurrence of the bacterium in rodents (Table 2). However, forest cover was the only significant variable ($p < 0.05$, Table 3).

Table 3. Results of the best GLMM (with logit link function, and locality as random factor) explaining the occurrence of *O. tsutsugamushi* in rodents, as a function of surrounding habitat characteristics (see Table 2 for the initial models and best top 3 selected models) (estimate of the logit function with SD = standard deviation, residual deviance with DF = degree of freedom).

Explanatory Surrounding Habitat Characteristics	Estimate (SD), *p*	Log Likelihood, Deviance (DF)
Forest cover	3.87 (1.25), 0.002	
Distance to agriculture on flat land	0.003 (0.001), 0.096	
Slope	−0.22 (0.14), 0.10	−160.6, 321.1 (1360)

Using Random Forest analysis, again forest cover was selected as the best explanatory variable, followed by cover of agriculture on flat land (Figure 3). However, the values of mean decrease accuracy and mean decrease Gini dropped from cover of agriculture on flat land (Figure 2). Although the accuracy of the Random Forest was high with a value of 0.991 (with 95% CI: 0.97–0.999), the *p* value was not significant ($p = 0.059$), due to the low number of infected rodents (9) compared to the negative ones (378).

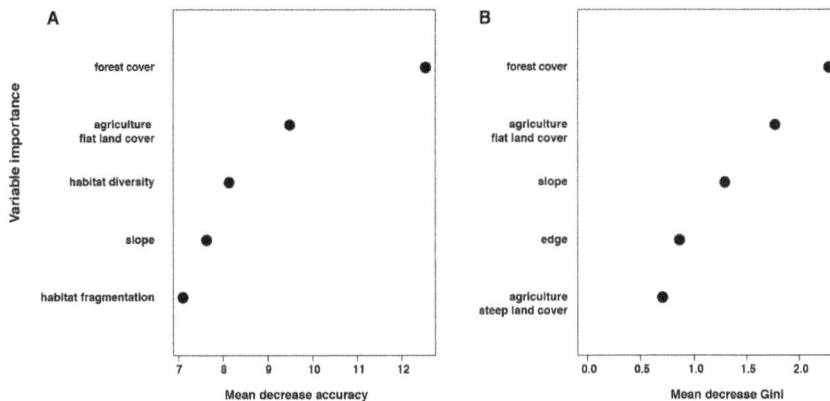

Figure 3. Results of Random Forest analysis with: (**a**) values of mean decrease accuracy; measuring the decrease of model accuracy when variables are dropped; (**b**) values of mean decrease Gini impurity index measuring the importance of each variable.

4. Discussion

The goal of this study was to investigate the relationship between the landscape structure of the three localities and the occurrence of the bacterium *O. tsutsugamushi* in wild rodents detected using the 16S rDNA amplicon sequencing approach. Our findings indicate that the prevalence of the bacterium is very low, with only nine out of the 387 micro-mammals investigated, positive (2.3%). The prevalence of bacterium in animals was higher on the site of Buriram than the sites of Nan and Loei, in contrast to the human scrub typhus incidence report, which gave higher human incidence in Nan and Loei than in Buriram [35]. However, the data were not obtained at the same scale; the whole province is represented in health surveillance, versus only a few square kilometers for the rodent survey.

We confirmed the presence of the bacterium in several known rodent host species, such as *B. savilei*, *R. exulans* and the two species of the *R. tanezumi* complex [24]. We confirmed that the *Mus* species

Trop. Med. Infect. Dis. **2017**, *2*, 53

did not appear as infected by *O. tsutsugamushi* [21]. We recorded two new infected rodent species in Thailand: *B. bowersi* and *L. edwardsi*. The positive rodents are either habitat specialists, such as the forest-dwelling *L. edwardsi*, or habitat generalists, such as *R. tanezumi* [29]. Moreover, our results showed the epidemiological importance of the two synanthropic species, *R. exulans* and *R. tanezumi*, which live in close association with humans [29,46,47].

Our results seem to support our hypotheses that rodents infected by *O. tsutsugamushi* were more likely to be found in environments with large forest cover using either GLMM or Random Forest analysis. Our results suggest that a rodent was likely infected in a habitat such as a house, a fallow, or a rice field, if these habitats were in the vicinity of a forested area. The low support values (w_r) for the overall models could be explained by the fact that the prevalence of the bacterium is very low with a low number of positive individuals for each land use land cover of the three localities. This low prevalence also explains why the accuracy of the Random Forest analysis was not significant (although close to significance).

The significance of forest cover for scrub typhus seropositivity was expected, as several studies conducted in Taiwan or in China showed that the incidence of scrub typhus is related to land use characterized by forested areas with abandonment of agriculture land and return to fallows and forests [28,30,31]. Southeast Asia is characterized by increased fragmentation and conversion of forest to agricultural land [48,49]). This new frontier of forest conversion is potentially risky habitat for scrub typhus infection.

4.1. Limitations of Our Study

There are some limitations of our study. First, we are just starting to obtain an evaluation on the sensitivity of 16S amplicon sequencing in the frame of epidemiological studies. Razzauti et al. [50] recently showed that the sensitivity of 16S rRNA amplicon sequencing on the MiSeq platform was equivalent to that of whole-RNA sequencing (RNA-seq) on the HiSeq platform for detecting bacteria in rodent samples. Galan et al. [36] revealed an excellent repeatability of bacterial detection (93%) using systematic replicates in 711 rodents. Finally, work in progress at our laboratory (unpublished result) shows that the sensitivity of the 16S rRNA amplicon sequencing approach used here is as good as the sensitivity of quantitative PCR (qPCR) performed with specific primers, the current gold standard for bacterial detection in biological samples. Thus, we are confident in our *Orientia* screening.

Second, more detailed information on human cases at high resolution, i.e., at the level of sub-district or villages, will help to accurately investigate accurately the relationship between human cases and rodent infection by *O. tsutsugamushi*.

Third, our study could not assess the impact of seasonality on the epidemiology of *O. tsutsugamushi*. Another limitation concerns the diversity and infection of chigger mites. All chigger mites were collected and preserved. Future studies are planned to explore this point.

4.2. Implications for Public Health

The incidence of scrub typhus is increasing in several countries of East Asia. Previous studies [30] showed that habitat fragmentation and extensive agriculture disrupt rodent habitats favoring generalist and synanthropic rodent species, which ultimately enhance rodent-borne transmission. The results of our study suggest that risky habitats for *O. tsutsugamushi* transmission are heterogenous forested areas, comprising conversed agriculture or reforested areas, fallow or abandoned agriculture. Surveillance of rodents' population dynamics in these habitats may help to prevent zoonotic transmission.

Acknowledgments: This study was funded by the French ANR CERoPath (www.ceropath.org) CP&ES, grant ANR 11 CPEL 002 BiodivHealthSEA project (www.biodivhealthsea.org). SM is supported by the Thailand International Cooperation Agency (TICA). Special thanks to Annelise Tran for the GIS development. We thank the CERoPath team and the drivers for their invaluable help during fieldwork.

Author Contributions: J.F.C. and S.M. conceived the trapping sampling and the design of the experiment; J.F.C. designed the screening of rodents; all authors analyzed the data; all authors contributed equally to the writing of the paper.

Conflicts of Interest: The authors declare no conflict of interest.

References

1. Kelly, D.J.; Fuerst, P.A.; Ching, W.M.; Richards, A.L. Scrub typhus: The geographic distribution of phenotypic and genotypic variants of *Orientia tsutsugamushi*. *Clin. Infect. Dis.* **2009**, *15*, S203–S230. [CrossRef] [PubMed]

2. Cosson, J.-F.; Galan, M.; Bard, E.; Razzauti, M.; Bernard, M.; Morand, S.; Brouat, C.; Dalecky, A.; Ba, K.; Charbonnel, N.; et al. Detection of *Orientia* sp. DNA in rodents from Asia, West Africa and Europe. *Parasites Vect.* **2015**, *8*, 172. [CrossRef] [PubMed]

3. Watt, G.; Parola, P. Scrub typhus and tropical rickettsioses. *Curr. Opinion Infect. Dis.* **2003**, *16*, 429–436. [CrossRef]

4. Walker, M.D. Scrub typhus—Scientific neglect, ever-widening impact. *N. Engl. J. Med.* **2016**, *375*, 913–915. [CrossRef] [PubMed]

5. Chaisiri, K.; McGarry, J.W.; Morand, S.; Makepeace, B.L. Symbiosis in an overlooked microcosm: A systematic review of the bacterial flora of mites. *Parasitology* **2015**, *142*, 1152–1156. [CrossRef] [PubMed]

6. Roberts, L.W.; Rapmund, G.; Gadigan, F.G. Sex ratios in *Rickettsia tsutsugamushi*-infected and noninfected colonies of *Leptotrombidium*. (Acari: Trombiculidae). *J. Med. Entomol.* **1977**, *14*, 89–92. [CrossRef] [PubMed]

7. Frances, S.P.; Watcharapichat, P.; Phulsuksombati, D. Vertical transmission of *Orientia tsutsugamushi* in two lines of naturally infected *Leptotrombidium deliense* (Acari: Trombiculidae). *J. Med. Entomol.* **2001**, *38*, 17–21. [CrossRef] [PubMed]

8. Phasomkusolsil, S.; Tanskul, P.; Ratanatham, S.; Watcharapichat, P.; Phulsuksombati, D.; Frances, S.P.; Lerdthusnee, K.; Linthicum, K.J. Influence of *Orientia tsutsugamushi* infection on the developmental biology of *Leptotrombidium imphalum* and *Leptotrombidium chiangraiensis* (Acari: Trombiculidae). *J. Med. Entomol.* **2012**, *49*, 1270–1275. [CrossRef]

9. Traub, R.; Wisseman, C.L.J. The ecology of chigger-borne rickettsiosis (scrub typhus). *J. Med. Entomol.* **1974**, *11*, 237–303. [CrossRef] [PubMed]

10. Stekolnikov, A.A. *Leptotrombidium* (Acari: Trombiculidae) of the world. *Zootaxa* **2013**, *3728*, zootaxa.3728.1.1. [CrossRef]

11. Santibanez, P.; Palomar, A.M.; Portillo, A.; Santibanez, S.; Oteo, J.A. The role of chiggers as human pathogens. Available online: https://www.intechopen.com/books/an-overview-of-tropical-diseases/the-role-of-chiggers-as-human-pathogens (accessed on 5 October 2017).

12. Coleman, R.E.; Monkanna, T.; Linthicum, K.J.; Strickman, D.A.; Frances, S.P.; Tanskul, P.; Kollars, T.M., Jr.; Inlao, I.; Watcharapichat, P.; Khlaimanee, N.; et al. Occurrence of *Orientia tsutsugamushi* in small mammals from Thailand. *Am. J. Trop. Med. Hyg.* **2003**, *69*, 519–524. [PubMed]

13. Paris, D.H.; Shelite, T.R.; Day, N.P.; Walker, D.H. Unresolved problems related to scrub typhus: A seriously neglected life-threatening disease. *Am. J. Trop. Med. Hyg.* **2013**, *89*, 301–307. [CrossRef] [PubMed]

14. Shatrov, A.B.; Kudryashova, N.I. Taxonomic ranking of major trombiculid subtaxa with remarks on the evolution of host-parasite relationships (Acariformes: Parasitengona: Trombiculidae). *Ann. Zool.* **2008**, *58*, 279–287. [CrossRef]

15. Zhang, M.; Zhao, Z.; Yang, H.L.; Zhang, A.H.; Xu, X.Q.; Meng, X.P.; Zhang, H.Y.; Wang, X.J.; Li, Z.; Ding, S.J.; et al. Molecular epidemiology of *Orientia tsutsugamushi* in chiggers and ticks from domestic rodents in Shandong, northern China. *Parasites Vect.* **2013**, *6*, 312. [CrossRef] [PubMed]

16. Chaisiri, K.; Stekolnikov, A.A.; Makepeace, B.L.; Morand, S. A Revised checklist of chigger mites (Acari: Trombiculidae) from Thailand, with the description of three new species. *J. Med. Entomol.* **2016**, *53*, 321–342. [CrossRef] [PubMed]

17. Peng, P.Y.; Guo, X.G.; Ren, T.G.; Song, W.Y.; Dong, W.G.; Fan, R. Species diversity of ectoparasitic chigger mites (Acari: Prostigmata) on small mammals in Yunnan Province, China. *Parasitol. Res.* **2016**, *15*, 3605–3618. [CrossRef] [PubMed]

18. Meerburg, B.G.; Singleton, G.R.; Kijlstra, A. Rodent-borne diseases and their risks for public health. *Crit. Rev. Microbiol.* **2009**, *35*, 221–270. [CrossRef] [PubMed]

19. Khuntirat, B.; Lerdthusnee, K.; Leepitakrat, W.; Kengleucha, A.; Wongkalasin, K.; Monkanna, T.; Mungviriya, S.; Jones, J.W.; Coleman, R.E. Characterization of *Orientia tsutsugamushi* isolated from wild-caught rodents and chiggers in northern Thailand. *Ann. N. Y. Acad. Sci.* **2003**, *990*, 205–212. [CrossRef]

20. Lerdthusnee, K.; Nigro, J.; Monkanna, T.; Leepitakrat, W.; Leepitakrat, S.; Insuan, S.; Charoensongsermkit, W.; Khlaimanee, N.; Akkagraisee, W.; Chayapum, K.; et al. Surveys of rodent-borne disease in Thailand with a focus on scrub typhus assessment. *Integrat. Zool.* **2008**, *3*, 267–273. [CrossRef] [PubMed]

21. Wangroongsarb, P.; Saengsongkong, W.; Petkanjanapong, W.; Mimgratok, M.; Panjai, D.; Wootta, W.; Hagiwara, T. An application of duplex PCR for detection of *Leptospira* spp. and *Orientia tsutsugamushi* from wild rodents. *Jpn. J. Inf. Dis.* **2008**, *61*, 407–409.

22. Rodkvamtook, W.; Gaywee, J.; Kanjanavanit, S.; Ruangareerate, T.; Richards, A.L.; Sangjun, N.; Jeamwattanalert, P.; Sirisopana, N. Scrub typhus outbreak, northern Thailand, 2006–2007. *Emerg. Inf. Dis.* **2013**, *19*, 774–777. [CrossRef] [PubMed]

23. Rodkvamtook, W.; Ruang-Areerate, T.; Gaywee, J.; Richards, A.L.; Jeamwattanalert, P.; Bodhidatta, D.; Sangjun, N.; Prasartvit, A.; Jatisatienr, A.; Jatisatienr, C. Isolation and Characterization of *Orientia tsutsugamushi* from rodents captured following a scrub typhus outbreak at a military training base, Bothong District, Chonburi Province, Central Thailand. *Am. J. Trop. Med. Hyg.* **2011**, *84*, 599–607. [CrossRef] [PubMed]

24. Herbreteau, V.; Bordes, F.; Jittapalapong, S.; Supputamongkol, Y.; Morand, S. Rodent-borne diseases in Thailand: Targeting rodent carriers and risky habitats. *Infect. Ecol. Epidemiol.* **2012**, *2*, 18637. [CrossRef] [PubMed]

25. Chareonviriyaphap, T.; Leepitakrat, W.; Lerdthusnee, K.; Chao, C.C.; Ching, W.M. Dual exposure of *Rickettsia typhi* and *Orientia tsutsugamushi* in the field-collected *Rattus* rodents from Thailand. *J. Vect. Ecol.* **2014**, *39*, 182–189. [CrossRef] [PubMed]

26. Hamady, M.; Knight, R. Microbial community profiling for human microbiome projects: Tools, techniques, and challenges. *Genome Res.* **2009**, *19*, 1141–1152. [CrossRef] [PubMed]

27. Muul, I.; Lim, B.L.; Walker, J.S. Scrub typhus infection in rats in four habitats in Peninsular Malaysia. *Trans. R Soc. Trop. Med. Hyg.* **1977**, *71*, 493–497. [CrossRef]

28. Wardrop, N.A.; Kuo, C.-C.; Wang, H.-C.; Clements, A.C.A.; Lee, P.-F.; Atkinson, P.M. Bayesian spatial modelling and the significance of agricultural land use to scrub typhus infection in Taiwan. *Geospatial Health* **2013**, *8*, 229–239. [CrossRef] [PubMed]

29. Morand, S.; Bordes, F.; Blasdell, K.; Pilosof, S.; Cornu, J.-F.; Chaisiri, K.; Chaval, Y.; Cosson, J.-F.; Claude, J.; Feyfant, T.; et al. Assessing the distribution of disease-bearing rodents in human-modified tropical landscapes. *J. Appl. Ecol.* **2015**, *52*, 784–794. [CrossRef]

30. Sun, Y.; Wei, Y.-H.; Yang, Y.; Ma, Y.; de Vlas, S.J.; Yao, H.W.; Huang, Y.; Ma, M.J.; Liu, K.; Li, X.N.; et al. Rapid increase of scrub typhus incidence in Guangzhou, southern China, 2006–2014. *BMC Inf. Dis.* **2017**, *17*, 13. [CrossRef] [PubMed]

31. Kuo, C.C.; Huang, J.L.; Shu, P.Y.; Lee, P.L.; Kelt, D.A.; Wang, H.C. Cascading effect of economic globalization on human risks of scrub typhus and tick-borne rickettsial diseases. *Ecol. Appl.* **2012**, *22*, 1803–1816. [CrossRef] [PubMed]

32. Bordes, F.; Morand, S.; Pilosof, S.; Claude, J.; Cosson, J.-F.; Chaval, Y.; Ribas, A.; Chaisiri, K.; Blasdell, K.; Tran, A. Habitat fragmentation alters the properties of a host-parasite network: Rodents and their helminths in South-East Asia. *J. Anim. Ecol.* **2015**, *84*, 1253–1263. [CrossRef] [PubMed]

33. Bordes, F.; Caron, A.; Blasdell, K.; de Garine Wichatitsky, M.; Morand, S. Forecasting potential emergence of zoonotic diseases in South-East Asia: Network analysis identifies key rodent hosts. *J. Appl. Ecol.* **2016**, *54*. [CrossRef]

34. Herbreteau, V.; Rerkamnuaychoke, W.; Jittapalapong, S.; Chaval, Y.; Cosson, J.-F.; Morand, S. Field and laboratory protocols for rodent studies. Kasetsart University. Available online: www.ceropath.org/FichiersComplementaires/Herbreteau_Rodents_protocols_2011.pdf (accessed on 6 October 2017).

35. Bureau of Epidemiology, Department of Disease Control, Ministry of Public Health, Thailand. Annual epidemiologic surveillance report 2007. Scrub typhus. Available online: http://www.boe.moph.go.th/Annual/ANNUAL2550/Part1/Annual_MenuPart1.html (accessed on 4 October 2017).

36. Galan, M.; Pagès, M.; Cosson, J.F. Next-generation sequencing for rodent barcoding: Species identification from fresh, degraded and environmental samples. *PLoS ONE* **2012**, *7*, e4837. [CrossRef] [PubMed]

37. Claesson, M.J.; Wang, Q.; O'Sullivan, O.; Greene-Diniz, R.; Cole, J.R.; Ross, R.P.; O'Toole, P.W. Comparison of two next-generation sequencing technologies for resolving highly complex microbiota composition using tandem variable 16S rRNA gene regions. *Nucleic Acids Res.* **2010**, *38*, e200. [CrossRef] [PubMed]

38. Kozich, J.J.; Westcott, S.L.; Baxter, N.T.; Highlander, S.K.; Schloss, P.D. Development of a dual-index sequencing strategy and curation pipeline for analyzing amplicon sequence data on the MiSeq Illumina sequencing platform. *Appl. Env. Microbiol.* **2013**, *79*, 5112–5120. [CrossRef] [PubMed]

39. Silva. Available online: http://www.arb-silva.de/projects/ssu-ref-nr/ (accessed on 6 October 2017).

40. Galan, M.; Razzauti, M.; Bard, E.; Bernard, M.; Brouat, C.; Charbonnel, N.; Dehne-Garcia, A.; Loiseau, A.; Tatard, C.; Tamisier, L.; et al. 16S rRNA amplicon sequencing for epidemiological surveys of bacteria in wildlife. *MSystems* **2016**, *1*, e00032-16. [CrossRef] [PubMed]

41. Bates, D.; Maechler, M.; Bolker, B.; Walker, S. Fitting linear mixed-effects models using lme4. *J. Stat. Software* **2015**, *67*, 1–48. [CrossRef]

42. R Development Core Team. The R project for statistical computing, R version 3.4.1, 2017. Available online: https://www.r-project.org (accessed on 4 October 2017).

43. Calcagno, V.; de Mazancourt, C. Glmulti: An R package for easy automated model selection with (generalized) linear models. *J. Stat. Software* **2010**, *34*, 12. [CrossRef]

44. Breiman, L. Random Forests. *Mach. Learn.* **2001**, *45*, 5–32. [CrossRef]

45. Liaw, A.; Wiener, M. Classification and regression by random Forest. *R News* **2002**, *2*, 18–22.

46. Bordes, F.; Blasdell, K.; Morand, S. Transmission ecology of rodent-borne diseases: New frontiers. *Integrat. Zool.* **2015**, *10*, 424–435. [CrossRef] [PubMed]

47. Kosoy, M.; Khlyap, L.; Cosson, J.-F.; Morand, S. Aboriginal and invasive rats of genus Rattus as hosts of infectious agents. *Vector-Borne Zoon Dis.* **2015**, *15*, 3–12. [CrossRef] [PubMed]

48. Wilcove, D.S.; Giam, X.; Edwards, D.P.; Fisher, B.; Koh, L.P. Navjot's nightmare revisited: Logging, agriculture, and biodiversity in Southeast Asia. *Trends Ecol. Evol.* **2013**, *28*, 531–540. [CrossRef] [PubMed]

49. Cornu, J.-F.; Lajaunie, C.; Laborde, H.; Morand, S. Landscape changes and policies for biodiversity and environment conservation in Southeast Asia. In *Biodiversity Conservation in Southeast Asia: Challenges in a Changing Environment*; Morand, S., Lajaunie, C., Satrawaha, R., Eds.; Routledge: Abingdon, UK, 2017; pp. 49–66.

50. Razzauti, M.; Galan, M.; Bernard, M.; Maman, S.; Klopp, C.; Charbonnel, N.; Vayssier-Taussat, M.; Eloit, M.; Cosson, J.F. A comparison between transcriptome sequencing and 16S metagenomics for detection of bacterial pathogens in wildlife. *PLoS Negl. Trop. Dis.* **2015**, *9*, e0003929. [CrossRef] [PubMed]

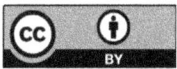

Tropical Medicine and Infectious Disease

MDPI

Perspective

Confronting the Emerging Threat to Public Health in Northern Australia of Neglected Indigenous Arboviruses

Narayan Gyawali [1,2] and Andrew W. Taylor-Robinson [3,*]

1   School of Health, Medical & Applied Sciences, Central Queensland University,
    Rockhampton, QLD 4702, Australia; n.gyawali@cqu.edu.au
2   Institute of Health & Biomedical Innovation, Queensland University of Technology,
    Brisbane, QLD 4059, Australia
3   School of Health, Medical & Applied Sciences, Central Queensland University,
    Brisbane, QLD 4000, Australia
*   Correspondence: a.taylor-robinson@cqu.edu.au; Tel: +61-7-3295-1185

Received: 11 September 2017; Accepted: 12 October 2017; Published: 17 October 2017

Abstract: In excess of 75 arboviruses have been identified in Australia, some of which are now well established as causative agents of debilitating diseases. These include Ross River virus, Barmah Forest virus, and Murray Valley encephalitis virus, each of which may be detected by both antibody-based recognition and molecular typing. However, for most of the remaining arboviruses that may be associated with pathology in humans, routine tests are not available to diagnose infection. A number of these so-called 'neglected' or 'orphan' arboviruses that are indigenous to Australia might have been infecting humans at a regular rate for decades. Some of them may be associated with undifferentiated febrile illness—fever, the cause of which is not obvious—for which around half of all cases each year remain undiagnosed. This is of particular relevance to Northern Australia, given the Commonwealth Government's transformative vision for the midterm future of massive infrastructure investment in this region. An expansion of the industrial and business development of this previously underpopulated region is predicted. This is set to bring into intimate proximity infection-naïve human hosts, native reservoir animals, and vector mosquitoes, thereby creating a perfect storm for increased prevalence of infection with neglected Australian arboviruses. Moreover, the escalating rate and effects of climate change that are increasingly observed in the tropical north of the country are likely to lead to elevated numbers of arbovirus-transmitting mosquitoes. As a commensurate response, continuing assiduous attention to vector monitoring and control is required. In this overall context, improved epidemiological surveillance and diagnostic screening, including establishing novel, rapid pan-viral tests to facilitate early diagnosis and appropriate treatment of febrile primary care patients, should be considered a public health priority. Investment in a rigorous identification program would reduce the possibility of significant outbreaks of these indigenous arboviruses at a time when population growth accelerates in Northern Australia.

Keywords: arbovirus; neglected; undifferentiated febrile illness; Northern Australia; diagnostics; control; prevention

1. Introduction

Arthropod-*borne viruses* (arboviruses) are by definition transmitted between vertebrate hosts by biting arthropods (mosquitoes, ticks, sandflies, midges and gnats) [1], and the infections that they cause pose a significant public health risk worldwide. The International Catalogue of Arboviruses currently lists 537 registered viruses on the basis of their known transmission by arthropods, known for potential infectivity to humans or domestic animals, and antigenic or phylogenetic relationships to known arboviruses [2].

At present, more than 130 arboviruses are recognised as causing mild to fulminant disease in humans [3]. Symptoms of uncomplicated arboviral infection generally occur between 3 and 15 days after exposure to the virus and may persist for a week or so. The most common clinical features of infection are the indistinct influenza-like symptoms of fever, headache, and malaise, which, without recourse to further information regarding a patient's clinical and exposure history, often preclude a correct diagnosis [4].

Australia is home to over 75 arboviruses that have been isolated from its native arthropods [2]. While so far only 13 of these are found to be associated with human infection, just Barmah Forest virus (BFV) and Ross River virus (RRV) are tested for routinely. Moreover, laboratory tests are available for Murray Valley encephalitis virus (MVEV) and West Nile Kunjin virus (KUNV) but test requests are made on patients with highly suggestive signs and symptoms [5]. The ecology and role of other arboviruses in humans, whether they are associated with any serious infections or undiagnosed undifferentiated febrile illness (UFI), are unknown and their study is not prioritised. An analysis of the notifications of BFV, RRV, MVEV, and KUNV in the last two decades has clearly shown a higher distribution of these viruses in Northern Australia [6] (reviewed in [5]).

In this article, we describe briefly the neglected Australian arboviruses that are most likely to emerge as significant agents of human disease. The arboviruses that we discuss have been found to infect humans—serological evidence of host immune responses has been found. It is implicitly understood that a virus that is associated with human infection could potentially be a pathogen, i.e. it may have been causing a disease, the aetiology of which is so far unknown, or it could cause disease under certain circumstances, such as in immunocompromised persons, during pregnancy, or upon secondary infection. We also consider what action should be taken to confront the potential threat of such neglected indigenous arboviruses in the particular environment of Northern Australia. This is a largely tropical climatic region where both mosquito vectors and vertebrate reservoir hosts are abundant and in which a future major expansion of a human population primarily comprising relocating, previously non-exposed individuals, is predicted.

2. Arbovirus Ecology and Epidemiology

Most arboviruses studied thus far are transmitted in zoonotic cycles, i.e. the principal vertebrate host is an animal other than human [7]. The distribution of an arbovirus is restricted to areas inhabited by vertebrate hosts that serve as its reservoirs and vectors. Thus, many arboviruses have clearly defined ecological zones, while some, distributed globally, cause diseases of considerable public health and veterinary importance (reviewed in [8]). Examples of the latter include dengue (worldwide, approximately between the Tropics of Cancer and Capricorn), yellow fever (Africa and South America), Japanese encephalitis (eastern and southeast Asia and Australia), West Nile encephalitis (North America, Europe and the Middle East), chikungunya (Asia, Central and South America, parts of the Pacific), eastern and western equine encephalitis (North America), and Venezuelan equine encephalitis (South America). Due to focal, global, environmental, societal and/or demographic changes, many of these viruses have either emerged or re-emerged in the first years of this century [9–11].

Notably, the non-segmented, positive-strand RNA viruses belonging to the genus *Flavivirus*, family *Flaviviridae*, or genus *Alphavirus*, family *Togaviridae*, are the aetiological agents of several major global infectious diseases such as dengue, yellow fever, chikungunya and Zika. Other related pathogens belong to the segmented, negative strand RNA *Orthobunyavirus* genus. The vast majority of arbovirus-associated epidemics occur in the tropics and subtropics due to the prevailing hot and humid climate which is conducive to the habitation of vector mosquitoes, including members of *Aedes*, *Anopheles*, *Culex*, *Haemagogus*, and *Ochlerotatus* genera [12]. To this growing list of real or potential public health threats posed by arboviruses Mayarocan now be added, identified recently in the Amazon and other tropical regions of South America [13]. The issue of whether neglected

Australian arboviruses similarly present an emerging, hitherto unrecognised challenge to humans is a subject of discussion.

3. Arboviruses in Australia

Australia is the sixth largest country in the world by area, the largest country without land borders, and the largest country overall in the southern hemisphere. Early European settlement, urbanisation, increased sea and air travel and trade, globalisation, pathogen evolution, and elevated mean global temperature are some of the factors that may have influenced the introduction and expanded geographical reach of infectious diseases, including those caused by arboviruses, in Australia [14]. Furthermore, Australia spans tropical and subtropical latitudes, where arboviruses have access to an abundant source of both reservoir hosts and vectors.

While only 13 of the more than 75 identified arboviruses indigenous to Australia are currently known to cause disease in humans, information is scarce as to the potential human pathogenicity of most others [15]. Of those that are recognised to cause infection in humans in Australia (Figure 1), the alphaviruses RRV and BFV are the most well-known, infection with either of which triggers an incapacitating and occasionally chronic polyarthritis with accompanying myalgia and lethargy [16,17]. The flaviviruses MVEV and KUNV cause encephalitis, an acute inflammation of the brain [18].

Infection with the flavivirus dengue (DENV) is typically characterised by a febrile illness but a small proportion of cases manifest as a life-threatening haemorrhagic fever or shock syndrome (reviewed in [19]). DENV may be acquired outside Australia and brought back by returning travellers, a significant proportion of whom are hospitalised with unrecognised warning signs of severe disease. As intercontinental travel from Australia, particularly to Asia, continues to increase, in order to avert serious outcomes it is crucial that clinicians anticipate, and can recognise and manage, such tropical infectious diseases. While DENV has a transglobal distribution, local outbreaks are also reported regularly in far north Queensland, with foci in the vicinities of Cairns and Townsville [20], where it is well recognised by the resident population as a not insignificant threat to their health [21].

Several other arboviruses that are indigenous to Australia (Figure 1), such as the alphavirus Sindbis (SINV), the flaviviruses Alfuy (ALFV), Edge Hill (EHV), Kokobera (KOKV) and Stratford (STRV), and the orthobunyaviruses Gan Gan (GGV), Kowanyama (KOWV) and Trubanaman (TRUV), are recognised through eliciting mild symptoms of febrile illness, corroborated by detection of serum antibodies to viral antigens, as being able to infect humans [17,22,23] (reviewed in [5]). There are occasional reports of human disease caused by SINV, EHV and KOKV [24–26], but these are not currently included individually in the list of Australian national notifiable diseases by disease type [27]. The magnitude of each of these arboviral infections raises the question as to what is an appropriate threshold for recording cases for the purposes of annual notification at state/territory and national levels. SINV is reportedly the arbovirus most frequently isolated from mosquitoes in Australia [23], but as an alphavirus it does not come under the 'flavivirus infection (unspecified)' umbrella presently used for nationwide notification [27].

Other arboviruses have been isolated from arthropods in the Australia-Pacific region [15]. These include the newly identified Bamaga (BGV) and Fitzroy River (FRV) flaviviruses [28,29], which are closely related to the disease-causing yellow fever virus (YFV) and EHV, but for each of which there is scant information about its capacity to infect humans or to cause disease in humans.

RRV
BFV
KUNV
MVEV
ALFV
EHV
KOKV
SINV
STRV
TRUV

DENV
RRV
BFV
KUNV
MVEV
ALFV
EHV
KOKV
KOWV
STRV
TRUV

RRV
BFV
KUNV
MVEV
ALFV
EHV
KOKV
SINV
STRV
TRUV

NT

QLD

WA

SA

NSW

RRV
BFV
KUNV
MVEV
STRV

RRV
BFV
KUNV
MVEV
EHV
KOKV
SINV
STRV
TRUV

VIC

RRV
BFV
KUNV
MVEV
EHV
GGV
KOKV
STRV
TRUV

TAS

RRV
BFV

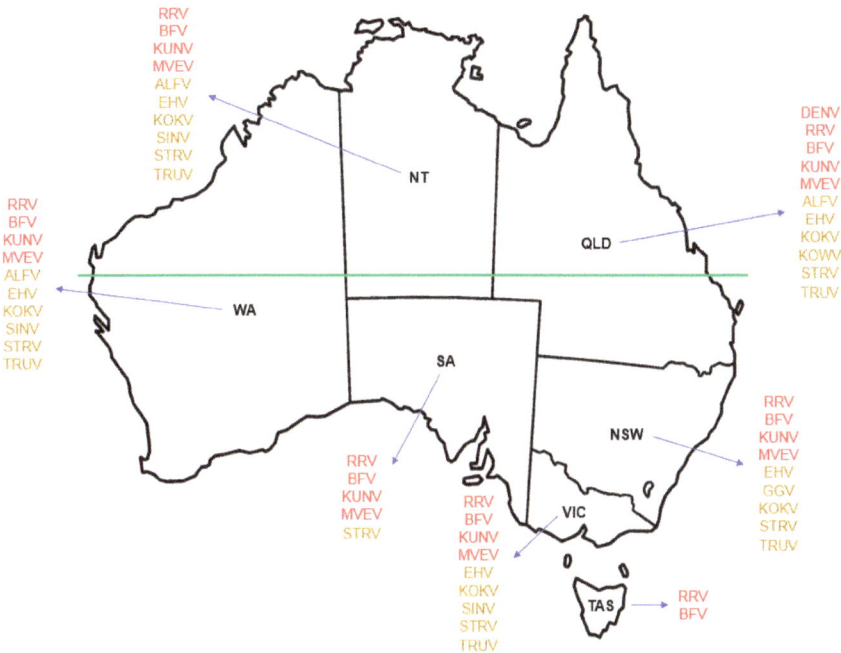

Figure 1. Geographical distribution of Australian indigenous arboviruses known to cause human infection. Use of red font for each named virus indicates the state or territory from which that virus is known to be recovered and the notifiable disease for which it is listed in the Australian National Notifiable Disease Surveillance System (ANNDSS). Use of amber font for each named virus indicates the reported recovery of that virus from mosquitoes during mosquito surveillance but that the corresponding virus-associated disease is not currently recorded in the ANNDSS. Named arboviruses: ALFV—Alfuy; BFV—Barmah Forest; DENV—Dengue; EHV—Edge Hill; GGV—Gan Gan; KOKV—Kokobera; KOWV—Kowanyama; KUNV—Kunjin; MVEV—Murray Valley encephalitis; RRV—Ross River; SINV—Sindbis; STRV—Stratford; Trubanaman—TRUV. The land mass above the horizontal green line, which marks the southern edge of the Pilbara Range (latitude 24° S, just south of the Tropic of Capricorn, 23.52° S), approximates to the region termed Northern Australia. States and territory: NSW—New South Wales; NT—Northern Territory; QLD—Queensland; SA—South Australia; TAS—Tasmania; VIC—Victoria; WA—Western Australia.

4. Undifferentiated Febrile Illness and Pyrexia of Unknown Origin

Fever, defined as an abnormally high body temperature (>100 °F, 37.8 °C), is a common symptom of patients seeking healthcare. Due to the non-specific clinical manifestations and a lack of positivity in initial laboratory testing, the cause of fever may not be identified. When the onset of fever is acute and no cause can be found after taking a full history and physical examination of the patient, it is called a UFI. If the UFI continues, it is classified as a pyrexia of unknown origin (PUO), defined in 1961 as an illness of more than three weeks' duration, with fever greater than 101 °F (38.3 °C) on several occasions, the cause of which is not identified after one week of in-hospital investigation [30]. Since this description does not include many self-limiting viral diseases, it was revised in 1991 [31]. The newer definition of PUO has four categories: classical; hospital-acquired; neutropenic (immune-deficient); and HIV-associated. Also, the revision proposed a minimum of three days of hospitalisation or at least three outpatient visits before this diagnosis may be made. Most commonly, PUO is the result of infection, malignancy, or non-malignant inflammatory diseases [32].

5. UFI/PUO as a Health Problem

Between 20% and 60% of UFI cases are attributed to infections [31,33–35]. The aetiological agents of UFI and PUO vary according to the geography and demography of the patients. For instance, in post-industrial countries, self-limited viral infections and infections with bacteria such as *Brucella* spp., *Leptospira* spp., and the atypical mycobacteria are major causes of UFI/PUO. In economically emerging nations, UFI/PUO include illnesses caused by a diverse range of human pathogens including *Mycobacterium tuberculosis*, *Neisseria meningitidis*, systemic *Salmonella enterica* infections, *Plasmodium* spp., DENV, Epstein-Barr virus, cytomegalovirus, and hantaviruses [36–38].

In a landmark prospective study in Belgium of patients hospitalised with febrile illness, depending on if and when a final diagnosis was in fact established, an estimated 12–35% were assessed to have died from PUO-associated complications [39]. The cause of the fever remained obscure in 48% of patients with episodic fever, compared to 26% of patients with continuous fever [39]. Prolonged febrile illnesses remain a diagnostic challenge; about one-third to half of PUO cases remain undiagnosed [40–42]. In developing countries, a diagnosis of UFI/PUO may result from a lack of laboratory resources but even in a high-income nation like Japan that has excellent diagnostic tools, 28.9% of PUO goes undiagnosed [43].

6. Diagnosis of Australian Arboviral Infection

For almost a decade after the identification of RRV in 1959 [44], only small numbers of patients were identified as having a clinical infection with this agent, because virological and serological diagnostic testing was available only within a research framework using an in-house test. Following the development of a commercial enzyme-linked immunosorbent assay (ELISA) to detect anti-RRV immunoglobulin (Ig)M antibody [45], the number of patients diagnosed annually rose to between 4000 and 6000 [46]. The number of localities from where RRV cases were reported increased almost two-fold from 1985 onwards [47].

Following its identification from northern Victoria in 1974 [48], a similar experience occurred with the diagnosis of BFV infection and its annual notification [49]. Epidemic polyarthritis, the now outmoded term that was then used to describe the autoimmune conditions associated with both RRV and BFV, became a nationally notifiable disease in 1990 [46]. While typically there are around 4500 notifications of epidemic polyarthritis per annum, 9554 cases were reported in 2015 [50].

Clinical infections with KUNV [51–54], EHV [25], GGV and KOKV [22,26] can now be confirmed in specialised laboratories, but only suspected KUNV infected cases undergo screening as standard.

7. A Causal Link between Neglected Arboviral Infections and UFI/PUO?

It has been proposed that arboviruses may be responsible for some cases of UFI observed in Australia [55]. While remarkably few systematic studies of UFI or PUO in an Australian setting have been undertaken, those that have been performed suggest that a large proportion of UFI/PUO cases remain undiagnosed (reviewed in [5]). This is despite the now-routine commercial testing for RRV and for BFV. A three-year retrospective study from 2008–2011 of a tertiary referral hospital in North Queensland found 58.8% of patients with UFI had no definitive diagnosis [56]. Neglected indigenous arboviruses may have infected humans regularly for decades, thereby being responsible for at least some of these UFI cases in this tropical north region. The possibility of arbovirus pathogens from Northern Australia causing more wide-scale outbreaks, such as the notified incidences of MVEV in 2001, 2008 and 2011, and the KUNV equine outbreak of 2011 in south-eastern Australia [57], should also be considered. While the horse derived WNVNSW2011 strain of KUNV not only differed to, but was more virulent than, other KUNV strains that circulated previously in Australia [57], it may be argued that the ecology of this arbovirus changed alongside the emergence of virulence.

The introduction of commercial screening for RRV and BFV led to a highly significant rise in their respective reported rates of infection when compared to historical records [46,49]; these conspicuous examples of unforeseen prevalence may also apply to other arboviral infections. Hence, it is possible that further, neglected, arboviruses—for which diagnostic tests are not yet available outside research laboratories—are a major underlying cause of undiagnosed UFI/PUO cases in Australia.

8. Transmission Cycles of Australian Arboviruses

Over several decades, many arboviruses have been identified in Australian mosquitoes, ticks, and biting midges [5,15]. Little is known about their transmission cycles, their pathogenicity for humans, or their potential to cause epidemics. Although large marsupials such as kangaroos and wallabies are considered potential reservoirs for RRV [58,59] and BFV [59,60], and waterbirds such as herons and egrets are regarded as hosts for MVEV, ALFV and SINV [61,62], there are many other arboviruses whose relationship with reservoirs and vectors, and their role in human infections or diseases, are yet to be defined.

While the epidemiology of these arboviruses is poorly understood, it is likely that they are maintained in zoonotic cycles rather than by human-to-human transmission. It may be that these neglected viruses are harboured by apathogenic, persistent infections in native Australian reservoir mammals and birds, with occasional spillover into humans [5].

9. Northern Australia's Climate Favours Arboviruses

Many of Australia's indigenous arboviruses that are known to cause human disease have been recovered from Northern Australia (Figure 1). Since it had no previous political purpose, the term 'Northern Australia' was defined formally only very recently with the passing of the Northern Australia Infrastructure Facility Act 2016 [63]. Although there are several minor qualifications, broadly speaking it is considered to comprise the Northern Territory and the areas of Queensland and Western Australia that are north of the Tropic of Capricorn (latitude 23.5 degrees south of the Equator).

The northern coastal fringe of the country is made up of northern Queensland, the Northern Territory, and the remote Kimberley and Pilbara Ranges of Western Australia. Uniquely for Australia, the region experiences a tropical, often monsoonal, wet season during the southern hemisphere summer months of November to April each year [59,64]. Moreover, if the mean annual air temperature continues to rise as a consequence of global climate change, the spatial range of mosquito species able to transmit arboviruses is likely to broaden [65]. While the presence of vectors does not necessarily mean the emergence of human pathogens, these factors contribute to favourable breeding conditions for mosquito species that are especially well-suited to maintaining arboviruses of potential public health importance [66].

10. Potential Public Health Threat

The Australian Commonwealth Government is actively promoting increased settlement and economic activity in the currently less populated areas that lie to the north of the Tropic of Capricorn as an integral part of its 'Developing Northern Australia' white paper for massive infrastructure investment in this region over the coming decades [67]. Although it comprises nearly half of the total land mass of the country, Northern Australia includes only about one-quarter of the current Australian population. It is therefore considered to be a region of largely untapped potential that is ripe for 21st century population growth outside of the urban densification in the major metropolitan conurbations to the south [67]. An incentivised expansion of the industrial, business and agricultural development of this vast tract of land is predicted, with an increase in the residential population from the current 1.33 million to up to 2.9 million people by 2050 projected [68]. The anticipated increased human activity in many areas of the tropical north of Australia will lead to fast-growing urbanisation that places relocated immune-naïve people into closer proximity to native reservoir wildlife, as well as to vector mosquitoes, for Australian indigenous arboviruses.

The growth in agriculture and other economic developments proposed for these localities will inevitably alter the ecology of the native animals and birds that act as reservoir hosts for numerous neglected Australian arboviruses, as well as affecting the mosquito vectors [5]. Additionally, sudden climatic and environmental variations [69], including the high rainfall, more frequent cyclones and resultant increased intensity of flooding associated with outbreaks of MVEV [70] and RRV [71], have occurred with alarming regularity in recent years [72], potentially generating an ecological expansion of Australian arboviruses. These circumstances therefore create a perfect storm for greater prevalence of infection with neglected Australian arboviruses, particularly in the tropical north of the country. It is perhaps worth considering that notable close relatives of these many indigenous arboviruses have already caused global pandemics in recent decades [73].

11. A Call to Arms for Novel Diagnostic Tests and Therapy Targets

In this circumstance, therefore, there is a pressing obligation to determine the geographical range and true disease burden of neglected indigenous arboviruses in Northern Australia. This may be accomplished by implementing a scheme of systematic, continual surveillance of vectors, reservoirs and viruses in order to address where, when, and how virus transmission to humans occurs as well as building up a picture of its likely impact. This may also be progressed through performing routine testing by designated public health laboratories of a systematic sub-sample of UFI/PUO patients for evidence of recent infection with neglected arboviruses as well as other potential causative agents of UFI/PUO. Furthermore, to screen patients with UFI/PUO and other suspected cases of arboviral infection, in addition to serology testing, the development of novel diagnostic tools should be given high research priority. Already available methods of detection of pan-alphaviruses and pan-flaviviruses include IgM antibody-based ELISA, quantitative reverse transcription PCR (RT-qPCR), and microarray [74–76]. Other state-of-the-art methods, for example RNA-seq metagenomics, which reveal an individual's virome [77], could also be applied to this setting.

Notwithstanding the striking exceptions of YFV, Japanese encephalitis virus, and tick-borne encephalitis virus [78], an obstacle to the successful control of infections caused by arboviruses is the lack of effective, authority-registered vaccines [79]. Strenuous efforts to yield a commercially available vaccine against DENV are ongoing but these are exacerbated by media-fuelled concerns over suitability and side-effects in pilot immunisation programs [80,81]. Also, the phenomenon of antibody-dependent enhancement of infection of humans that has been shown for many flaviviruses and alphaviruses [82] is an impediment to any future potential consideration of therapeutic antibodies as an alternative treatment [83]. Given this scenario, there is a dire need to accelerate the quest for novel options for both diagnosis and therapy.

Therapy regimens that are syndrome-based are currently common practice, frequently informing the prescription of antibiotics in empirical treatment. Such antibacterial pharmaceutical agents are ineffective when the UFI/PUO is caused by arboviruses; indeed, their inappropriate use may contribute to the worsening problem of antimicrobial resistance. Early, on-site, and rapid screening for neglected Australian arboviruses could help to identify the cause of infection and thus reduce the often ill-informed perceived obligation to provide antibiotics. Adoption of this measure would also expedite early detection of outbreak foci, thereby facilitating a prompt, efficient and proportionate response. This would have the effect of limiting the spread of disease, as hindsight suggests public health policymakers could have achieved better during the recent epidemic in Latin America of the flavivirus Zika [84,85].

The existing funding model for diagnostic pathology services in Australia does not foster requests by a general practitioner or hospital clinician to test for infection with a little-known arbovirus, even if they are aware of its possible role in disease. Hence, many UFI/PUO cases are not diagnosed correctly as the treating clinicians may consider the cost of testing is not warranted or because samples for testing were collected at an inappropriate time or from an incorrect site. They also may go undiagnosed on account of the causative agent being novel, not known to cause human disease, or because there are no routine diagnostic tests available.

For cases of UFI/PUO, for reasons of both practical feasibility and cost, it is not a realistic proposition to recommend multiple, individual laboratory tests in order to detect most or all neglected arboviruses. In light of this, development of a generic assay that would provide for many pathogens and which may be applied in a broad range of settings should be prioritised. For example, routine testing by designated public health laboratories of a two-step protocol could be envisaged, starting with pan-flavivirus and pan-alphavirus IgM antibody rapid tests and, as required of a sub-sample of patients, followed by confirmatory detection of viral RNA by RT-qPCR [76]. Along with the ability to screen for multiple arboviruses in a short space of time there is a saving in resources for the testing laboratory by virtue of a quicker diagnosis. This means that any future decision not to request sample analysis may ultimately prove a false economy.

12. One Component of a 'One Health' Approach to Combating Arboviruses

The One Health approach is a currently promulgated systems-based movement in which biomedical researchers and professionals in public health, veterinary medicine, and ecology combine their expertise in order to monitor and control the threat of infectious diseases and determine how pathogens spread among people, animals, and the environment [86]. Involvement of biomedical researchers, pathologists, and clinicians in this transdisciplinary model may lead to more efficient diagnosis of, and improved outcomes for, patients with arboviral infections.

In order to achieve success in preventing outbreaks of neglected arboviruses within the context of Northern Australia, it will be necessary to engage all relevant stakeholders, from federal, state and local authorities, via tertiary care and general practice centres, to local neighbourhoods, schools, and households. Risk of outbreak is always amplified when people are unaware of a disease or its route of transmission. As with the ongoing threat posed by DENV in Queensland [21], raising awareness levels among residents of regional communities is an extremely important component of a future public health policy for Northern Australia. Well-targeted information campaigns would aim to increase individual knowledge of the symptoms and possible sequelae of UFI/PUO and, with regard to mosquito transmission of arboviral infections, personal preventive methods and vector control.

13. Conclusions and Future Directions

For the neglected arboviruses that are indigenous to Australia there is an inadequate understanding of their distribution, epidemiology, and transmission ecology. Information is also lacking with respect to theimmunopathology and true disease burden, including undiagnosed cases UFI/PUO, which they cause. This knowledge gap exists despite the potential for these neglected arboviruses to become significant human pathogens in the rapidly developing region of Northern Australia, thereby presenting a major challenge to the public health of the nation, and conceivably also globally [87]. Future research into the areas discussed herein, combined with production of diagnostic tools to include first-line screening of a suite of indigenous arboviruses, would help greatly to limit the impact of this emerging threat to human health and wellbeing in the tropical north of Australia. Preferably, this would form a key component of a holistic, transdisciplinary strategy to improve environmental health in order to prevent mosquito-borne diseases in Northern Australia [88].

Acknowledgments: We warmly thank Richard Bradbury (Central Queensland University, Rockhampton, Australia) and John Aaskov (Queensland University of Technology, Brisbane, Australia) for advice and insightful discussion throughout the conceptualisation of this study. Narayan Gyawali is in receipt of an International Postgraduate Research Scholarship and an Australian Postgraduate Award administered by Central Queensland University. Our research is supported in part through a Health Collaborative Research Network Merit Grant.

Author Contributions: Narayan Gyawali conceived the paper and Andrew Taylor-Robinson helped to refine ideas. Narayan Gyawali prepared the first draft and Andrew Taylor-Robinson critically reviewed and revised various versions. Both authors contributed to preparation of the final version and agreed to its submission.

Conflicts of Interest: The authors declare no conflict of interest.

References

1. World Health Organization. *Arboviruses and Human Disease: Report of a WHO Scientific Group*; Technical Report Series No. 369; WHO: Geneva, Switzerland, 1967.
2. Centers for Disease Control and Prevention. Arbovirus Catalog. Available online: https://wwwn.cdc.gov/arbocat/ (accessed on 11 September 2017).
3. Centers for Disease Control and Prevention. National Notifiable Diseases Surveillance System (NNDSS)—Arboviral Diseases, Neuroinvasive and Non-neuroinvasive 2015 Case Definition. Available online: https://wwwn.cdc.gov/nndss/conditions/arboviral-diseases-neuroinvasive-and-non-neuroinvasive/case-definition/2015/ (accessed on 11 September 2017).
4. Beckham, J.D.; Tyler, K.L. Arbovirus infections. *Continuum (Minneapolis, Minn)* **2015**, *21*, 1599–1611. [CrossRef] [PubMed]
5. Gyawali, N.; Bradbury, R.S.; Aaskov, J.G.; Taylor-Robinson, A.W. Neglected Australian arboviruses: Quam gravis? *Microbes Infect.* **2017**, *19*, 388–401. [CrossRef] [PubMed]
6. Australian Government Department of Health. National Notifiable Diseases Surveillance System. Notifications for All Diseases by State & Territory and Year. Available online: http://www9.health.gov.au/cda/source/rpt_2_sel.cfm (accessed on 11 September 2017).
7. Weaver, S.C.; Barrett, A.D. Transmission cycles, host range, evolution and emergence of arboviral disease. *Nat. Rev. Microbiol.* **2004**, *2*, 789–801. [CrossRef] [PubMed]
8. Young, P.R.; Ng, L.F.P.; Hall, R.A.; Smith, D.W.; Johansen, C.A. Arbovirus infection. In *Manson's Tropical Diseases*, 23rd ed.; Farrar, J., Hotez, P.J., Junghanss, T., Kang, G., Lalloo, D., White, N.J., Eds.; Elsevier: Amsterdam, The Netherlands, 2013; pp. 129–161.
9. Morens, D.M.; Fauci, A.S. Emerging infectious diseases: Threats to human health and global stability. *PLoS Pathog.* **2013**, *9*, e1003467. [CrossRef] [PubMed]
10. Cao-Lormeau, V.-M.; Musso, D. Emerging arboviruses in the Pacific. *Lancet* **2014**, *384*, 1571–1572. [CrossRef]
11. Gubler, D.J. Dengue viruses: Their evolution, history and emergence as a global public health problem. In *Dengue and Dengue Hemorrhagic Fever*; Gubler, D.J., Ooi, E., Vasudevan, S., Farrar, J., Eds.; CAB International: Wallingford, UK, 2014; pp. 1–29.
12. Mackenzie, J.S.; Gubler, D.J.; Peterson, L.R. Emerging flaviviruses: The spread and resurgence of Japanese encephalitis, West Nile and dengue viruses. *Nat. Med.* **2004**, *10*, S98–S109. [CrossRef] [PubMed]
13. Hotez, P.J.; Murray, K.O. Dengue, West Nile virus, chikungunya, Zika and now Mayaro? *PLoS Negl. Trop. Dis.* **2017**, *11*, e0005462. [CrossRef] [PubMed]
14. Sutherst, R.W. Global change and human vulnerability to vector-borne diseases. *Clin. Microbiol. Rev.* **2004**, *17*, 136–173. [CrossRef] [PubMed]
15. Russell, R.C. Mosquito-borne disease and climate change in Australia: Time for a reality check. *Aust. J. Entomol.* **2009**, *48*, 1–7. [CrossRef]
16. Fraser, J.R. Epidemic polyarthritis and Ross River virus disease. *Clin. Rheum. Dis.* **1986**, *12*, 369–388. [PubMed]
17. Vale, T.G.; Carter, I.W.; McPhie, K.A.; James, G.; Cloonan, M.J. Human arbovirus infections along the south coast of New South Wales. *Aust. J. Exp. Biol. Med. Sci.* **1986**, *64*, 307–309. [CrossRef] [PubMed]
18. Russell, R.C. Arboviruses and their vectors in Australia: An update on the ecology and epidemiology of some mosquito-borne arboviruses. *Rev. Med. Vet. Entomol.* **1995**, *83*, 141–158.
19. Gyawali, N.; Bradbury, R.S.; Taylor-Robinson, A.W. The epidemiology of dengue infection: Harnessing past experience and current knowledge to support implementation of future control strategies. *J. Vector Borne Dis.* **2016**, *53*, 293–304. [PubMed]
20. Naish, S.; Tong, S. Hot spot detection and spatio-temporal dynamics of dengue in Queensland, Australia. In Proceedings of the ISPRS Technical Commission VIII Symposium, Hyderabad, India, 9–12 December 2014; Dadhwal, V.K., Diwakar, P.G., Seshasai, M.V.R., Raju, P.L.N., Hakeem, A., Eds.; International Society of Photogrammetry and Remote Sensing. pp. 197–204.
21. Gyawali, N.; Bradbury, R.S.; Taylor-Robinson, A.W. Knowledge, attitude and recommendations for practice regarding dengue among the resident population of Queensland, Australia. *Asian Pac. J. Trop. Biomed.* **2016**, *6*, 360–366. [CrossRef]

22. Hawkes, R.A.; Boughton, C.R.; Naim, H.M.; Wild, J.; Chapman, B. Arbovirus infections of humans in New South Wales. Seroepidemiology of the flavivirus group of togaviruses. *Med. J. Aust.* **1985**, *143*, 555–561. [PubMed]

23. Mackenzie, J.; Lindsay, M.; Coelen, R.; Broom, A.; Hall, R.; Smith, D. Arboviruses causing human disease in the Australasian zoogeographic region. *Arch. Virol.* **1994**, *136*, 447–467. [CrossRef] [PubMed]

24. Guard, R.W.; McAuliffe, M.; Stallman, N.; Bramston, B. Haemorrhagic manifestations with Sindbis infection. Case report. *Pathology* **1982**, *14*, 89–90. [CrossRef] [PubMed]

25. Aaskov, J.G.; Phillips, D.A.; Wiemers, M.A. Possible clinical infection with Edge Hill virus. *Trans. R. Soc. Trop. Med. Hyg.* **1993**, *87*, 452–453. [CrossRef]

26. Boughton, C.R.; Hawkes, R.A.; Naim, H.M. Illness caused by a Kokobera-like virus in south-eastern Australia. *Med. J. Aust.* **1986**, *145*, 90–92. [PubMed]

27. Australian Government Department of Health. Australian National Notifiable Diseases by Disease Type. Available online: http://www.health.gov.au/internet/main/publishing.nsf/Content/cda-surveil-nndss-casedefs-distype.htm (accessed on 11 September 2017).

28. Colmant, A.M.; Bielefeldt-Ohmann, H.; Hobson-Peters, J.; Suen, W.W.; O'Brien, C.A.; van den Hurk, A.F.; Hall, R.A. A newly discovered flavivirus in the yellow fever virus group displays restricted replication in vertebrates. *J. Gen. Virol.* **2016**, *97*, 1087–1093. [CrossRef] [PubMed]

29. Johansen, C.A.; Williams, S.H.; Melville, L.F.; Nicholson, J.; Hall, R.A.; Bielefeldt-Ohmann, H.; Prow, N.A.; Chidlow, G.R.; Wong, S.; Sinha, R.; et al. Characterization of Fitzroy River virus and serologic evidence of human and animal infection. *Emerg. Infect. Dis.* **2017**, *23*, 1289–1299. [CrossRef] [PubMed]

30. Petersdorf, R.G.; Beeson, P.B. Fever of unexplained origin: Report on 100 cases. *Medicine* **1961**, *40*, 1–30. [CrossRef] [PubMed]

31. Durack, D.T.; Street, A.C. Fever of unknown origin—Reexamined and redefined. *Curr. Clin. Top. Infect. Dis.* **1991**, *11*, 35–51. [PubMed]

32. Mourad, O.; Palda, V.; Detsky, A.S. A comprehensive evidence-based approach to fever of unknown origin. *Arch. Intern. Med.* **2003**, *163*, 545–551. [CrossRef] [PubMed]

33. Jacoby, G.A.; Swartz, M.N. Fever of undetermined origin. *N. Engl. J. Med.* **1973**, *289*, 1407–1410. [CrossRef] [PubMed]

34. Larson, E.B.; Featherstone, H.J.; Petersdorf, R.G. Fever of undetermined origin: diagnosis and follow-up of 105 cases, 1970–1980. *Medicine* **1982**, *61*, 269–292. [CrossRef] [PubMed]

35. De Kleijn, E.M.; Vandenbroucke, J.P.; van der Meer, J.W.; Group, N.F.S. Fever of unknown origin (FUO): I. A prospective multicenter study of 167 patients with FUO, using fixed epidemiologic entry criteria. *Medicine* **1997**, *76*, 392–400. [CrossRef] [PubMed]

36. Boivin, G.; Hardy, I.; Tellier, G.; Maziade, J. Predicting influenza infections during epidemics with use of a clinical case definition. *Clin. Infect. Dis.* **2000**, *31*, 1166–1169. [CrossRef] [PubMed]

37. Rongrungruang, Y.; Leelarasamee, A. Characteristics and outcomes of adult patients with symptomatic dengue virus infections. *J. Infect. Dis. Antimicrob. Agents* **2001**, *18*, 19–23.

38. Efstathiou, S.P.; Pefanis, A.V.; Tsiakou, A.G.; Skeva, I.I.; Tsioulos, D.I.; Achimastos, A.D.; Mountokalakis, T.D. Fever of unknown origin: Discrimination between infectious and non-infectious causes. *Eur. J. Intern. Med.* **2010**, *21*, 137–143. [CrossRef] [PubMed]

39. Vanderschueren, S.; Knockaert, D.; Adriaenssens, T.; Demey, W.; Durnez, A.; Blockmans, D.; Bobbaers, H. From prolonged febrile illness to fever of unknown origin: The challenge continues. *Arch. Intern. Med.* **2003**, *163*, 1033–1041. [CrossRef] [PubMed]

40. Buysschaert, I.; Vanderschueren, S.; Blockmans, D.; Mortelmans, L.; Knockaert, D. Contribution of [18]fluoro-deoxyglucose positron emission tomography to the work-up of patients with fever of unknown origin. *Eur. J. Intern. Med.* **2004**, *15*, 151–156. [CrossRef] [PubMed]

41. Bleeker-Rovers, C.P.; Vos, F.J.; de Kleijn, E.M.; Mudde, A.H.; Dofferhoff, T.S.; Richter, C.; Smilde, T.J.; Krabbe, P.F.; Oyen, W.J.; van der Meer, J.W. A prospective multicenter study on fever of unknown origin: The yield of a structured diagnostic protocol. *Medicine* **2007**, *86*, 26–38. [CrossRef] [PubMed]

42. Robine, A.; Hot, A.; Maucort-Boulch, D.; Iwaz, J.; Broussolle, C.; Sève, P. Fever of unknown origin in the 2000s: Evaluation of 103 cases over eleven years. *Presse Méd.* **2014**, *43*, e233–e240. [CrossRef] [PubMed]

43. Yamanouchi, M.; Uehara, Y.; Yokokawa, H.; Hosoda, T.; Watanabe, Y.; Shiga, T.; Inui, A.; Otsuki, Y.; Fujibayashi, K.; Isonuma, H.; Naito, T. Analysis of 256 cases of classic fever of unknown origin. *Intern. Med.* **2013**, *53*, 2471–2475. [CrossRef]

44. Doherty, R.L.; Whitehead, R.H.; Gorman, B.M.; O'Gower, A.K. The isolation of a third group A arbovirus in Australia, with preliminary observations on its relationship to epidemic polyarthritis. *Aust. J. Sci.* **1963**, *26*, 183–184.

45. Oseni, R.A.; Donaldson, M.D.; Dalglish, D.A.; Aaskov, J.G. Detection by ELISA of IgM antibodies to Ross River virus in serum from patients with suspected epidemic polyarthritis. *Bull. World Health Organ.* **1983**, *61*, 703–708. [PubMed]

46. Hargreaves, J.; Longbottom, H.; Myint, H.; Herceg, A.; Oliver, G.; Curran, M.; Evans, D. Annual report of the National Notifiable Diseases Surveillance System, 1994. *Commun. Dis. Intell.* **1995**, *19*, 542–574.

47. Tong, S.; Bi, P.; Hayes, J.; Donald, K.; Mackenzie, J. Geographic variation of notified Ross River virus infections in Queensland, Australia, 1985–1996. *Am. J. Trop. Med. Hyg.* **2001**, *65*, 171–176. [CrossRef] [PubMed]

48. Marshall, I.D.; Woodroofe, G.M.; Hirsch, S. Viruses recovered from mosquitoes and wildlife serum collected in the Murray Valley of south-eastern Australia, February 1974, during an epidemic of encephalitis. *Aust. J. Exp. Biol. Med. Sci.* **1982**, *60*, 457–470. [CrossRef] [PubMed]

49. Jacups, S.P.; Whelan, P.I.; Currie, B.J. Ross River virus and Barmah Forest virus infections: A review of history, ecology, and predictive models, with implications for tropical northern Australia. *Vector Borne Zoonotic Dis.* **2008**, *8*, 283–298. [CrossRef] [PubMed]

50. Australian Government Department of Health. National Notifiable Diseases: Australia's Notifiable Diseases Status. Annual Reports of the National Notifiable Diseases Surveillance System, 1994–2014. Available online: http://www.health.gov.au/internet/main/publishing.nsf/Content/cda-pubs-annlrpt-nndssar.htm (accessed on 11 September 2017).

51. Doherty, R.L.; Carley, J.G.; Filippich, C.; White, J.; Gust, I.D. Murray Valley encephalitis in Australia, 1974: Antibody response in cases and community. *Aust. N.Z. J. Med.* **1976**, *6*, 446–453. [CrossRef] [PubMed]

52. Phillips, D.A.; Aaskov, J.G.; Atkin, C.; Wiemers, M.A. Isolation of Kunjin virus from a patient with a naturally acquired infection. *Med. J. Aust.* **1992**, *157*, 190–191. [PubMed]

53. Mackenzie, J.; Smith, D.; Broom, A.; Bucens, M. Australian encephalitis in Western Australia, 1978–1991. *Med. J. Aust.* **1993**, *158*, 591–595. [PubMed]

54. Broom, A.; Whelan, P.; Smith, D.; Lindsay, M.; Melville, L.; Bolisetty, S.; Wheaton, G.; Brown, A.; Higgins, G. An outbreak of Australian encephalitis in Western Australia and Central Australia (Northern Territory and South Australia) during the 2000 wet season. *Arbovirus Res. Aust.* **2001**, *8*, 37–42.

55. Doherty, R.L. Arthropod-borne viruses in Australia and their relation to infection and disease. *Prog. Med. Virol.* **1974**, *17*, 136–192. [PubMed]

56. Susilawati, T.N.; McBride, W.J.H. Undiagnosed undifferentiated fever in far north Queensland, Australia: A retrospective study. *Int. J. Infect. Dis.* **2014**, *27*, 59–64. [CrossRef] [PubMed]

57. Frost, M.J.; Zhang, J.; Edmonds, J.H.; Prow, N.A.; Gu, X.; Davis, R.; Hornitzky, C.; Arzey, K.E.; Finlaison, D.; Hick, P.; et al. Characterization of virulent West Nile virus Kunjin strain, Australia, 2011. *Emerg. Infect. Dis.* **2012**, *18*, 792–800. [CrossRef] [PubMed]

58. Doherty, R.L.; Gorman, B.M.; Whitehead, R.H.; Carley, J.G. Studies of arthropod-borne virus infections in Queensland. V. Survey of antibodies to group A arboviruses in man and other animals. *Aust. J. Exp. Biol. Med. Sci.* **1966**, *44*, 365–377. [CrossRef] [PubMed]

59. Inglis, T.J.; Bradbury, R.S.; McInnes, R.L.; Frances, S.P.; Merritt, A.J.; Levy, A.; Nicholson, J.; Neville, P.J.; Lindsay, M.; Smith, D.W. Deployable molecular detection of arboviruses in the Australian Outback. *Am. J. Trop. Med. Hyg.* **2016**, *95*, 633–638. [CrossRef] [PubMed]

60. Vale, T.G.; Spratt, D.M.; Cloonan, M.J. Serological evidence of arbovirus infection in native and domesticated mammals on the south coast of New South Wales. *Aust. J. Zool.* **1991**, *39*, 1–7. [CrossRef]

61. Anderson, S.G. Murray Valley encephalitis and Australian X disease. *Epidemiol. Infect.* **1954**, *52*, 447–468. [CrossRef]

62. Doherty, R. Arboviruses of Australia. *Aust. Vet. J.* **1972**, *48*, 172–180. [CrossRef] [PubMed]

63. Australian Government. Northern Australia Infrastructure Facility Act 2016. Available online: https://www.legislation.gov.au/Details/C2016A00041 (accessed on 11 September 2017).

64. Australian Government. Australian Weather and Seasons—A Variety of Climates. Available online: http://www.australia.gov.au/about-australia/australian-story/austn-weather-and-the-seasons (accessed on 11 September 2017).

65. Parham, P.E.; Waldock, J.; Christophides, G.K.; Hemming, D.; Agusto, F.; Evans, K.J.; Fefferman, N.; Gaff, H.; Gumel, A.; LaDeau, S.; et al. Climate, environmental and socio-economic change: Weighing up the balance in vector-borne disease transmission. *Philos. Trans. R. Soc. Lond. B Biol. Sci.* **2015**, *370*, 20130551. [CrossRef] [PubMed]

66. Van den Hurk, A.F.; Craig, S.B.; Tulsiani, S.M.; Jansen, C.C. Emerging tropical diseases in Australia. Part 4. Mosquito-borne diseases. *Ann. Trop. Med. Parasitol.* **2010**, *104*, 623–640. [CrossRef] [PubMed]

67. Australian Government. Our North, Our Future: White Paper on Developing Northern Australia. Available online: http://northernaustralia.gov.au/sites/prod.office-northern-australia.gov.au/files/files/NAWP-FullReport.pdf (accessed on 11 September 2017).

68. Cummings Economics, March 2015. Long-Term Population Growth in Northern Australia. Available online: http://www.cummings.net.au/pdf/recent/J2806NthnAusLongTermPopulationGrowth.pdf (accessed on 11 September 2017).

69. Inglis, T.J. Climate change and infectious diseases in Australia. *Aust. Prescr.* **2009**, *32*, 58–59. [CrossRef]

70. Selvey, L.A.; Johansen, C.A.; Broom, A.K.; Antão, C.; Lindsay, M.D.; Mackenzie, J.S.; Smith, D.W. Rainfall and sentinel chicken seroconversions predict human cases of Murray Valley encephalitis in the north of Western Australia. *BMC Infect. Dis.* **2014**, *14*, 672. [CrossRef] [PubMed]

71. Tall, J.A.; Gatton, M.L.; Tong, S. Ross River virus disease activity associated with naturally occurring nontidal flood events in Australia: A systematic review. *J. Med. Entomol.* **2014**, *51*, 1097–1108. [CrossRef] [PubMed]

72. Knutson, T.R.; McBride, J.L.; Chan, J.; Emanuel, K.; Holland, G.; Landsea, C.; Held, I.; Kossin, J.P.; Srivastava, A.K.; Sugi, M. Tropical cyclones and climate change. *Nat. Geosci.* **2010**, *3*, 157–163. [CrossRef]

73. Mayer, S.V.; Tesh, R.B.; Vasilakis, N. The emergence of arthropod-borne viral diseases: A global prospective on dengue, chikungunya and Zika fevers. *Acta Trop.* **2017**, *166*, 155–163. [CrossRef] [PubMed]

74. Palacios, G.; Quan, P.L.; Jabado, O.J.; Conlan, S.; Hirschberg, D.L.; Liu, Y.; Zhai, J.; Renwick, N.; Hui, J.; Hegyi, H.; et al. Panmicrobial oligonucleotide array for diagnosis of infectious diseases. *Emerg. Infect. Dis.* **2007**, *13*, 73–81. [CrossRef] [PubMed]

75. Giry, C.; Roquebert, B.; Li-Pat-Yuen, G.; Gasque, P.; Jaffar-Bandjee, M.C. Improved detection of genus-specific *Alphavirus* using a generic TaqMan®assay. *BMC Microbiol.* **2017**, *17*, 164. [CrossRef] [PubMed]

76. Vina-Rodriguez, A.; Sachse, K.; Ziegler, U.; Chaintoutis, S.C.; Keller, M.; Groschup, M.H.; Eiden, M. A novel pan-*Flavivirus* detection and identification assay based on RT-qPCR and microarray. *Biomed. Res. Int.* **2017**, *4248756*. [CrossRef] [PubMed]

77. Rosani, U.; Gerdol, M. A bioinformatics approach reveals seven nearly-complete RNA-virus genomes in bivalve RNA-seq data. *Virus Res.* **2017**, *239*, 33–42. [CrossRef] [PubMed]

78. Khou, C.; Pardigon, N. Identifying attenuating mutations: Tools for a new vaccine design against flaviviruses. *Intervirology* **2017**, *60*, 8–18. [CrossRef] [PubMed]

79. Gautam, R.; Mishra, S.; Milhotra, A.; Nagpal, R.; Mohan, M.; Singhal, A.; Kumari, P. Challenges with mosquito-borne viral diseases: Outbreak of the monsters. *Curr. Top. Med. Chem.* **2017**, *17*, 2199–2214. [CrossRef] [PubMed]

80. Sun Star Manila, 25 April 2016. DOH Records 362 Adverse Reactions of Dengue Vaccine. Available online: http://www.sunstar.com.ph/manila/local-news/2016/04/25/doh-records-362-adverse-effects-dengue-vaccine-469921 (accessed on 11 September 2017).

81. Malay Mail Online, 7 April 2017. Controversial Dengue Vaccine Approved for Further Trials in Malaysia. Available online: http://www.themalaymailonline.com/malaysia/article/controversial-dengue-vaccine-approved-for-further-trials-in-malaysia#sErjCc1APGerWKmy.99 (accessed on 11 September 2017).

82. Pierson, T.C.; Fremont, D.H.; Kuhn, R.J.; Diamond, M.S. Structural insights into the mechanisms of antibody-mediated neutralization of flavivirus infection: Implications for vaccine development. *Cell Host Microbe* **2008**, *4*, 229–238. [CrossRef] [PubMed]

83. Gautam, S.; Subedi, D.; Taylor-Robinson, A.W. Anti-idiotype antibody against pre-membrane-specific antibody as an adjunct to current dengue vaccination strategy. *Immun. Dis.* **2015**, *3*, 1–7.

84. Fauci, A.S.; Morens, D.M. Zika virus in the Americas—Yet another arbovirus threat. *N. Engl. J. Med.* **2016**, *374*, 601–604. [CrossRef] [PubMed]

85. Lazear, H.M.; Stringer, E.M.; de Silva, A.M. The emerging Zika virus epidemic in the Americas: Research priorities. *JAMA* **2016**, *315*, 1945–1946. [CrossRef] [PubMed]

86. Rüegg, S.R.; McMahon, B.J.; Häsler, B.; Esposito, R.; Nielsen, L.R.; Ifejika Speranza, C.; Ehlinger, T.; Peyre, M.; Aragrande, M.; Zinsstag, J.; et al. A blueprint to evaluate One Health. *Front. Public Health* **2017**, *5*, 20.

87. Gyawali, N.; Bradbury, R.S.; Taylor-Robinson, A.W. Do neglected Australian arboviruses pose a global epidemic threat? *Aust. N. Z. J. Public Health* **2016**, *40*, 596. [CrossRef] [PubMed]

88. Hardy, M.C.; Barrington, D.J. A transdisciplinary approach to managing emerging and resurging mosquito-borne diseases in the Western Pacific Region. *Trop. Med. Infect. Dis.* **2017**, *2*, 1. [CrossRef]

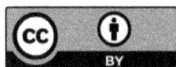

MDPI

St. Alban-Anlage 66

4052 Basel

Switzerland

Tel. +41 61 683 77 34

Fax +41 61 302 89 18

www.mdpi.com

Tropical Medicine and Infectious Disease Editorial Office

E-mail: tropicalmed@mdpi.com

www.mdpi.com/journal/tropicalmed

www.ingramcontent.com/pod-product-compliance
Lightning Source LLC
Chambersburg PA
CBHW051904210326
41597CB00033B/6015